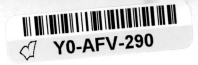

ARE YOU REALLY SAFE?

PROTECTING YOURSELF IN AMERICA TODAY

LARRY TALLEY

LONGSTREET PRESS
Atlanta, Georgia

This book is dedicated to all the people
who have suffered as victims of crime and to my
loving wife, Karen, whose love and compassion for
others inspired me to write this book.

Published by
LONGSTREET PRESS, INC.
A subsidiary of Cox Newspapers,
A division of Cox Enterprises, Inc.
2140 Newmarket Parkway
Suite 118
Marietta, GA 30067

Printed in the United States of America

1st printing 1994

Library of Congress Catalog Number 93-81137

ISBN 1-56352-129-6

This book was printed by R. R. Donnelley & Sons, Harrisonburg, Virginia.

Jacket design by Jill Dible
Jacket photograph courtesy H. Armstrong Roberts, Inc.
Book design by Laura McDonald

CONTENTS

Preface

This book contains true stories about real people who had the misfortune of being victims of violent crimes, who had to suffer, and, if they survived their attack, who had to live with the ugliness of the event for the rest of their lives. My intention, by including profanity and graphic detail in the descriptions of these events, is to instill in the reader's mind a lasting impression of the crimes and the reasons which made it possible for them to take place. I sincerely hope I do not offend anyone with my frank recounting of these victims' stories; my intent, rather, is to help people avoid the same tragedy in their own lives.

The names and the locations of the people in the case histories have been changed to protect their privacy; I have recreated their experiences in story form, but the facts of the cases are all true.

Unfortunately, reading this book and following all of the suggested security and safety tips will not guarantee that you or one of your family members won't become a victim of a crime. However, if you seek to learn from the tragic events suffered by the victims described in this book and follow reasonable security measures, the likelihood that you will be a victim will be greatly diminished.

If this book helps save one person from a brutal and vicious crime, I will know that all the proverbial blood, sweat, and tears that I poured into it were worth the effort.

May all of your life's travels be successful—and safe.

Larry Talley

Introduction

A plague has descended upon our country which has the likelihood of affecting every man, woman, and child. This plague is not a disease, but claims more victims than the most deadly diseases. Even more frightening, this plague shows no signs of abating, but continues to increase each year. There are no teams of research scientists working around the clock to find a cure or a vaccine to decrease or curb its growth.

The plague is crime in our society. The possibility of becoming a victim of crime in America has increased tenfold during the past decade. The Uniform Crime Report, released annually by the Federal Bureau of Investigation to address the seriousness of the problem, shows that approximately 5,800 out of every 100,000 people become the victims of a violent or property-related crime during any given year. During this same period, nearly 36 million Americans are victims of serious crimes. This includes nearly 19,000 who are murdered.

With poor economic conditions facing our nation, law enforcement officials are faced with budget cuts which further hamper their efforts to fight crime. This scenario exacerbates the concern that crime will continue to increase during the rest of the 1990s and into the next century.

Drug trafficking appears to have a direct correlation to increases in crime. The use of illegal drugs by criminals while they commit violent crimes has increased dramatically. It has become commonplace for criminals to commit senseless acts of violence against their victims in the course of a street rip-off or break-in or car-jacking. Juvenile crimes increased 10 percent from 1980 to 1989. The number of arrests for violent crimes among young males (10-17 years old) increased 40 percent from 1987 to 1991; among females in the same age group the increase was 49 percent.

We are reminded of the crime problem every day through newspaper, radio, and television accounts of gruesome assaults occurring in our communities. However, even with this increased awareness, a casual attitude about crime prevails: Most people feel it is something they only hear about. They find it hard to imagine that they or any of their loved ones could become a victim.

There is no question that crime is a serious problem across our country and in our communities. Most of us would be shocked to learn that in our society, the possibilities of becoming a victim increase dramatically under conditions many of us face daily. When we stay in hotels or motels, while we are out shopping in malls, when we travel, when we rent an apartment home, or when we go to a bar or health club, we may be at much greater risk than we ever imagined.

Statistics from lawsuits filed show that you are especially prone to a criminal attack while staying at a hotel/motel or while living in an apartment complex, to cite two particular instances. This may be news to you, but business leaders in these industries have known it for years.

During the past fifteen to twenty years, thousands of lawsuits have been filed against hotels/motels and apartment owners for their failure to provide reasonable security to guests or tenants. These industries and their insurance carriers would prefer to keep these suits quiet. In most cases they reach out-of-court settlements and have the court records sealed, which prevents the public from discovering how much money they are willing to pay for their negligent acts.

The lodging and apartment industries would like for the public to believe that these businesses are doing everything possible to prevent crimes from occurring and should not be held liable for crimes committed on their premises by third parties. After all, as they like to state, "No matter what measures we take to prevent crimes from occurring on our premises, they still can occur." They ask that if society cannot prevent or curb crimes, then why should they be held accountable for these types of acts?

The problem is that most of these businesses do not want to commit the necessary funds to address security-related problems on their premises. The main reason is that money spent on security directly affects the bottom line. They would much rather spend money on "curb appeal" items—how an apartment complex, hotel/motel, or shopping center looks—than on security.

These industries have often chosen to ignore crimes committed on their premises and the surrounding areas. The process is simple. A risk analyst considers the cost of deterrent measures versus the cost of insurance to cover the risk. Since insurance is necessary and costs less in up-front funds, most businesses purchase more of it and assume the risk of being sued. So the chances increase that a person may become a victim of a crime while on their premises.

Deterrents may not prevent all crimes from occurring, but they may often prevent guests or tenants from being raped, robbed, assaulted, or, in some instances, murdered.

To better understand the effects and the frequency of crime, we should look at the national crime clock. According to the latest FBI Uniform Crime Report, the national crime clock ticks as follows:

- A crime is committed in America every 2 seconds.
- One violent crime occurs every 19 seconds.
- One property crime is committed every 3 seconds.
- A murder is committed every 24 minutes.
- A forcible rape occurs every 6 minutes.
- A robbery is committed every 55 seconds.
- An aggravated assault is committed every 33 seconds.
- A burglary occurs every 10 seconds.
- A motor vehicle theft occurs every 20 seconds.

Over the years the causes and origins of crime have been studied by experts in many disciplines, and they have identified some basic factors for the causes of crimes:

- Economic conditions
- Population density
- Degree and size of urbanization
- Composition of the population, particularly the youth concentration
- Transient factors
- Highway systems and modes of transportation
- Climate
- Family conditions
- Attitudes and crime-reporting practices of citizens
- Drugs

Recently, experts have become more convinced that crime is anything but a random event. Many believe that crime is conditioned by the environment; that is, a criminal may select where he is going to commit a crime. He will carefully choose surroundings that suggest he has a chance of getting away with the crime.

This factor in the crime problem takes on a special meaning to industries such as hotels, motels, apartments, and shopping centers, all of which invite people onto their premises to conduct business or live. If these businesses have experienced several crimes committed against their customers, then those crimes could be determined a foreseeable event. This means that business owners should take reasonable measures to deter and prevent crimes from occurring and reoccurring upon their premises. Otherwise, they could be held liable if sued by a crime victim.

The effects of being a victim of a crime can leave long-lasting physical and emotional scars. These scars not only affect the victims but their families as well. I have encountered firsthand the aftermath of these tragedies, and it is horrible—families torn apart and scars that won't heal.

According to an article by Dr. Theodore H. Blau in the *Diagnostic and Statistical Manual of Mental Orders* published by the American Psychiatric Association, victims of assault can suffer afterwards from "post-traumatic stress disorder." They reexperience the traumatic event in a variety of ways. "Commonly the person has recurrent and intrusive recollections of the event or recurrent distressing dreams during which the event is reexperienced. . . . In addition to the reexperiencing of the trauma, there is persistent avoidance of stimuli associated with it, or a numbing of general responsiveness that was not present before the trauma. The person commonly makes deliberate efforts to avoid thoughts or feelings about the traumatic event and about activities or situations that arouse recollections of it." Dr. Blau further states that a person may complain of feeling detached or alienated from other people, that he or she has lost the ability to become interested in previously enjoyed activities, or that the ability to feel emotions of any type, especially those associated with intimacy, tenderness, and sexuality, is "markedly decreased." Frequent symptoms include difficulty in falling or staying asleep, difficulty in concentrating or completing tasks, irritability with fears of losing control, and an inability to express angry feelings.

In the following chapters, you will read what the hotel/motel, apartment, and other industries are and are not doing to protect you. You will read about actual case histories of crimes committed in hotels/motels and apartment communities in which I have worked as a security expert. You will see how, in each case, the crime affected the victims and their families, and what lasting effects it left on their lives.

In the later chapters, I offer security tips for traveling, shopping, and choosing an apartment and living in it, tips which will help you protect yourself from becoming a victim of a crime. I also suggest what to do if you are assaulted in your apartment or while shopping or traveling.

Most of all, I hope this book will influence the hotel/motel, apartment, and shopping industries to take seriously the problem of crime committed against persons on their premises. I hope they will put aside the lure of increased profits for what is morally right: to offer you and me the degree of security and safety we deserve.

ARE YOU REALLY SAFE?

■ ■ ■

Crime Trends in Hotels and Apartments

TWO OF THE LARGEST AND MOST CRIME-PRONE INDUSTRIES IN America are lodging and apartments. In fact, according to Liability Consultants, Inc., a security consulting firm based in Framingham, Massachusetts, residential apartment buildings and hotels/motels were the top defendants in law suits from 1983 to 1992 which alleged inadequate security at commercial sites of violent crime. The lodging industry is one of the largest service industries in the United States. There are more than 40,000 hotels and motels operating across the nation, and these facilities provide tens of thousands of jobs. The style and cost of lodging accommodations range from the small "mom and pop" motel, in which you may be required to change your own sheets, to the full-service luxury hotel, which pampers you with service at every turn. The one thing a "mom and pop" motel *may* have in common with a fancy luxury hotel is the degree of security and safety it is providing the guest.

During the mid–1900s, the lodging industry saw a new concept springing up across the country—the creation of hotel and motel chains. At first, most were solely owned by the company developing them. However, they soon saw a new opportunity through franchising, which gave investors the opportunity to enter the lodging industry by following the successful standards used by the major chain.

The chain offering the franchise would provide the franchisee with training and strict standards by which to operate his or her businesses. These standards would include matters ranging from the type and color of room decorations to how to fold toilet paper after it had been placed on the roller. Two of the major benefits that a franchisee received from the parent company would be the mass-marketing programs of the major chain and the use of a national reservation system.

Today, names such as Holiday Inns, Days Inns, Best Western, and Motel 6 are etched in our minds as we travel. The outer appearance and the basic services provided at hotel/motel chains are pretty consistent due to strict requirements set by the parent company. Most of the traveling public has no way of knowing if they are staying at a company-owned unit or a franchise unit. From a security and safety standpoint, however, this could make a great deal of difference in whether you have a safe and pleasant trip or become a crime statistic.

The majority of major hotel/motel chains have in-house security departments headed up by professional security managers. These departments are responsible for designing and implementing security programs to protect their guests and assets. To insure that security standards are being met, the security department will conduct security audits once or twice a year.

This approach seems very reasonable, but these programs are only mandatory at company-owned units. Security measures at franchise units are thus left totally to the owner's discretion. It is not uncommon to find better security-trained employees and more physical security measures in place at company-owned hotels than at franchise units bearing the same sign and logo. Thus a person may be better protected from crime when staying in a company-owned hotel or motel rather than a franchise.

The lodging industry has known of the dangers facing its guests for years. It is also aware of tremendous exposure to liability lawsuits brought by guests who became victims while staying on its premises. However, most lodging companies have chosen to purchase more insurance to cover this risk rather than budget money for security measures which could offer more protection for guests.

The results? Hotels and motels are among the largest defendants in civil actions, according to the ten-year survey by Liability Consultants, Inc. Settlements and verdicts for rape averaged nearly $.7 million dollars, $1.5 million for robbery, $.4 million and $.7 million for assault and battery, and $1.2 million for wrongful death. The top ten claims states were Texas, New York, Florida, California, Nevada, Massachusetts, Washington, D.C., Georgia, Arizona, and Illinois.

At Days Inns of America, Inc., where I was employed from 1976 to 1986 as vice president of risk management, the corporate security department tracks such crimes at company-owned hotels. During the period of 1981 to 1984, a total of 4,978 crimes was reported to have been committed against guests. They included murder, rape, armed robbery, and assault.

The trend in hotel/motel assaults was apparent as far back as 1974 when entertainer Connie Francis filed a landmark liability lawsuit against a hotel. She was a victim of sexual assault while staying at a Howard Johnson's Motor Lodge in Westbury, Long Island, New York.

In 1974, Ms. Francis had been in the Westbury area performing. She had given her last performance for the evening and had retired to what she thought was the safety of her room. During the night, an intruder gained entry into her room through a sliding glass door. She had checked the door prior to going to bed and it had given the appearance of being locked. In reality, outside entry was relatively easy.

Ms. Francis was brutally beaten, raped, and robbed. The resulting physical and mental anguish almost ended her life and career.

After a long trial and several appeals, Ms. Francis and her husband settled the case with Howard Johnson's for $1.5 million. But that amount is "small potatoes" compared to figures being awarded today as the number and gruesomeness of crimes increase.

The publicity the Francis case received had a major impact on the lodging industry. Other people who had been victims of similar crimes came forward and filed lawsuits. The case also put the lodging industry on notice that it needed to address security issues in order to offer its guests a reasonable degree of safety.

After the Connie Francis case, many major chains hired security professionals. They sought both to design security programs to protect their guests and to reduce the kind of liability risk highlighted by the Connie Francis case. The American Hotel and Motel Association, which has more than 10,000 members nationwide, formed a committee to examine security problems facing the lodging industry. But since these efforts during the mid-1970s and early 1980s, the economics of the lodging industry has brought cutbacks in security staffs or deletion of them altogether. These cutbacks, along with the increase of crimes across the nation, have placed hotel and motel guests at greater risk.

Staying at a luxury hotel is no guarantee of safety. Most of the hotel crime reported in a new study in *Corporate Travel Magazine* involved thefts from rooms, and 69 percent of those thefts were in chain-affiliated hotels. Only 4 percent of the victims were staying in economy lodgings, while 41 percent were in luxury hotels.

Days Inns of America, Inc., formerly headquartered in Atlanta, Georgia, is a case in point. During my employment, this organization had a very highly recognized security and safety program which set many standards that other chains follow today. Up until 1984, Days Inns operated 150 company-owned units and franchised more than 350 hotels and motels nationwide.

In 1976, Richard Kessler, Days Inns' president and chief executive officer, was one of the first lodging executives to sense the need for an internal department to address issues of guest safety. Due to his support, security and safety issues became an important part in the day-to-day operation of a Days Inns motel. Mr. Kessler encouraged all franchise owners to conform with the security policies followed by the corporate-owned units but left the final decisions up to them.

An incident-reporting system was initiated in 1976 which tracked all crimes occurring on the premises of a corporate Days Inn. It required the general manager of the hotel/motel to report all crimes within twenty-four hours of their occurrence and to follow up with a detailed written report.

When I first started to work at Days Inns, I found one of the biggest threats to security and safety of hotel guests was the accountability of guest room keys. This problem is unique to the entire lodging industry and remains so today. I was amazed to find no uniform policies concerning key control, especially in an industry that is centuries old.

In Days Inns, some properties had not been rekeyed or had an accounting of the room keys made since they were constructed in 1970. It was very common then, and still remains a practice in some hotels and motels, for the maids, maintenance men, managers, and, in some cases, outside service personnel, to have master keys to the entire property. Amazingly, in these cases there are often no requirements for keys to be turned in at the end of the day or any effort made to collect keys from terminated employees.

We immediately set up strict key control policies that if violated resulted in an employee's termination. The guest rooms were keyed in sub-master stations with no more than fifteen guest rooms per station. If a sub-master key were lost or stolen, the integrity of the guest rooms could be regained fairly easily without having to rekey the entire property. A program was also established which required each company-owned property to be rekeyed annually.

But programs this comprehensive are the exception. Take the simple matter of carelessness with room keys. A majority of the travelers surveyed by *Corporate Travel* said they had been able to get duplicate keys without providing identification. Nearly two-thirds said that they had been given a key to a room already occupied. Another 38 percent said another person had been given a key to their rooms.

The reductio ad absurdum of this helter-skelter key practice is that many keys from years past will still open a hotel or motel door. Indeed, one couple who had honeymooned in a certain San Diego hotel right after World War II held on to the room key as a keepsake. Forty years later, the couple returned to the room for a second honeymoon. The original key still worked. Later, the couple was to be brutalized and assaulted by an assailant who took advantage of lax security.

Today, many chains have started installing electronic locking systems which issue a new guest key each time the room is rented. These systems can also track the identity of any hotel employee who enters a guest room. The problem is that these systems are flawed, and most owners of hotels and motels are not willing to pay the price for increased guest security. More than 90 percent of the hotel/motel guest rooms across the country still have the older key and knob locking systems. More frightening, they also have thousands of keys unaccounted for.

Have you ever been rushed for time when checking out of a hotel and forgotten to turn in your room key? Did you ever wonder what the hotel did about this when it discovered the room key was missing? Did you or somebody you know ever get a letter or call from a hotel informing you that you had failed to turn your key in and requesting you send it back? The ugly truth is that most hotels/motels don't ever know when a key is missing.

If you have any "forgotten" hotel/motel keys lying around, you, too, may be surprised to find they would still open the same room door. It is not rare to find hotels and motels which have not been rekeyed since they were opened for business decades ago and which have no system for tracking lost or stolen keys.

Another danger of using the standard hotel/motel locks with brass keys is the threat of professional hotel/motel criminals. These criminals devise ways of duplicating master keys which allow them access to every guest room on a property.

Several years ago, a group of criminals traveled throughout the United States targeting hotels and motels that used standard locking systems. This band of criminals would travel in groups of men, women, and children. They appeared to be the typical American family on vacation.

Once they had selected their target, they would register in groups of three or four families. Each group would ask for a room in different parts of the hotel/motel. This would be necessary for their master plan to work. As part of their luggage, they would bring along a complete locksmith kit and a key-making machine.

When the entire gang had checked into the hotel/motel, they were ready to begin their work. The trained locksmith in the gang would go to each member's room and remove the door lock. By looking at the positions of the pin settings in three or four doors, he could figure out the master key code. This would enable him to make a master key which opened every guest room on the property.

After making the master key, they were ready to begin identifying prospective victims. One of their favorite methods was for the women and children of the gang to go out and sit beside the pool. There, they could spot families leaving for the day. They would then notify their male counterparts as to what rooms were targets. This tactic would also enable them to be lookouts for returning guests or hotel employees.

Another method they used was to knock on room doors and announce they were with the hotel's housekeeping or maintenance staff. If they received no response, they would use their master key to enter and commit their crime.

Later, when the hotel guests returned, they would discover their room had been burglarized. Because there would be no sign of forced entry, the guests would immediately blame the theft on members of the hotel staff.

Police officials in the Orlando, Tampa, and Daytona Beach, Florida, areas estimated a band of thieves of this type was responsible for hundreds of room burglaries and the theft of millions of dollars in personal property from hotel/motel guests. When leaders of this group were finally arrested, police found in their possession briefcases containing hundreds of master keys fitting hotels/motels from Texas to Florida. Each key was tagged and identified by hotel/motel and city in which it was located.

Other forms of inadequate security have led to more violent crimes—like those committed by a man now in custody and accused of terrorizing, robbing, and raping women in a slew of motel attacks along interstate highways from Virginia to Florida.

One would think that the lodging industry, knowing the danger of using standard locking systems, would make it mandatory that all hotels and motels in the country be equipped with the new electronic systems. However, electronic systems will not be installed universally unless public outcry demands them or insurance companies require them before they write any coverage for the property.

The lodging industry is currently faced with tremendous economic problems. Largely because of the overbuilt condition of the industry created in the early and mid-eighties, hotels and motels are being forced to be more competitive, and strict budget tightening is going on throughout the industry. One of the first areas to suffer during these times is the security and safety budgets. Recently, in fact, several major hotel/motel chains made severe cuts in their security operations. With this present economic condition and the ever-increasing crime rate, the traveling public is most likely to suffer.

The security situation in apartments is just as revolting. There are several reasons. Few businesses in America have experienced the explosive growth of the apartment industry. Today, more than 36 million people live in apartments. In many cities and suburbs, over half of their population lives in apartments, and for many of us an apartment is our first home.

Like their cousins in the hotel/motel industry, many apartment owners have experienced extreme increases in crimes occurring on their premises—resulting in irreparable harm to tenants and multi-million dollar lawsuits. On February 10, 1993, for instance, a suburban Atlanta property owner was ordered to pay $2.5 million to a woman who was raped in her apartment complex in 1989. That case is only the tip of the iceberg.

Until recently, however, apartments had a much greater veil of protection from being sued by their tenants. They took the position that a tenant's security and safety was the sole responsibility of the tenant. Apartment owners are generally more concerned with items they call "curb appeal," such as tennis courts, swimming pools, and landscaping. Adequate door and window locks or lighting are not things that most people initially look for when renting an apartment.

In recent years, apartments have become prime targets for criminals. One reason is the lax attitude of apartment owners toward spending money on security measures, which possibly would deter or prevent tenants from becoming victims of a burglary, robbery, or sexual assault, all crimes that could result in serious injury or loss of life.

Another reason criminals are attracted to apartments is that most tenants are naive about their personal safety. They have a false sense of security caused in part by overzealous leasing agents. Most leasing agents work on commission and bonus programs based on the number of new apartments they lease each month. It is not uncommon for a leasing agent, in an effort to close a sale, to relate to a prospective tenant that a complex is safe when the agent knows the opposite is true.

For whatever reason, apartment complex owners were sued more often than any other business in recent years, according to Liability Consultants, Inc. Apartment unit crimes far outpaced even those in hotels and motels, and the average settlement and verdict in "residential areas" was $.5 million and $1.5 million respectively, far more than hotels and motels.

In 1989, Susan E. Lunn and Lisa E. Kiersky conducted a survey of tenants living in apartment complexes in metropolitan Atlanta. The survey was published in the July 1989 issue of *Counterpart* magazine. Of the respondents, 53 percent reported that they moved out of a previous apartment complex because they felt unsafe; 86 percent stated that they felt their present apartment complex was unsafe.

The following questions were posed to the respondents, and their answers and comments were:

1. Are all possible precautions taken for tenant safety at your complex?

Answer: 14 percent said yes; 86 percent said no.

Comment: "Our main outdoor lights go out often and the failure to fix them immediately is upsetting."

....

2. Does your complex notify you about burglaries or other incidents?

Answer: 13 percent said yes; 87 percent said no.

Comment: "No, they cover up."

....

3. If management informed you about burglaries or other incidents in your complex, how would you react?

Answer: 64 percent said they would appreciate the warning and stay in the complex; 34 percent said they would appreciate the warning but would move when the lease was up.

Comment: No one said they would prefer not to know.

4. Does management of your complex suggest safety precautions?

Answer: 40 percent said yes; 60 percent said no.

5. When you moved in, did management change your locks?

Answer: 25 percent said yes; 60 percent said no.

6. Did you inquire about crime when you moved into the complex?

Answer: 47 percent said yes; 53 percent said no.

Comment: "My new complex wouldn't give me the number of incidents, but they have a police officer living on the premises."

7. Have the following incidents ever happened to you at your complex?

Burglary: 20 percent said yes.

Robbery: None reported.

Rape: 7 percent said yes.

Assault outside the apartment: 20 percent said yes.

Assault inside the apartment: 7 percent said yes.

8. If you answered any of the above "yes," did you report the incident to management?

Answer: 71 percent said yes; 29 percent said no.

....

9. If yes, what was management's response?

Answer:
0 percent said management notified other residents;
17 percent said management added window or extra door locks;
17 percent said management hired security guards;
17 percent suggested that they keep it quiet;
67 percent said they got no response.

Comment: "No one has ever come to help when I called. Another time, the management office told me to call the police because they didn't want any of their security staff to take any risks."

"I filed a police report, no locks were changed, no extra security was hired, and I was asked to keep quiet for fear of scaring off other tenants."

....

In recent years, tenants have placed increasing pressures on apartment owners to provide security services. Apartment owners in search of finding "cost-effective" means of providing these services have devised a clever way to answer these demands. They find one or two local police officers willing to accept free rent in exchange for their services in their off-duty time. This is fairly simple to do since most police officers, due to their low pay, are forced to work part-time jobs just to make ends meet. Apartment owners like this arrangement since it does not require any outlay of working capital but provides them with a business deduction for the free apartment.

Instead of being called security officers, the apartments' staff are instructed to refer to the police officers as "courtesy officers." On the surface, this practice would appear to be very effective. However, in reality, it amounts to no more than "window dressing" and has many inherent problems and little or no deterrent or preventive effect on crime.

One of the major problems is the working schedules of the police offi-

cers. Most work on rotating schedules which take them away from the apartments during the most vulnerable times. Secondly, after working a full shift,
their "courtesy" patrols may amount to no more than a five- to ten-minute
drive-through inspection of the premises. However, the biggest problem
is how leasing managers and agents will use the presence of "courtesy officers" to their advantage in renting apartments.

A prospective tenant may inquire about any security services the complex may provide. Leasing personnel are ever too ready to respond by saying, "Oh, we have police officers living on site. That takes care of all our
security." This is very appealing to most people, since they have a higher degree of confidence in police officers than private security services.

Another practice which many apartment owners employ is the hiring
of a "security patrol" to protect tenants. What this means is a private security company will drive through the complex two or three times during
the evening hours in a marked patrol vehicle. The security service will normally place signs at the entrance and throughout the premises announcing they are being patrolled. In theory, these random patrols and signs offer
a deterrent to crime. These services normally cost the apartment owner
no more than $150 to $250 per month.

Both of these practices are grossly misleading and lure tenants into a false
sense of security. For example, a single female, living alone, arrives home
after working late only to find her normal parking space has been taken.
This requires her to park several spaces away and to walk through a
dimly lit parking lot. Under normal circumstances, she may be fearful, but
knowing her apartment complex has off-duty police officers or security
patrols, she walks the distance with a carefree attitude, never realizing her
safety depends on such careless practices by apartment owners.

However, when faced with a liability lawsuit due to a tenant having been
robbed, assaulted, or raped on their premises, apartment owners will
deny that the police officer was there to perform any security duties. They
will insist that the "courtesy officer" was there only to provide assistance
to tenants who may have locked themselves out of their apartments,
answer loud music complaints, or lock the pool at closing time.

All of these practices no doubt increase their ability to rent apartments. However, it may very well be placing an unsuspecting person in
harm's way at the hands of a criminal.

■ ■ ■

New Year's in New York

WHILE THE STATISTICS OF INCREASED VIOLENT CRIME AGAINST travelers, renters, and others speak volumes, it takes a case like Mary Kenner's to bring the agony home.

New York City, with its population of more than nine million persons, is the largest city in the United States and the ninth largest in the world. The very sight of the Statue of Liberty in Upper New York Bay is electrifying, especially when you stop and think of all the immigrants who have sailed into the harbor with hope in their hearts as they set out in a new life in a free land.

Much of what happens in New York City affects the lives of people throughout the United States and around the world. Because of its prominence as an entertainment and cultural center, the city is sometimes fondly referred to as "The Big Apple," and many people consider it to be the most fascinating city in the world. People often say, "If you can't find it in New York, it doesn't exist."

With all of its greatness, New York City is faced with some very serious problems. With more than one million people on welfare, poverty is pandemic, and the city has one of the highest crime rates, particularly for violent crime, in the nation. Nevertheless, thousands upon thousands of people travel to New York weekly on vacation or on business. Despite all the negative publicity—in 1992, for example, *Time* magazine featured a rotting apple on its cover to represent the city—New York remains one of the country's most frequent tourist destinations.

While in New York City, however, bad things can happen to the unwary tourist. In an internationally publicized case several years ago, a young man from Utah visiting New York for the U.S. Open Tennis Tournament, was fatally stabbed on a subway platform by a group of muggers who were ripping off his parents. And, with crime a contagion, it's not surprising that some of the most crime-prone locales in the Big Apple are hotel/motels.

Visitors are unaware of New York City's hidden problems—problems that could turn a trip into a nightmare as they did for Mary Kenner, an attractive, 45-year-old divorcee with stylishly coiffed graying hair, a ramrod-straight carriage, and a bent for "numbers crunching." She came to New York City in January 1985 on business with General Electric. She had worked as an account specialist for the past thirteen years and was in line for a promotion to a job that paid just under six figures. Mary grew up in nearby New Jersey and had visited New York City many times, both for pleasure and business. She wasn't at all naive about life in the big city. At least that's what she thought.

In mid-December, Mary had been notified by her supervisor that he wanted her to head up a special year-end accounting team at the New York headquarters in midtown Manhattan. She was told the project would probably take several weeks. Mary was very excited about being picked to head up this special audit team. She was sure it would enhance her chances for promotion. And it would be fun to spend New Year's Eve in New York. What could go wrong?

The company arranged for her and the other members of the audit team to stay at the Peak Hotel, conveniently located right down the street from their offices in Manhattan. Mary had stayed there on other visits to their New York City office and was always very pleased with the accommodations. The Peak Hotel is one of Manhattan's best known hotels; its more than 800 guest rooms are almost always filled because of its prime location. An average room per night costs about $175. The management of the Peak Hotel projects pride when it speaks of its hotel and the efforts it makes to provide its guests with the finest service.

The general manager knew that hotel security was a necessity in downtown New York and that various undesirables, including burglars and worse, had made life miserable for the guests of other hotels. In 1983, he hired a retired New York City police detective to head up his in-house security program. Feeling confident that he had hired a qualified security director, the general manager left the day-to-day operation up to him and rarely came in contact with the security department.

Mary checked into the Peak Hotel on the afternoon of December 31, 1984, and was assigned room 312 on the third floor. She provided the desk clerk with the names of the other people who would be working on the audit team. Most of them had already arrived, and the desk clerk gave her a listing of their room numbers. After getting settled in her room, Mary called the other team members, and they agreed to meet later in the bar for happy hour.

The hotel lounge was in an especially festive mood since it was New Year's Eve. Mary's group talked about going down to Times Square and being part of the "Big Apple" descent as the New Year came in. However, the bartender talked them out of that by saying it was a mob scene and not very safe. Besides, he said, they were going to have a big party in the lounge and they could watch the Times Square celebration on the wide-screen television set the bar was setting up.

Over the next five days, the routine was pretty much the same. Mary and her cohorts would arise early and meet in the hotel restaurant by 7:00 a.m. for breakfast. They would then walk the short distance to General Electric's office to begin work for the day. Once there, they were faced with mounds of paperwork, and the sound of calculators filled the air. Due to the enormous work load and a pressing timetable, they normally skipped lunch or had light lunches sent up from a local deli. They would continue to work long into the night, even after the local office staff had quit. During the first four days, it was common for the small working group not to sign out with the building's security officer before 10:30 or 11:00 p.m.

They would then normally catch a bite to eat at an all-night deli next to the hotel. By the time they finished eating and winding down, they would get in around 1:00 a.m. The next morning the routine would begin again.

The fifth day of January 1985 fell on a Saturday. Mary and the other members of the audit team had hoped to be able to take the weekend off and go sightseeing. However, late Friday night Mary realized they were several days behind schedule for finishing the project. She had the unpleasant task of informing the others they would have to work over the weekend.

Saturday started off the same as the previous mornings for the special audit team. Mary could hear some of the team members moaning about working the weekend. She didn't say anything, though, sadly realizing that the rest of New York was sleeping in and looking forward to the second weekend of the new year.

After finishing breakfast, they walked the short distance to their company's office building. The day was bright and amazingly warm for the first week in January. As they signed in with the security guard—an ever-friendly middle-aged man with a broad face and a ready smile—a couple of the team members commented that they were glad someone else had to work on such a beautiful Saturday.

The day seemed especially long since they were the only ones working in the entire building. They skipped lunch altogether while they continued to slave over the tedious job of crunching numbers.

Mary had a difficult time keeping her team's attention as the day wore on. Everyone, including herself, would catch themselves daydreaming while they looked out the windows at the rest of New York enjoying such a beautiful day.

Mary had intended to quit early so they could go to a movie and eat dinner at a decent hour. However, time slipped away and when she looked at her watch it was already 9:00 p.m. Mary apologized to everyone and told them how much she appreciated their hard work. She asked if they wanted to go for Mexican food—her treat. The stress of the long week was showing as she only had one taker, Larry Johnson, a studious man in horn-rimmed glasses who had worked diligently and quietly ever since the group arrived in New York.

Someone in the office had told Mary about a popular Mexican restaurant a short taxi ride from the Peak Hotel. Larry and Mary walked back across the street to their hotel to freshen up and agreed to meet in the lobby in thirty minutes. Meanwhile, Gene Smith, another member of their team, decided to remain in the office and continue to work.

The bellman had no trouble hailing Mary and Larry a taxi, and they arrived at the restaurant around ten o'clock. Typically for a Saturday night, the restaurant was packed, so they decided to wait in the lounge until their table was ready.

After a couple of margaritas, neither Mary nor Larry cared much about the long wait. When they finally were seated, the food was excellent and well worth the wait. Mary was pleased to discover that, behind his horn rims and usually stolid expressions, Larry had a previously disguised quick wit. Despite all the hours of hard work, she was wondering just how the trip could have gone any better.

After finishing dinner, they decided to get some exercise by walking the short distance back to the hotel. It was a little after midnight, but the sidewalks were full of people of all types. There were nicely dressed people like themselves, and street people trying to hustle everything from Rolex watches to X-rated photos. As always, there were the ladies of the night offering their services to every male passing by. On one corner a street preacher was ranting that the end of the world was coming. He was standing in front of a bookstore which had huge posters and display racks with a new, best-selling book concerning the year 2000 and beyond. Mary thought to herself, only in New York.

By the time they arrived back at the entrance to the hotel, Mary and Larry wished they had taken a taxi, but they had made it back safe and sound. Mary wanted a cup of hot coffee to take the chill off the evening before going to bed. She walked over to the corner coffee shop and got a cup of coffee to take back to her room. On her way back to the hotel, Mary heard the scream of sirens as a procession of police cars sped past her down the avenue. Like everyone else in her vicinity, she turned and followed the flashing blue lights with her gaze. She felt nervous.

As Mary entered the lobby, she had a passing thought of just how easy it would be for anyone to simply walk off the street and go into the hotel. The employees of the hotel seemed not to even notice her as she walked through the lobby and headed toward the elevator bank.

She caught the elevator and felt relieved when no one else got on with her. As the elevator started up, she chided herself for suddenly feeling scared. She thought it must have been the walk back from the restaurant amid the street people that had made her nervous.

The elevator came to a stop on the third floor, and Mary stepped off. The hallway lights seemed dimmer than previous nights, and she jumped as she heard a room door closing. "Stop this," she said to herself as she fished her room key from her purse. She opened her room door, reached in and flipped the light switch, but it would not come on. She leaned over, while holding the room door open to allow the light from the hallway to shine through. She reached for and found the light switch in the bathroom. She flipped it and the bathroom lights came on. Feeling safe and secure for the first time since she entered the hotel, she breathed deeply and slumped against the door for a minute. As she did, she became angry at herself for spooking so easily. She was sure it was because of the exhausting week she had just experienced.

As she caught her breath, Mary could smell the antiseptic-like aroma from where the maids had cleaned her room earlier in the day. Mary stood for a second and looked around the room. Everything appeared to be okay, so she walked over and placed her purse and coffee down on the dresser. She removed her coat and walked back over to the closet which was located to the right of the room door.

The closet door had double sliding mirror doors. When she first approached the closet doors, Mary again felt frightened as she noticed the position of the doors. She was sure they were in the reverse order from the way she had left them that morning. "Don't be silly," she said to herself. "The maids cleaned the room and they would have moved the doors while cleaning." She reached in the closet, removed a hanger, and hung up her coat.

Mary realized she had not turned the dead-bolt on the door as she entered, so she turned to her right and did so. She walked back over to the dresser, opened her coffee, and took a sip. As she stood there drinking her coffee, the position of the closet doors still bothered her. She had hidden some of her jewelry in her garment bag. For her own peace of mind, she walked back over to the closet and slid the closet doors to the position in which she had left them that morning.

She reached into the closet and grabbed her hanging garment bag and pulled it toward her. She put her coffee cup down on the floor and unzipped the compartment where she had hidden her jewelry, and reached inside to pull out the clear plastic bag that contained her precious jewels, including a broach handed down in her family for three generations. She was relieved to see that it was all there. She pushed the smaller bag back into its compartment, zipped it, and let the bag fall backwards into the closet.

As the bag fell back into the closet, it bounced as if it had hit something behind it. Mary leaned slightly into the closet to see what the bag had hit. It was then that she saw a black man slouched down in the rear corner of the closet. In a state of total terror and hysteria, she quickly turned and attempted to unlock the room door and run, knocking over the coffee cup in the process.

She heard the closet doors slamming open as the assailant forced them to one side. Everything seemed to be in slow motion as if she were daydreaming. She could feel herself screaming, but could hear no sounds coming from her mouth.

The man ran straight toward her. He swung his arm, knocking her hands away from the room door locks. He ran into her and the force of his body knocked her against the wall. She hit the wall hard and slid down the corner of the wall onto the floor. Half-dazed and breathless, she looked up to see her assailant was wearing a white mask, which she later described to the police as the kind the "Lone Ranger" had worn.

Mary would later testify that, as she had long heard it described, her whole life was flashing before her eyes, and there were no words which could describe the horror she was experiencing at that moment. She cried uncontrollably.

The assailant pulled a pistol from his pocket and placed it next to her temple, screaming, "Stop crying or I'll kill you." While resisting her attacker, she instinctively reached up and grabbed the barrel of the gun, knocking it aside.

She thought it was odd that it wasn't cold like she would have expected a gun barrel to be. Mary held on for dear life while she fought with the assailant. As they fought, the gun barrel broke, and she realized it was a plastic toy gun. In anger, the assailant threw the toy gun across the room.

The man was madder than ever. He began yelling profanities at her as he grabbed for a hunting knife which was in his belt. He placed the knife at her throat. He reached around to the back of her head and grabbed a handful of her hair. He violently jerked her head backwards as he raised the knife to her throat. Seeing that she was not going to stop fighting him, he slid the blade of the knife deftly across her throat. Mary then realized he didn't want to kill her, but he wanted to gain control. The cut was applied with just enough pressure to cause her to start bleeding slightly.

Feeling the warmth of the blood streaming down her neck sent Mary into a mild state of shock. She felt her body going limp, and there was no more fight left in her. She was becoming light-headed and fought with herself not to pass out.

She could barely talk, but later remembered asking the man, "Why are you doing this to me?" She repeatedly begged him not to hurt her anymore. He told her to shut up, that all he wanted was her money and jewelry.

He slowly lifted her from the floor while he held the knife tightly pressed to her throat. Once she was on her feet, he walked her slowly over to the dresser where her purse was sitting. He loosened the grip he had on her arm but still kept the knife at her throat.

He ordered her to remove all the money she had in her wallet and to take her rings and watch off. She complied, and he grabbed the items from her and shoved them into his pants pocket. He then walked her back over to the closet and told her to get the plastic bag, which contained her other jewelry, from her garment bag. He took the bag from her and shoved it into his pants.

He then removed the knife from her throat, but grabbed her by the hair and walked her over to the bed. He shoved her and she landed half on the bed and half off.

Mary lay there sobbing and shaking all over. She looked up at her assailant and for the first time saw him clearly. He was approximately 5' 11" tall, about 175 pounds, with a full beard. Besides the white mask, he was wearing a winter hat with earflaps. He wasn't wearing a coat but had on a red turtleneck sweater and black slacks. She glanced down at his feet and saw he had on white, high-top tennis shoes. Through her daze, she wondered to herself how such an oddly dressed man could walk through the lobby of an expensive downtown hotel without being noticed and challenged.

He reached over and pushed the rest of her body onto the bed and turned her over onto her stomach. He then removed a piece of rope from one of his pants pockets and wrapped it around her left wrist, pulling it so tightly she could feel the circulation being cut off.

Mary's sobbing had turned into uncontrollable crying. This appeared to provoke him more, and he began slapping her on the back of her head. "Shut up, bitch," he demanded. Fearful that he was going to rape her, she begged him not to or to hurt her anymore. He told her that if she did not quit crying and fighting with him, he was going to kill her.

He grabbed her other arm and twisted it across her back and began tying her two hands together. When she wouldn't stop crying, he leaned over and bit her right cheek so hard that it left his teeth marks, and blood rushed to the surface. He sucked on the wound and when he had a mouthful of blood, he spit it in her face. He then backhanded her and held the knife up to her face. "If you don't stop crying, I'm going to cut your tongue out," he screamed.

He then started slapping her across the face, causing her head to jerk back and forth. Mary knew that if she didn't stop crying, he was more than likely going to kill her. In order to stop crying, she began biting her lower lip to help her regain control. This helped, but she bit it so hard it would later require stitches to close the wound. Mary did not cry or utter another sound. She just lay there waiting to see what he was going to do next.

Seeing that she had stopped fighting, he took his knife and started cutting off her clothes—first her blouse and bra, then her slacks, panty hose, and panties.

Once he had cut all of her clothes off, he stood up and removed his pants. He then mounted Mary and entered her from the rear. Mary felt a sick feeling coming over her and she wanted to scream, but she didn't dare move or make a sound.

After he ejaculated, he turned her over and began kissing and running his tongue over her breasts. He bit her nipples so hard that she was sure he was going to bite them off.

He started saying, "I know you like this, bitch, why don't you tell me you like it." He then raped her a second time.

When he was finished, he sat across her chest and told her that he was going to give her something to remember him by. He took his knife and began poking the tip of the blade all around both of her breasts. He did this with such care as to make each wound superficial, yet deep enough to bleed.

The total assault and rape of Mary lasted about one and a half hours.

The assailant decided it was time to leave. He got up from the bed, picked up his pants from the floor, and went into the bathroom. Mary could hear the water running and his using the toilet. When he was finished, he walked back into the bedroom area fully dressed.

He walked over and stood next to the bed. Mary, still lying on her back, looked up at him with a dazed expression on her face. He stared back and said, "I know, bitch, it was as good for you as it was for me." He then yanked the phone out of the wall and threw it across the room. He told her he was leaving now, but if she tried to follow him or call the police, he would come back and kill her. After he made sure the ropes on her wrists were still secure, he left.

As soon as she heard the door shut, Mary burst into tears again. Her body began shaking so hard that the headboard was hitting the wall. It was too late to prevent the rape, she later remembered thinking, but why hadn't anyone come? Why couldn't anyone come after all the noise? She wanted to stop crying, afraid that the rapist would hear her and come back to kill her.

Mary's mind was racing a mile a minute. She started to wonder how he had been able to get into her room. The doors were self-closing and closed tightly when you left the room. She thought he must be an employee of the hotel or had gotten a key from somewhere.

She lay there for at least thirty minutes before trying to work her way free. But it seemed like the more she tugged on the ropes, the more they cut into her wrists, making the bleeding increase. Finally, she was successful in working her way out.

The first thing she did was jump off the bed and run over to the door. She twisted the dead-bolt latch into its slot and put the safety chain up. Mary wanted to scream for help or run out into the hallway and start knocking on doors until she found someone to help her. But she thought her attacker might still be out there and would surely kill her. She was still sobbing occasionally, and she felt numb from head to toe.

Mary paced frantically back and forth. She stopped in front of the dresser and, for the first time, looked at herself. She was horrified at what she saw. There was blood all over her face and neck. Her cheek was swollen and blue where he had bitten her. Blood was smeared and dripping down her body from the wounds he had inflicted on her breasts. As she stood there looking in the mirror, she began to feel ashamed and disgusted with herself. She dreaded the thought of facing her family and friends.

She walked over to the corner near the door and sat down. She pulled her knees up into her chest and wrapped her arms around her body. There she sat crying and wondering if she would ever be able to leave that room.

Some time passed, and Mary could feel herself becoming weaker and weaker. The blood seemed to be oozing out at a faster pace. She knew she had to get help, even at further risk to herself.

She got up and walked over to the bed. She tore off the sheet and wrapped it around her nude body. She walked over to the door, shaking, and very slowly cracked it open. She took a deep breath and peeked out into the hallway in search of her assailant.

Seeing the hallway was clear, she ran from the room. The bed sheet, which she had wrapped around her, was now soaked with her blood. Instead of waiting for the elevator, she ran to the emergency stairwell.

She ran down the stairs and into the lobby. Mary could see figures of people, but everything seemed hazy to her. She could hear people yelling at her, but she could not understand what they were saying and wasn't about to stop. "He must still be in here," she thought.

Mary ran through the lobby and out the main lobby doors, thinking she would be safe if she could get to the security guard at her office building. She ran across the street and was almost run down by a New York City police car. The two policemen jumped from their car and yelled for her to stop. Mary continued to run toward her office building in her bloody sheet with the two officers chasing behind.

She reached the lobby doors of her office building and swung them open. She ran inside and collapsed at the foot of the desk, where the startled security officer sat reading a book—which he dropped in shock when he saw her.

The two police officers reached her side, saw her condition, and immediately called for an ambulance. While awaiting its arrival, the police officers tried to ask her what had happened. But Mary was in a total state of hysteria, and the only words coming out of her mouth were, "Someone was in my room."

Gene Smith, Mary's co-worker, came down to sign out for the night. He could not believe his eyes. He told the police who Mary was and where they were staying and recounted to them when he had last seen her. The ambulance arrived and transported Mary to the local hospital for treatment.

The two patrol officers called for a crime scene and detective unit to meet them at the Peak Hotel to process the crime scene. The two policemen thought it interesting that no one from the hotel had called the police department to report a bloody lady wrapped in a bed sheet running through the lobby.

At the hospital, Mary was treated for the multiple stab wounds she received at the hands of her attacker. The doctors treating Mary counted more than one hundred puncture wounds around her breasts.

Fortunately, the physical wounds caused very little damage and healed in a couple of weeks. However, Mary's release from the hospital only marked the beginning of her real pain and suffering.

Mary returned home to New Jersey and immediately gave up her apartment and moved in with her mother. Mary's father had passed away several years before. Mary felt safer with her mother than living alone again; the familiar surroundings held so many fond memories.

Mary could not bring herself to go back to work. She talked with her boss, and he agreed to continue to pay her while she was on an extended leave of absence.

Mary sought treatment at the local rape crisis center, and her family doctor prescribed tranquilizers to calm her nerves and help her sleep. The people at the rape crisis center, realizing that she needed more help than they could provide, recommended she see a local psychologist. She continued to see the psychologist every week for some time, but was not feeling any better.

She turned to her priest for comfort. Yet no matter what she did, she could not shake the frightened feelings built up inside her. She constantly looked over her shoulder, thinking the black man was following her, and she had nightmares where he was brutalizing her and cutting her breasts again.

She started calling the police detective in New York City who had been assigned to investigate her case. She would always ask the same question, "Have you arrested the man who raped me?" The answer was always negative, but she continued to call daily until she realized the officer was treating her like a crank. Once while shopping, she saw a black man who, she was convinced, was her assailant. She was horrified that he had come to kill her. She ran from the store, got into her car, sped home, locked the doors, and kept a watch out the window to see if she had been followed.

Later that night, as she lay in bed, she thought she heard a noise coming from the kitchen. She called the local police, screaming into the phone, "He's going to get into my room and kill me." The police arrived and searched the entire house and grounds, but they could find no evidence that anyone had tried to get into the house.

After that incident, Mary had a dead-bolt lock installed on her bedroom door and began sleeping with all the lights on. She found herself not trusting anyone and becoming more distant from her mother and friends. She could not sleep at night and would lie there listening for her assailant to come back.

After six months, Mary received a letter from her employer stating that it would be necessary for her to come back to work or risk being terminated. Mary had known it was only a matter of time until she would have to face that decision. She met with her psychologist, who suggested that it might be good for her to go back to work.

On the day she was to report, it actually felt good to Mary to have a reason to get up. Her mother fixed her a big breakfast and they both were optimistic over Mary's cheerful mood. Mary's mother offered to drive her to work, but Mary wanted to drive herself.

It was about a thirty-minute drive to her office, and Mary, for the first time in ages, felt great. She pulled into the employee parking lot and parked. She shut the motor off, removed the keys, and started to get out of the car. As she opened the door, she glanced over toward the entrance and saw a black man dressed in a maintenance uniform. She froze.

Around lunchtime, a co-worker of Mary's crossed the parking lot on the way to his car and was surprised to find Mary sitting mummy-like behind the steering wheel of her car. The doors were locked and her hands were wrapped so tightly around the steering wheel that her knuckles had turned white. He tried to get her attention, but she would only stare ahead. He went back into the building and called the police and an ambulance.

Mary was hospitalized for several months while undergoing intensive psychotherapy. When she was finally released from the hospital, she realized she was going to have to undergo a lot of expensive therapy before she would be able to cope with everyday life again. Now faced with unemployment, she sought the help of an attorney.

A little more than a year and a half after Mary's attack, her attorney filed a multi-million dollar lawsuit against the Peak Hotel. The suit alleged the hotel failed to provide adequate security for the protection of its guests. The suit also alleged that this failure was the proximate cause of Mary's injuries. Having earned a reputation as an expert in the field of hotel/motel security, I was retained by the attorneys representing the Peak Hotel.

An expert's role is to evaluate the security program in place at the hotel on the date of the occurrence that has brought about the litigation. For me, this meant a thorough examination of the security policies and procedures, staffing, training, pre-employment screening, security hardware, management's role, and local police support and an analysis of past crimes committed on the premises and in the surrounding area.

The latter responsibility is extremely important, especially to ascertain crimes of a similar nature. In the case of Mary Kenner, these included sexual assault, robberies, and room burglaries, with special attention paid to any guest rooms entered where there were no signs of forced entry.

The evaluation process also includes reading all depositions or statements taken from possible witnesses and all other materials obtained during the discovery stages of the litigation. After these steps are accomplished, a two- to three-day on-site evaluation is conducted during which interviews are held with potential witnesses. Close attention is also paid to the day-to-day operation of the hotel.

The security measures other hotels in the area were providing for their guests is another important point of investigation. If, for instance, a hotel a block away is offering a higher degree of security than the property where the crime occurred, this could become a major issue. The question to answer is why the hotel being sued is not affording their guests the same level of protection.

Once an expert has completed the evaluation, he or she should then be able to render an opinion as to the adequacy of the security. This opinion would relate only to the time frame of the incident for which the business is being sued and prior to that time.

It is possible the expert may render an opinion which may be adverse to the client's position. If this occurs, the case will normally settle out of court. An out-of-court settlement in most cases allows the business being sued to escape the publicity associated with a courtroom trial. In some cases, this could prove to be contrary to public interest. It may allow the business owner merely to insure his risk by purchasing more insurance rather than fix security problems.

In due time, I spoke to the Peak Hotel's director of security. He admitted that, on the night of Mary Kenner's assault and rape, there were no security personnel on duty in the lobby. He further admitted that during the eighteen months prior to Mary's attack, more than 350 guest rooms had been illegally entered. The guests were either robbed in person or items were stolen from their rooms while they were out. At the time of his deposition, he stated that he could not recall how entry had been gained into these rooms.

The security director revealed that he had recommended the hotel install a closed circuit television (CCTV) system throughout the premises. This would have augmented his security staff and allowed for better surveillance of the hotel. He had also recommended that the hotel place safes in guest rooms and that extra security officers be added during evening hours. Most of the crimes, after all, were occurring during the evening hours.

I questioned him about the hotel's rekeying policy after a guest-room crime has been reported. He said the hotel's policy was to rekey the lock prior to renting the room to another guest.

During my on-site evaluation, I reviewed the hotel's incident reports concerning crimes that had been committed in the guest rooms. I found more than fifty reports written by the hotel's security staff which indicated "no signs of forced entry, outside hotel key used." I asked what that meant. The security director said it meant entry had been gained by someone with a key to the room. I asked him if this were possible. He then confided to me that rooms were not always rekeyed if a guest failed to turn in a key when checking out. In fact, the hotel's engineering staff had not even rekeyed all the rooms where crimes had been committed. He said he always reported this to the general manager, but did not know if the manager took any action to correct the problem.

Having received the information about the keys from the director of security, I interviewed the hotel's chief engineer. He related there had been several occasions where a breakdown of communication had existed between his staff and the security staff. He admitted it was true that all rooms had not been rekeyed according to policy.

When I asked if the hotel guest rooms had ever been rekeyed, he replied, "The hotel has not been rekeyed since it opened some twenty-five years ago." I then asked if they had ever switched guest-room locks from one floor to another. In the absence of rekeying, this would have somewhat maintained the security of the guest rooms. He replied, "We never thought of that."

I then requested that he produce hotel records for all brass key blanks purchased by the hotel in the two years prior to Mary Kenner's attack. I also requested that he conduct an inventory of the guest-room keys presently in use by the hotel. I knew this would be a monumental task, but a necessary one if we were going to defend the lawsuit.

While waiting for the information, I went about completing my evaluation. One item that had been overlooked and which I felt was critical was the report prepared by the crime scene unit of the New York City Police Department. A copy of this report confirmed what I suspected—that on the night of the attack against Mary, the officer on the scene had removed the lock from room 312 and sent it to the crime lab for examination. The crime lab's report showed there were no signs of forced entry into the lock taken from Mary's room. There were no signs that someone had attempted to pick the lock. Therefore, it was the lab's opinion that either a key had been used or someone had opened the door, allowing the assailant to enter.

All I could think about on my way back to the hotel were the reports I had read: "No signs of forced entry, outside hotel key used."

On my third day at the Peak Hotel, I received a phone call from the chief engineer. He requested that we meet to go over the results of his study concerning the status of the hotel guest-room keys. When he arrived in my room, I noticed he was very nervous and upset. He told me that during the two years prior to Mary Kenner's attack, more than 20,000 room keys could not be accounted for. He also informed me there were no records kept to show when additional keys had been made to guest rooms. This simply meant the hotel could not, with any degree of certainty, testify as to how many keys were missing to Mary's room on the night of January 5, 1987. I was depressed after this conversation. I felt for Mary, whom I had never met but whose brutal attack colored my investigation for the hotel. She didn't have a chance.

After completing my on-site evaluation, I rendered the following opinions in the case of *Mary Kenner v. Peak Hotel:*

1. That key control at the Peak Hotel on the night of January 5, 1987, was inadequate. In fact, the hotel could not account for 20,000 keys within a two-year period prior to the assault and rape of Mary Kenner.

2. That access into the hotel was unrestricted and the staffing level of hotel security was not adequate for a hotel of its size and location.

3. That the Peak Hotel violated its own policies in the area of key control and the rekeying of guest rooms.

4. That the crime committed against Mary Kenner was foreseeable due to the numerous entries into guest rooms by what the hotel security staff termed "outside hotel keys." This in itself was enough proof that the hotel had notice that a crime of this nature was going to occur.

5. That the Peak Hotel ignored the advice of its own inhouse security expert as to staffing and recommendations concerning security hardware devices needed to insure reasonable guest security.

6. That the Peak Hotel did not provide its guests with reasonable security measures.

Based upon these opinions, I informed the attorneys that I would not be able to testify on their behalf. I strongly recommended that they seek an out-of-court settlement. Within a week after my report to the Peak Hotel's attorneys, an out-of-court settlement was reached between the parties to the lawsuit. The court ordered the records sealed (thus the Peak would never receive the negative publicity it deserved from the incident) and the dollar amount of the settlement kept confidential.

I am sure the dollar amount was substantial. However, no dollar amount could compensate Mary Kenner for the pain and suffering she sustained on the night of January 5, 1987. Her assailant was never identified nor arrested for the savage crime he committed.

Mary still has recurring nightmares of her attack. She still cannot leave her house unattended. She is unemployed. I don't know if Mary's life will ever be normal again.

What You Should Learn from This Crime

If you are traveling alone, consider having a member of the hotel staff escort you to your room. If you are traveling with others, ask that one of the male members of your group escort you to your room. Also, always trust that inner voice inside of you; if you feel something is out of place or does not feel right, *immediately* go to the front desk and report your suspicions to the hotel staff. They should be willing to check your room. Do not return to your room alone; insist on assistance.

■ ■ ■

A New Beginning Lost

THE SWEAT WAS DRIPPING OFF HER FOREHEAD, AND MUSCLES were aching in parts of her body that she had long ago forgotten she had, as she sat straddling the lifecycle and pumping away.

Betty Jo Keller stared into the full-length mirror facing her in the health club. However, she was not thinking about her body. Like most recently divorced women, she was wondering what had gone wrong with her marriage. She had been brought up in a family that believed that once you are married, it is "until death do us part." In fact, she was the first in the history of her line of the McDonald family to ever be divorced—a realization that only increased her concern. She desperately needed her family's support, but whenever she spoke to her mother, father, brothers, or sisters it was like a broken record: "Have you figured out what you did wrong?" And, "How are you ever going to raise those two children by yourself?" It seemed like Ricky, her ex-husband, received more sympathy from her own family members than she did.

Betty Jo had married Ricky Keller when she was seventeen years old. Ricky had been the quarterback of their high school football team, and from the time they had been in junior high they had been inseparable. People could have easily mistaken Ricky as part of the McDonald family because of the amount of time he spent at the house. Indeed, Betty Jo's father and mother both referred to Ricky as "our son."

Ricky Keller had a strong but likable personality. After high school he had enlisted in the Army, where he was trained as a heavy equipment operator. Those were tough times for the newly married Kellers. They were always having to borrow money from her parents to make ends meet, and it didn't help any when Betty Jo got pregnant. Ricky thought she was taking birth control pills, but she confessed that, trying to save money, she had not gotten her last prescription filled. "Besides, nobody gets pregnant that easily," she exclaimed passionately. Nine months later their first son was born.

While Ricky was overjoyed at the time, he never quite got over Betty Jo's irresponsible decision concerning the birth control pills. It was hard enough trying to feed two mouths on a private's pay, much less three. Somehow, they made it through the next two years. Upon Ricky's discharge they immediately went back home to Memphis. Ricky had no problem landing a high-paying construction job based on the training he had received in the military. It wasn't long afterwards that Betty Jo became pregnant with their second unplanned child; at least they could afford it now.

Throughout the course of their marriage, Ricky made all the decisions without even once discussing anything with Betty Jo. Her jobs were to take care of the kids, go grocery shopping (with a list prepared by Ricky), get up at 5:30 in the morning to fix his breakfast and pack his lunch, and have his dinner on the table when he walked in the door at 6:00 p.m.

After dinner, Ricky would take his dirty work clothes and boots off, pile them on the floor for Betty Jo to pick up, take a shower, and settle into his recliner. He would read the paper, watch the local news, then tune into the sports channel and view it until dozing off to sleep.

In the early years of the marriage, Betty Jo would wake him up around 10:00 p.m. to go bed. Later, after years of hearing him curse because she had awakened him, she would just let him sleep many a night away in his chair.

The weekends were all pretty much the same. Ricky played on two different softball teams, one on Friday nights and the other on Saturday afternoons. By the time the beer party after the game was over, it would be too late to ever take in a movie. In the off season, Ricky would be preoccupied with college football games on the television all day Saturday and pro football all day Sunday.

This scenario pretty much accounted for their marriage over the next seven years, until Ricky started staying out all Friday and Saturday nights with "the boys." It didn't take long for Betty Jo to pick up on the tell-tale signs like lipstick on the collar of his shirts and the smell of cheap perfume all over his clothes. They had never had much of a sex life after their second child was born, but since Ricky started staying out all night, their sex life became nonexistent. If Betty Jo tried to protest his behavior, he would become very angry and start yelling and screaming at her—"Bitch, bitch, bitch, that's all you ever do. Can't you ever be happy?"

This went on for about a year and a half. Then one day, after piling up his dirty work clothes and boots, Ricky announced that he wanted to have a talk with Betty Jo after she had cleaned up the kitchen and he had finished his shower. Before getting into the shower, Ricky told her to put the kids to bed early; this must be a private conversation.

When they finally talked, Ricky told her that the way he saw it they had grown apart. Betty Jo thought to herself, "What the hell does that mean?"

He continued, "It's just not the same between us. I want a divorce."

Betty Jo started crying and wanted to ask him why, but as always, Ricky dominated the conversation. He wanted the divorce and nothing she said was going to change his mind.

Not surprisingly, things would turn out Ricky's way. Betty Jo agreed to sign the divorce papers without hiring her own attorney. She would take the sum of money he offered for child support. Since Betty Jo had never worked or paid bills, she had no earthly idea what kind of money it took to live on. However, they had managed to save a little over the years. Ricky agreed to give her half of it, along with half of the proceeds from the sale of their house, to help her get started in her new life.

Betty Jo called on emotional resources she wasn't aware she had. She realized that for most of her life she had been a shy, almost frightened, person and had depended first on her parents and then on Ricky to make all her decisions for her. But now it was just her and the two children. Somehow they must survive. Somehow they *would* survive.

Within the next six months, Betty Jo had graduated from beautician's school and had landed a well-paying job. It had taken longer than Ricky and she had thought to sell the house. Naturally, he blamed the delay on her—as if she had something to do with the slow economy. But they finally received a contract, and now she was faced with the task of finding a suitable apartment in which she and the two boys could live.

All the apartments she really liked that appeared to be in a nice section of town were too expensive for her. She finally settled on a nice little complex just south of town called the Southern Arms Apartments. It would take her forty-five minutes to drive each way to and from work, but Southern Arms appeared to be clean and well maintained. The two-bedroom apartment she selected was spacious with new carpet; it had recently been painted. There was a pool and playground for the kids, and the surrounding neighborhood appeared to be very nice. Besides, if she worked hard and saved her money, she would be able to afford to buy another house in a year or so. The complex's resident managers, Jane and Billy Crew, told her they, too, had recently moved in. Jane assured Betty Jo that Southern Arms was a nice, safe place to live; they were on call twenty-four hours a day if she had any problems whatsoever.

The buzzer finally sounded on the lifecycle and not a minute too soon. Betty Jo sort of rolled off the seat and had to catch her balance to keep from falling. She stood there for a few minutes to catch her breath while again looking at herself in the mirror. Not a bad figure for a 28-year-old mother of two. A lot had happened over the past couple of years, and she could not remember when she had been happy. But all that was changing. She was getting in shape, had begun dressing as well as the other women where she worked, and for the first time in her life she was in control of her own destiny.

Betty Jo tossed her long blonde hair from side to side and said to herself, "Enough of this daydreaming." She needed to take a shower, and the movers would arrive at the house at noon to move them to their new apartment home.

As usual, it took much longer to get everything out of the house than planned. She had already dropped off a lot of belongings at a local storage company because they wouldn't fit into the apartment. Several of the girls from work along with their husbands or boyfriends came over and helped. They finally finished about 10:00 p.m., and then they ordered pizza. Betty Jo had promised there would be plenty of cold beer for everyone after they had finished.

Earlier in the evening Jane and Billy Crew, the apartment managers, had stopped by for a few minutes to see if everything was okay with the new apartment. Betty Jo thanked them for their concern, and they left.

When she first met the couple, Betty Jo had immediately liked Jane. However, Billy was a little strange, to say the least. He always seemed to dress the same: black shirt, black pants, black cowboy boots, and a black belt with a big shiny silver buckle. Betty Jo also couldn't help but notice the tattoos all over both of his arms and hands; she had seen a lot of guys with tattoos when Ricky was in the army, but these looked totally different—as if they had been put on by someone who did not know what he was doing. On top of everything else, Billy had the annoying habit of constantly sniffing as if he needed to blow his nose. His eyes were extremely bloodshot and watery, and he never said much. He just kind of stared at her as if he were undressing her. But enough of this, she thought; it was probably just her imagination running wild from these new "love novels" the girls at the shop were always passing around.

The moving party continued until about 1:00 a.m., when the beer finally ran out and half of the guests were falling asleep on the floor. It was about 1:45 when Betty Jo finally got the last of them out the door, locking the dead bolt behind her. She looked around at the mess and thought, what the hell—she had all day tomorrow to get everything cleaned up and in place before Ricky brought the kids home. She sat down on the sofa, took the last drink out of her beer can, and fell fast asleep sitting up.

Two buildings away, Jane and Billy Crew had just finished having a knock-down, drag-out fight over Jane's accusations that Billy had been staring at Betty Jo. The latter had been dressed in a low-cut shirt, which made it obvious she was not wearing a bra, and tight, cut-off shorts, which Jane thought showed too much of Betty Jo's backside.

"If you like blondes so goddamn much, I could dye my hair," Jane screamed at Billy.

The fight itself was nothing new between the two of them. They had been going at it ever since they had met about a year ago in a country & western bar where Billy was a bouncer. They had dated a few times, then moved in together and started telling people they were married. But the truth was, they were not married and legally couldn't be since Billy was still married to a woman back in Texas. Billy kept promising Jane he would get a divorce but never made any effort to do so. Whenever Jane would bring up the subject, he would make the excuse that he couldn't afford a divorce on what he was making. Jane thought she had solved that problem when she found them their new jobs.

About a month previously, Jane had come across an advertisement in the Sunday paper for a couple to manage an apartment complex for good pay, a free apartment, and excellent benefits. The only drawback: the ad stated extensive prior apartment management experience was required. Jane had worked as an apartment leasing agent years ago in Georgia, so maybe she could lie her way through the interview. Besides, this would be the break she and Billy needed. She told Billy about the ad, and they applied the next day.

The Maxwell Apartment Management Company owned and operated more than 150 apartments in twenty states. Like most apartment management firms, its biggest problem was finding qualified managers to run the various apartments—and then keeping them. There was a large turnover problem. So the owners decided to hire strong district managers to oversee multiple complexes. Under them, less-qualified people would be hired at the property level. These lower-level managers would then just more or less babysit a property, lease the apartments, and perform minor maintenance work. All the other decisions would be left up to the district managers.

So when Jane and Billy Crew showed up for their interview, they were just what the doctor ordered—or so it seemed. Jane lied about the extent of her management experience on her employment application, while Billy, in the meantime, falsified his application by listing all kinds of previous maintenance experience and training. The truth was, he barely knew how to change a light bulb, and the only training he had received was how to make license plates in the Texas State Prison System— something which he also omitted from his application. In fact, Billy had been ordered by a state court judge, at age 17, either to enter the army for three years or go to prison for three years for burglary. He chose the army, but later hit an officer, went AWOL, was captured, and was given a dishonorable discharge. But his three years of military service, with a tour in Vietnam, looked good on the application.

"Yes, indeed," the interviewer said, as he looked over their applications, "you people are made for Maxwell Management Company." They were offered the job at a combined salary of $35,000 a year and were to receive medical insurance and a free apartment without any reference checks or background investigation. Jane would take care of the office work and Billy the maintenance and any security problems that might crop up. Their first assignment would be the Southern Arms Apartments in south Memphis.

"Me, security," Billy chuckled as they left the office.

Their fight early Sunday morning ended like most, with Billy slapping Jane senseless and her running and locking herself in the bathroom. By that time of the morning, Billy had normally drunk so much beer and snorted so much cocaine that he wouldn't have the strength to kick the door in. He would just wander off, fall across the bed, and pass out. The next morning he rarely remembered what happened and would ask, "Did I do that?" as Jane tried to cover up the cuts and bruises on her face.

Jane would always reply, "Yes, you son of a bitch, and if you ever hit me again, I will leave you." But, that was easier said than done—she loved him. However, she worried that with each fight he was becoming more violent. He was snorting more and more cocaine.

The next morning, Betty Jo was half awakened by the sun shining through the sliding glass doors and by a noise within the apartment. She forced open one eye and then the other, and she was taken aback for a moment by the strange surroundings. She was now lying stretched out on the sofa under a blanket. That's strange, she thought. She didn't remember lying down, much less getting up and finding a blanket in this mess.

Betty Jo lay there a minute trying to regain her senses, when she heard the same noise that had awakened her in the first place. It was coming from the kitchen, and it sounded like someone was opening and closing the oven door. How could that be? Then she heard the noise again. She jumped to her feet, wrapped the blanket around her, and slowly walked over to the doorway of the kitchen. She let out a scream when she saw the figure of a man, dressed in black and bent over in front of her stove—it was Billy Crew. The scream scared him half to death. He jumped up, hitting his head on the front of the stove and dropping a long-handle screwdriver he was holding in his hand.

Betty Jo yelled, "What the hell are you doing in my apartment?" Billy Crew replied that he had noted that the light was not working in her oven and he had come to fix it. He added that he had noticed that she wasn't covered up, so he had taken a blanket out of the bedroom and covered her. "Besides," he said, "it looked like you had a party here last night and I figured you didn't want me to wake you up." He then apologized over and over again for frightening her, sniffling between each word, and asked if he could go and get her some coffee or something.

Betty Jo told him she didn't want anything, but for him to leave and to never come into her apartment again without first getting her permission. Besides, "How did you get in with the dead bolt locked?" she asked. Billy Crew explained to her that, as the maintenance man, he had a pass key to all of the apartments; he promised that he would call her in the future before coming into her apartment to make repairs.

Billy gathered his tools, put them back into his waist tool belt, and walked toward the front door. "I was just trying to be helpful, being that you just moved in and all," he said.

"That's fine and I appreciate your kindness," Betty Jo responded gingerly, as she was having second thoughts; maybe she had overreacted. "You just scared me, and I'm sorry for yelling at you. Just please call me the next time you plan on coming to make any repairs."

Billy Crew retorted, "Fine, no problem," and walked out the door. Betty Jo leaned against the door and engaged the dead bolt. Little good that does, she thought, if someone has a pass key.

Billy Crew was seething mad as he walked down the steps from her apartment. "I thought she might be different than the rest of them," he said to himself. "But she is just like all the rest of those fucking bitches—get what they can out of a man, then fuck him. Besides, her ass wasn't that nice."

Over the next few weeks, Betty Jo saw very little of Billy or Jane Crew. Only occasionally would she see them out in the parking lot or at the mailbox. As always, Billy was sniffing and wearing all black. "My God," she thought, "doesn't he have anything else to wear?"

Her days all started and ended about the same. In the morning, get the kids up, run around like crazy trying to get them off to school, and then get ready for work. At night, she would fix dinner, help with homework, get the kids ready for bed, read or watch television for awhile, then go to bed.

Ricky would pick the boys up every other weekend, and that would give her some time to herself. Occasionally, she would go out with some of the girls from work. She had not dated yet—she was just not quite ready for that—but maybe soon, she thought. She was gaining more and more self-confidence, and, for the first time that she could remember, she was happy.

Betty Jo was really looking forward to the upcoming Fourth of July weekend. It was Ricky's turn to have the boys, and she had been invited to three different parties. She was especially excited about her plans for the Fourth. One of the girls at work had fixed her up with Betty Jo's first date since she and Ricky had split. Since the Fourth fell on a Monday this year, she would have all day Saturday and Sunday to get ready—or so she thought.

On the night of June 30, Betty Jo had been awakened by police and ambulance sirens as the vehicles pulled into the apartment complex. The sliding glass door in her bedroom faced the leasing office and overlooked the parking lot. She looked at the digital clock on the bedside table next to her bed, and it was blinking 4:00 a.m. She pulled herself out of bed and looked out the blinds. In the parking lot below there were five or six police cars and two ambulances, all with their blue and red lights flashing. She could see someone being loaded onto one of the ambulances on a stretcher. She could also make out that several police officers were fighting with a man as they tried to get him in the back seat of one of the police cars. The man suddenly turned and appeared to be staring directly at her. But that had to be nonsense, she thought. She was too far away, and besides how could he see her? Since the lighting in the parking lot was so dim, she couldn't even make out who he was.

After a few minutes, all the emergency vehicles began pulling out. She went to bed and had trouble falling back to sleep, wondering what had been going on. "Well, it's none of my business," she thought. Jane and Billy would handle the problem, whatever it was; she soon fell asleep.

However, the problem was Jane and Billy Crew. After an all-night bout drinking beer with whiskey shooters and snorting an "eight ball" (3.5 grams of cocaine), Billy started fighting with Jane. But this time was different. In addition to slapping and kicking her, he had run out to the maintenance shed and picked up an ax when she ran and locked herself in the bathroom. He then got a knife from the kitchen drawer and, armed with his two weapons, banged on the bathroom door.

"Open the goddamn door, you bitch, or I'll chop it down and cut your goddamn heart out," he yelled as he pummelled the door with his fist. Thinking there was nothing new about this conduct—Billy would eventually pass out—Jane sat on the toilet and taunted him.

"Yeah, yeah, you worthless son of a bitch, you couldn't kill a fucking chicken," she slurred, barely able to talk herself after having matched him drink for drink and snort for snort for most of the night.

This is the last time she is going to insult my manhood, Billy thought as he raised the ax in the air. She doesn't know just how fucking bad I am and who she is fucking with. The first swing he took missed the whole bathroom door, but took a nice chunk out of the wall. The ax was embedded in the wall, and, in his drunken and drugged condition, Billy fell down three times trying to pull it free.

Meanwhile, inside the bathroom Jane was thinking maybe he was serious about killing her this time. However, she couldn't help but laugh when she heard him cursing and falling down.

"Yeah, yeah, you drunken son of a bitch, you can't even stand up, much less knock a door down." Jane had just gotten those words out of her mouth when the ax came crashing through the door, sending wood splinters all over the bathroom and her. She wasn't laughing anymore.

After about the tenth swing of the ax, the door was completely in ruins. Billy threw the ax down and pulled the butcher knife from his belt where he had stuck it while chopping away at the door. He whacked away at what remained of the door and entered the bathroom. Jane by this time had crawled over into the tub—as if that was going to offer her some type of protection.

"Now, I'm going to kill you, bitch," he yelled as he raised the knife over his head and came down with it. The blade of the knife caught the side of her left arm, inflicting a five-inch gash from which blood poured. Jane was now sober and terrified. As Billy raised the knife once again, she reached over with her right hand and turned the hot water on. She then grabbed the lever to transfer the water to the showerhead. The first burst of hot water hit her, but that was better than being stabbed to death. She reached up, grabbed the showerhead, and aimed it at Billy. The hot water hit him squarely in the eyes and face. He screamed, and, blinded temporarily, stumbled back a few steps and dropped his knife. Jane took the opportunity and bolted from the tub and out of the bathroom. She ran out into the parking lot and started screaming at the top of her lungs, "He's trying to kill me."

The neighbor next door, who by now was accustomed to being awakened by Jane and Billy's weekly fights, was no longer amused. He told his wife to call the police as he slipped his clothes on. He went out to the parking lot where Jane was standing, dressed only in her panties and bra, covered in blood, and still screaming with all the energy she had left, "The crazy son of a bitch is going to kill me."

About that time, Billy had recovered from his "shower" and came running out of their apartment, knife in hand and screaming, "You're right about one thing, bitch, I'm going to kill you."

The neighbor stepped in front of Jane and tried to talk Billy into putting the knife down. "Let's talk," the neighbor soothed.

Billy kept advancing. He didn't want to talk—he was going to kill Jane. He raised the knife, swung, and caught the neighbor in the shoulder.

Now the scene looked like something from hell to the other apartment tenants who had heard the disturbance and by now were standing on their patios or balconies. There was Jane in nothing but her underwear, covered with and dripping blood, hands waving in the air over her head, running around and around two parked cars screaming "He's going to kill us!"

There was the neighbor—barefooted with only his jeans on, and he too was covered in blood, screaming "He's going to kill us." And there was the man in black in hot pursuit.

By now the Memphis Police Department's 911 switchboard had lit up like a Christmas tree. Yes, they told numerous callers, they had received a call about a man with a knife chasing two people in the parking lot of the Southern Arms Apartments. Yes, they had cars en route to a man dressed in black killing people in the parking lot of the Southern Arms Apartments. Yes, it had been reported that a naked woman was running around in the parking lot with two men chasing her with knives. Cars and ambulances are en route—thank you for calling.

Betty Jo Keller had caught the tail end of the episode. As it turned out, Billy Crew had indeed, in that split second, spotted her looking out the sliding glass door. He hadn't seen the twenty to thirty other people standing outside their apartments or looking out their doors or windows, but he had seen her. As he lay on the back seat of the police car en route to jail he thought, "That no-good bitch. First, she talks to me like a dog—now she sticks her nose into my business by calling the police on me. Maybe some day I can return the favor."

At the police station, Billy Crew was charged with two counts of aggravated assault and drunk and disorderly conduct, and it was noted on his book-in sheet that he appeared to be under the influence of cocaine. When the investigating officer keyed Billy's name, social security number, and date of birth into the computer, he found Billy Lee Crew was no stranger to police stations or jail cells.

The print-out showed Billy had first been arrested at the age of 15 for breaking and entering the home of a 75-year-old woman whom he threatened with a knife after not being able to find any money. Billy spent two years in a juvenile detention center. After being released, he soon found himself back in front of the judge who had given him the military-prison options. After his brief stay in the army, Billy ended up in Dallas. After only three days there, Billy was arrested for trying to sell marijuana to an undercover police officer. He made bail for that charge, but, two nights later, after drinking and snorting cocaine, he started flirting with a local cowboy's girlfriend. When the cowboy voiced his anger, Billy pulled a knife and cut the cowboy so many times that his own parents had a hard time identifying him. Through a miracle the victim survived, and Billy was sentenced to twenty years in the Texas State Prison.

After being released ten years later, Billy drifted from state to state and ended up in Memphis. He found a job in a local honky-tonk as a doorman checking for under-age people trying to gain admittance. Of course Billy liked to tell the "honky-tonk queens" who came into the club that he was a bouncer. That's where Billy meet Jane Newton, who soon became his common-law wife.

Billy was allowed to make a phone call the next morning when he came down off of the cocaine and began to sober up from the "boilermakers" he had gulped down the night he attacked Jane and the neighbor. He called his brother who lived in Colorado and, after much blubbering and crying, convinced him to wire the money for his bail. The money arrived two days later at the bonding company, and Billy was released on bail.

When Billy arrived back at the apartment complex, he found an empty apartment and a "Dear John" note from Jane, who had made good on her promise to leave him. He walked up to the leasing office to find a temporary employee answering the phones and showing apartments. Billy introduced himself, and she handed him a message to call the district manager.

Billy phoned the district manager and was surprised to find his mood pleasant and understanding. The man said that Jane had come by the office and told him of their fight. She said she was quitting and moving back home with her mother. The assault on the tenant who had tried to come to Jane's aid was never mentioned. The district manager did add that it was company policy to have a husband-and-wife team manage the apartments, but asked him if he would remain to oversee maintenance until they could find a suitable replacement team. "Of course we will maintain your pay and the use of the apartment until that time," the district manager told Billy.

"Well, maybe there is a God watching after old Billy after all," Billy said to himself.

When Jane had reported their problems to the district office, it was very obvious from the large bandage on her arm and the cuts and bruises about her face that they had been engaged in a violent fight. Jane also mentioned the tenant who came to her aid. But the district manager had more pressing problems—the new annual budgets were due and the owners were on his back over rent-collection problems and for being over budget. The last thing he needed was to lose both of his managers at the Southern Arms. Besides, Billy had seemed like a nice enough guy. Hey, occasionally domestic situations get a little out of hand, but it happens to a lot of people, he thought. The district manager expressed his concerns to Jane, then bade her good-bye and good luck. Now that half of the problem is gone, Billy can hold the place together until I have time to find replacements, the district manger thought.

He made that decision without any follow-up investigation with the police which would have revealed Billy's long criminal history and his propensities toward violence. If the manager had been interested, he would also have found out about the large rash of burglaries reported from tenants of the Southern Arms, all of which had some similarities: money, jewelry, or small appliances were being stolen (jewelry and small appliances being items easily pawned), and all the crimes were committed without any signs of forced entry.

Over the next few days, Billy tried hard to drown his self-pity in as much beer, whiskey, and cocaine as he could consume while trying to keep up with the maintenance problems around the apartments. The Fourth of July weekend was coming up, and he was going to be all alone.

As it turned out, it didn't matter whether Billy had been alone or not. He woke up Sunday morning, and his head felt like it was the size of a watermelon. His body ached all over. He thought it was appropriate that blaring from the radio was Johnny Cash's old song "Sunday Morning Coming Down." Yes, like the words of the song, he, too, couldn't hold his head to where it didn't hurt. He knew he had started drinking and snorting cocaine some time on Friday afternoon with some newfound friends he had met at the liquor store, but that was about all he could remember—damn, what happened to Saturday?

Billy pulled himself up off the sofa and staggered toward the kitchen. Damn, it felt like somebody had stuck a wad of cotton in his mouth, he thought. He managed to open the refrigerator door to find two slices of three-day-old pizza, some stale sandwich meat, moldy bread, one can of tomato juice, and a can of beer. He reached for the tomato juice, but opted instead for the beer. He popped the top and drank about half the can in one gulp. He then walked over to the kitchen table and managed to scrape together a line of cocaine which had been scattered about the table and a piece of broken mirror on which he and his friends had been snorting Friday night. He leaned over, placed his right nostril on the piece of broken mirror where the line of cocaine began, held his finger to his left nostril and inhaled. "Wow! Now that is a way to start a day!" he thought.

Billy managed to shower, get dressed, and walk down to the leasing office. The temporary employee commented on how bad he looked and handed him a stack of work orders. He walked outside the office and thumbed through them. He saw one for a light bulb that needed to be replaced in some hallway, stuck it in his pocket, and threw the rest of them into the trash can. Taking care of the light bulb would be enough work for today. Besides, there were two more days left of the Fourth of July weekend, and he needed some more money.

In walking around the complex, Billy spotted several parking spaces vacant, and he assumed that those tenants would be away for the weekend. He pulled out his pass key and entered the first of four apartments he would break into that day. He quickly searched the apartments and took any money, jewelry, or small appliances he knew he could pawn or sell on the corner near his favorite liquor store.

Billy's "score" was good. He managed to sell or pawn his loot for more than $300, plenty to get him through the Fourth. He then drove around the projects until he found his "connection." He purchased three "eight balls" (over ten grams) of cocaine. He then went to the liquor store, bought two cases of beer and two half gallons of Jack Daniel's, and drove back to the apartments. He might have some people over later, and he needed to be prepared.

It had been a hard day at work and he needed to take a nap.

When Billy woke up it was nearly 7:00 p.m. At least he felt much better. He walked to the kitchen, opened a beer, and looked out the window. Across the parking lot, Betty Jo was getting in her car to go over to a friend's house for the pool party and cookout. Billy saw her getting into her car and said aloud, "That's the bitch that started all this trouble and called the police."

Betty Jo got into her car and drove off.

Billy got on the phone, called his newfound friends from Friday night and invited them over. Billy broke out his "Waylon and Willie" outlaw songs and cranked up the volume. He could identify with the lines in the songs about bad men and outlaws—yes, he was a bad man and an outlaw, too, he guessed.

His friends arrived, and over the next few hours they put a serious dent in the beer, Jack Daniel's, and cocaine. Everybody was sitting around talking about how bad they were until Billy went into the kitchen, got a knife, and began waving it around in the air and shouting, "I'm going to kill me somebody tonight."

Not wanting to be the one killed, each of Billy's visitors started making excuses and left Billy to his own misery. As the last one went out the door, Billy was slumped over the kitchen table, Jack Daniel's bottle in one hand and the knife in the other. In front of him sat an open, half-emptied beer, and his head rested near a line of cocaine. When the door closed for the last time, he was still mumbling something about killing somebody tonight.

Meanwhile, Betty Jo couldn't remember when she had had such a good time. She had met the nicest guy at the party, and he also had recently gone through a divorce. They talked throughout the evening and found they liked many of the same things. The party started breaking up shortly after midnight. Before leaving, Betty Jo gave her new friend her phone number and he promised to call. She hoped so.

Betty Jo drove back to her apartment, and when she got out of the car she could hear the loud music coming from across the parking lot in the direction of Jane and Billy's apartment. At the time, she did not know Billy had been locked up and Jane had quit her job and moved out. Betty Jo just figured it was another wild night in Dodge.

It was around 1:30 a.m. when Betty Jo finally got in bed. She was very tired, and it didn't take her long to fall asleep. Her final thought before fading away was that her life was finally coming back together.

Billy lifted his head up and looked at his watch—it was 4:00 a.m. He looked around and wondered where in the hell did the rest of the people go. Goddamn them, he was alone again. It was the fault of that bitch who lived across the parking lot.

Billy got to his feet, but was very unsteady. He sat back down in the chair and snorted another line of cocaine. It seemed to give him the strength he needed to stand up. He shoved the knife into his belt and looked out the window. Her car was back; it was time he paid a little visit to Ms. Betty Jo.

He walked out the front door of his apartment and stumbled and fell twice in the parking lot before reaching Betty Jo's apartment door. He fumbled with the key ring on the side of his belt, but finally managed to get it off, locate the pass key, and open Betty Jo's door.

Betty Jo had a habit of leaving the light on in the hallway bathroom in case one of her children needed to get up in the middle of the night to use the bathroom. Even though the kids were with their father, she had still turned on the light before going to bed. She can't remember if it was the stench of the alcohol mixed with his body odor, or the feeling that someone was standing over her, that awoke her.

At first she thought it was one of her kids and she called out the oldest child's name, but then she realized the kids where gone.

A voice answered, "It's not Jimmy, goddamn it, it's me, Billy Lee Crew, and I want to talk to your fucking ass."

Betty Jo jumped straight up in the bed and screamed. Billy reached over, slapped her across the mouth, grabbed a pillow and placed it over her face. "Don't scream, you no-good whore, or I'll kill you now," Billy said.

He lifted the pillow off her head so she could breathe better and talk. She tried asking Billy what he wanted, but she could only understand half of what he was saying. He pulled her from the bed and told her to remove her nightgown. Afraid not to do what he wanted, Betty Jo removed it and stood in front of him naked. Billy reached over and started fondling her breasts and making comments about her body. Then all of a sudden he stopped and said he needed a beer. Betty Jo told him there was beer in the kitchen, and he grabbed her by the arm and pulled her along with him. Betty Jo opened the refrigerator and handed him a beer. He stood there holding her with one hand and used the free hand to gulp the beer down. When he finished, he tossed the empty beer can across the kitchen. Billy then dragged her into the living room.

Betty Jo had to think of something to prevent him from raping her, or even killing her. She lied to him by telling him that her two children were asleep in the other room and that they would wake up if they heard any more noise.

"You lying, no-good bitch, I've been watching you all day, and I know your kids aren't at home. You think I am stupid," he shouted.

"I want to know why you broke up my home, then called the police on me," he yelled at her.

"I don't know what you are talking about, Billy, I swear I don't," Betty Jo responded.

"You are just like all the rest of them, you no-good bitch," he thundered, slapping her again with the back of his hand. The force of the blow knocked Betty Jo backwards, and she fell onto the floor.

Billy reached for his knife and said ominously, "Now I'm going to show you just how bad old Billy Lee is, I'm going to kill you."

Billy straddled Betty Jo and wildly started wielding the knife up and down, each time striking Betty Jo in a different part of her upper body. First her chest, then her shoulders, arms and head. Blood was flying everywhere as Billy continued his wild, insane rage.

Somehow, Betty Jo managed to wiggle out from under Billy, get to her feet and run toward the front door. Blood was running down her forehead, and blinding her. Not being able to see where she was going, she ran head-on into the wall next to the door and was almost knocked down. She reached out, grabbed the doorknob, and swung the door open. She ran outside with Billy close behind her, screaming, "Stop, bitch, I ain't finished killing you yet!"

Billy caught up to her and grabbed her by the hair, which was by now matted with blood. He yanked back and she fell onto the ground. He stomped her on the head with his cowboy boots, then leaned over her and started stabbing her again. Betty Jo let out bloodcurdling screams, and lights began switching on.

Billy continued to stab her until he broke the handle of the knife off, leaving the six-inch blade of the knife protruding out of her chest. Flustered by losing his knife, Billy leaned closer to Betty Jo and asked, "Are you dead yet, bitch?"

Betty Jo couldn't understand what was being said, but rolled her eyes up at the sound.

Seeing this, Billy bent down and started choking her, screaming at the top of his lungs, "Die, bitch, hurry up and die, bitch." Miraculously, Betty Jo managed a burst of strength and slammed her knee into Billy's groin. Billy yelled in pain and rolled over onto the ground. Betty Jo crawled on all fours to a nearby apartment door and clawed on it until the residents opened the door and jerked her inside.

Numerous people had phoned the police department to report the unbelievable events they had witnessed outside of the apartments.

Billy Lee Crew was still rolling around the grass when he first heard the sounds of the distant sirens. He got up on his knees and then stood up. He ran across the parking lot and back into his apartment. He was dripping blood, head to toe. Knowing he had been seen, he pushed the cover off of the attic entrance and climbed up, pulling the cover shut behind him.

As the police pulled up in front of the leasing office, twenty or so people were standing outside in the parking lot, most still dressed in their night clothes. There was no lack of witnesses to point out where the assailant had run.

An ambulance arrived, and the police and the paramedics immediately transported Betty Jo to the nearest hospital for treatment.

In the meantime, a team of police officers followed the trail of blood from the parking lot into Billy Crew's apartment. They searched the apartment, but there was no sign of Billy Crew. As the officers were getting ready to leave, one felt a drop of something hit his uniform shirt. He reached up and touched it and saw that it was blood. He looked up to discover he was standing right below the attic door from which blood was dripping. He motioned for his fellow officers, and, with guns drawn, they demanded that the suspect come out. Slowly, the attic cover moved, and dripping blood, Billy Lee Crew dropped out of the ceiling. At first, one of the officers thought that Billy had been cut also due to the large amount of blood on his body, but it turned out to be all Betty Jo's blood.

Betty Jo was treated for more than ten hours in emergency surgery by a team of four doctors. One of her lungs had collapsed, and several other major organs required repairing. She had been stabbed forty-three times and required more than 250 stitches to close up her wounds. She had lost over one-third of her blood supply. It would be touch and go if she lived or died.

A seasoned police detective and former Vietnam veteran who investigated the crime scene testified later, at Billy Lee Crew's criminal trial, that he had not seen *that* much blood during two tours in Vietnam.

With a lot of prayers and love from her family and an excellent medical staff, Betty Jo did survive. She spent more than two months in the hospital and will require extensive medical care for the remainder of her life, not to mention treatment for the accompanying psychological problems.

Billy Lee Crew was tried and convicted for the attempted murder of Betty Jo and the burglary of her apartment. During the investigation, police also were able to tie Billy to fifteen other burglaries he had committed at the Southern Arms Apartments to support his cocaine habit.

Betty Jo's parents hired the services of a personal injury attorney and filed suit against the apartment complex. As Betty Jo's security consultant, I had to do little work to build a case of negligence against the complex. Settlement conferences are under way as this book is written.

Betty Jo is coping with her mental and physical injuries as best as she can, but she will need many more years of care, love, and understanding to begin to recover.

Billy Lee Crew received a life prison sentence without parole—and is once again, hopefully forever, all alone.

What You Should Learn from This Crime

Apartment maintenance personnel should not show up at your apartment unannounced and should never enter your apartment without your permission, especially if you are at home. If you feel a staff member has done something improper or has made an improper remark or gesture toward you, immediately report it to the management office. If, as in this case, the maintenance person is also part of the on-site management team, call the management company or owners of the apartments and report to them what occurred.

■ ■ ■

A Tragic Holiday Trip to the Mall

THE TRAFFIC WAS BUMPER TO BUMPER, OVERCROWDING Charleston's streets, and a light rain didn't help matters any. It was only two weeks before Christmas, and shoppers were out in earnest.

Tammy Aaron sat in the traffic, tapping her fingers on the steering wheel and waiting for the light to change. It was 2:45 p.m., and she just knew she was going to be late picking up her two children, Tim and Robin, at school. The light changed, but only four cars made it through before it changed back to red. This was the fourth time, and she knew the children would be in a panic if she weren't there when they got out of school.

Tammy thought that maybe she was overprotective of her children. However, because of the way she had been raised and because their father, who was a Navy pilot, was away at sea duty for six months at a time, she felt she was doing the right thing. She was going to be a loving and protective mother.

The light changed again, and this time only two cars made it through before it changed back to red, stranding two more cars in the intersection; that immediately prompted the drivers going in the opposite direction to begin blowing their horns. A few of them rolled down their windows and yelled curse words and flashed their middle fingers at the drivers of the two cars sitting in the middle of the intersection—as if the whole traffic problem were their fault.

Tammy told herself the kids would be fine; this was simply one of life's minor set-backs that people let upset them more than they should. Besides, she had a lot for which to be thankful. Ronnie, her husband of eleven years, was returning from a six-month tour of duty on an aircraft carrier. The ship was due back at the Charleston Naval Station three days before Christmas.

This would be Ronnie's last tour after serving ten years in the Navy, about five of which were spent away from his wife and children. He had decided to get out and accept a job as a first officer with a major airline in Atlanta. All that was left was for him to be processed out of the Navy three days after Christmas. Tammy and Ronnie had spent months making the decision for him to leave the Navy. It was by no means an easy decision, but later it felt right. The children were excited about moving to Atlanta and having a real house in a real neighborhood, not a drab old officer's quarters on a Navy base. But, best of all, they would have their father at home more, and they knew that would make Mom happier.

The light changed, traffic began to move, and Tammy arrived at the front of the school at 3:05, only five minutes late. It was all lost on the children, who were busy talking to friends, and she had to blow the horn to get their attention.

Now off to football practice for Tim and Girl Scouts for Robin. "Being a mom is great," Tammy said to herself. "All I have to do is find time to finish my Christmas shopping."

The Civil War took a heavy toll on Charleston, as it did on other parts of the South. Gone were the rich plantations and factories of war. A decision to locate a naval yard in Charleston in the late 1800s was a turning point in its recovery, and it would bring the Aarons to Charleston more than a hundred years later. During the 1970s, Charleston saw better economic times; the city began to grow and the downtown area was modernized. In 1981, one of the first regional shopping malls opened in Charleston, and several followed. With all this growth, came another battle to fight: crime.

In October 1989 the first of a series of armed robberies was reported to the Charleston police. Clara Jones, a 58-year-old department store employee at one of the regional malls, had gotten off work around 9:00 p.m. on October 29. She walked out of the rear entrance of the mall and to the area of the parking lot which had been designated for employee parking. She opened her car door and sat down behind the steering wheel to wait on her friend who rode to and from work with her. The lighting was dim in that area of the parking lot, so Clara turned on the dome light to glance at a *Home & Garden* magazine to pass some time. The night was warmer than most for that time of the year, and she had rolled down the window to let fresh air in.

A noise, like the shuffling of feet, startled Clara. She looked up from her magazine and glanced to her left in the direction of the sound. As she turned, she found herself looking down the barrel of a sawed-off rifle. The man holding it was black and about 25 years old. His hair was cropped close, and he had on what appeared to be a warm-up suit. The assailant demanded that Clara give him her purse, and she immediately complied. He reached out with his left hand and grabbed the purse from her. The robber turned as if he was going to walk away, stopped, turned back toward Clara, and shot her in the face. The bullet entered the left side of her cheek, knocked out six teeth, pierced her tongue, and lodged in the base of her neck. Clara fell over in the seat. A mall maintenance employee, who had been picking up trash in the parking lot, heard the shot and took off running in its direction. He was able to see a light blue car with tinted windows racing through the parking lot at a high rate of speed. He went over to Clara's car and found her lying in the seat and bleeding very badly. He radioed for security personnel, who summoned the police and a rescue squad.

Clara Jones underwent six hours of surgery and stayed in the intensive care unit of the hospital until December 1. She was unable to give much of a description of her assailant to the police because of the suddenness of her attack.

The mall manager called the police department's public affairs officer the morning after and requested that the police not release news of the shooting and robbery to the press. The holiday season was just a few weeks away, and the news might scare people off unnecessarily, he said. Besides, the mall manager argued, this was just an isolated incident. The police agreed not to release the report, and the next call the manager made was to a local florist to order Clara Jones some flowers.

On November 5, 1989, Louise Collins, a co-worker of Clara Jones, got off work at 5:00 p.m. She clocked out, exited the employee entrance, and walked toward her car, which was parked in the same area as Clara Jones's car a few weeks previously.

The mall and store management had passed around a flyer shortly after Clara's shooting which basically said that she had been a victim of a random robbery and that the police were investigating. The flyer gave no description of the suspect or the car which had been seen speeding away from the scene. It did reassure readers that the mall was a safe place to work and shop.

Louise didn't notice the small light blue car with tinted windows parked opposite her when she set her purse atop her car to remove her car keys. She opened the door, and the last thing she remembered was a loud boom like somebody had set a cherry bomb off next to her head. Louise was found about ten minutes later by a co-worker, who was going to her car. The victim was lying half in the car and half on the pavement of the parking lot.

Rescue squad members rushed Louise Collins to the same hospital where Clara Jones lay in the intensive care unit recovering from her own wounds. The doctors removed a rifle bullet from the base of her skull and declared that only through the grace of God had she survived.

A story the following day in the local newspaper quoted the mall manager:

> I don't think the two shootings are connected. There are no motives or witnesses to the two shootings. It appears that this was just another random act of violence and we are damn mad about it. The Mall is a safe place and shoppers should not be scared. We have good security and the police hope to make an arrest soon. Our hearts and prayers go out to our employees and their families. We are very upset, but don't think we could have prevented it.

What the mall manager failed to mention during his interview was that in both cases the victims had been robbed of their purses, both had been shot in the head with a rifle, and in both cases witnesses had seen a small light blue car with tinted windows speed away.

Around 12:30 p.m. on November 28 of that year, Nancy Sue Carson had just finished fighting the early Christmas crowds at a mall located about five miles from where Clara Jones and Louise Collins had been shot and robbed. Nancy Sue had parked her car at the rear of the shopping center. Carrying three large shopping bags, she struggled through the lot to her car. She sat the bags down near the left rear tire, removed her keys from her purse, and opened the driver's door. She threw her purse onto the seat and reached in and pushed the automatic door-lock switch to unlock the doors. Nancy Sue then opened the left rear passenger's door to load her shopping bags. She had placed the first of the three bags in the rear seat when she heard a nearby car door slam shut. Nancy Sue looked over her shoulder in the direction of the noise and saw a nicely dressed black man getting out of a small light blue car with tinted windows. Thinking he was just another Christmas shopper, she reached down and picked up the two remaining bags and placed them in the rear seat with the other one.

As Nancy Sue closed the passenger's door, she felt the presence of someone standing behind her. Frightened, she jumped and let out a small scream. When she turned around, there was a sawed-off rifle pointing at her head. The same man she had seen getting out of the car ordered her to give him her purse. Nancy Sue explained that it was lying on the car seat.

"Please take whatever you want, just don't shoot me," Nancy Sue said.

The robber bent over and reached inside her car and grabbed the purse. He turned as if he was leaving. He stopped, then turned again, and raised the gun at Nancy Sue's head.

Nancy Sue Carson screamed, "Don't! Please, for God's sake, don't shoot me!"

The assailant squeezed the trigger of the sawed-off rifle—but it misfired. Not having time to eject the round and slide a new one into its place, the robber cursed and swung the butt of the rifle with all his strength, striking Nancy Sue on the side of the head.

Nancy Sue fell to the ground unconscious. Her assailant fled the scene after taking her purse and two of the shopping bags from the rear seat.

This incident never made the newspapers, and the two mall managers, while talking almost weekly about seasonal shopping patterns at their malls, never discussed the three robbery incidents.

Tony Nelson was a few minutes late getting back to work after his lunch break. He pulled his light blue Mustang with tinted windows through the gate of the trucking yard and waved at the security guard as he passed. Tony parked his car and ran over to the loading dock and told his supervisor he was sorry for being late.

"The traffic around the mall was murder, must have been the Christmas shoppers," Tony told his boss.

Tony's boss replied, "Don't worry about it, just get back to work."

What a prick, Tony thought.

At 22 years of age, Tony Nelson had already spent five years in jail for armed robbery of a liquor store at age 16. When his parole officer got him the job at the trucking company, the officer warned Tony that he had better stay out of trouble. Tony had long since decided that there would be no more liquor stores for him. They had hold-up buttons and cameras, as he found out when they played the videotape in court of his robbing the clerk. No, there would be no more liquor store robberies; people on the street were much easier. One of his convict friends had told him that if you are going to rob people, don't leave witnesses. That was the advice he had been trying to follow, but both the ladies he had shot had lived, according to the papers, and his gun had jammed during his last robbery. All he wanted was a couple of more good scores, and he was heading for the West Coast where he could start his life over. Besides, people were stupid at Christmas time, carrying all that extra money around.

Tony picked up another box and tossed it into the back of the trailer parked at the loading dock. He glanced over in the direction of his boss and mumbled under his breath, "What a prick. They're all pricks."

On Saturday morning, December 9, 1989, Tammy Aaron was busy cleaning the morning dishes and trying to straighten up the house before going to the mall to finish the last of her Christmas shopping. Ronnie's carrier was docking tomorrow, and they would start packing the following week. Both children had gone with the neighbor's kids to the soccer match and wouldn't be back until late in the afternoon. That would give her time to finish her shopping before they got home.

Tammy left the house later than she had planned, but she hoped the crowds would not be that bad and she could still beat the kids home. Before leaving, she had written them a note and attached it to the refrigerator. It read, "Tim & Robin: I hope you won the soccer match. There are snacks in the frig. I have gone shopping, will be back soon, if I am not already here when you get back. If I am not here, lock the doors and I will be close behind. Will go for pizza later. Love you both, Mommy. P.S.: Daddy's home tomorrow."

As Tammy got into her car, she turned on the radio. The announcer said that it was 1:00 p.m. and time for the area news. His first story was about the arrival of Santa Claus scheduled for 2:00 p.m. at South Lake Mall; the crowds were estimated to be the largest ever. "Damn," Tammy said to herself. This was just what she needed—to get caught up with Santa Claus and his reindeers. She slowed down and started to turn around, postponing her shopping trip until later in the week. But she talked herself out of giving up and decided to go ahead. She could pull around back and park and maybe beat some of the crowd that would be in front waiting on Santa Claus.

Tony Nelson had got up early that morning, deciding that it would be an excellent day to select another victim. The night before he had cleaned his new sawed-off 12-gauge shotgun and oiled it, hoping that it would not let him down like his old rifle had.

About eleven that morning, he drove out to South Lake Mall and cruised through the parking lots looking for a victim, but never saw anybody that looked inviting. Most of the people had kids or were couples shopping together. After a couple of passes through the front and back lots, he decided he would get some lunch and come back later. Maybe the pickings would be better.

Tammy drove into the main entrance of the mall and could not see a parking space anywhere. A large group of mothers, fathers, and children had already crowded around the front entrance of the mall awaiting the arrival of Santa. She hoped that she was right, and the back would be better. Sure enough, she found plenty of open parking spaces there.

Tammy had paid no attention to the small light blue car with tinted windows that was following close behind her from the time she had pulled into the main entrance of the mall. Nor did she think anything about it when she pulled into the parking space behind the mall, and the same car that had been following her pulled into the space next to hers.

She placed the gear shift into park. She reached over and pulled the rear view mirror over toward her and checked her lipstick and makeup. At 31, she was tall and slim and rather attractive. Tammy reached into her purse and removed her lipstick and hairbrush. She neatly applied a fresh coat of lipstick and brushed her hair into place. She placed the lipstick and brush back into her purse. She looked at her watch then reached over and opened the door. Tammy started to step out.

The last thing Tammy Aaron must have seen was the blinding flash of

Tony Nelson's new shotgun. The force of the blast almost decapitated her. Blood, splinters of bone and brain matter splattered the inside of the car and splashed in the face of Tony Nelson. Tammy's body, limp as a wet dishrag, slumped onto the pavement of the parking lot less than ten feet from where Clara Jones and Louise Collins had been robbed and shot just weeks before.

Tony Nelson stood there for a minute almost in disbelief at what the blast of his new gun had done. "Damn, what a mess," he said aloud, as if Tammy could hear him. "Oh well, you won't be needing this," he said out loud again, as he reached over and grabbed her purse. He ran over to his car, jumped in, and sped off.

A mall maintenance employee was standing near the storage shed located at the rear of the mall when he heard what at first sounded like a loud backfiring of a truck or motorcycle. He looked in the direction of the noise and saw a tall black man dressed in a jogging suit running away from a car with its driver door open. The man was carrying something in his right hand that from the distance looked like a stick or a baseball bat. The man jumped into a small light blue car and sped toward him. As the car passed him, the maintenance employee tried to look inside, but couldn't see due to the dark tinted windows. He took a notebook from his shirt pocket and scribbled down the license number.

The maintenance employee started to walk over to check the open car door but stopped when he received a call over the two-way radio. All employees were needed at the front of the mall. About that time, the sound of the whirring of a helicopter and sirens from police cars and fire trucks filled the air, signaling the arrival of Santa Claus.

I can always check the car later, if it is still there, the maintenance man thought. Besides, if the guy stole the person's stereo or something, he had his tag number. He pushed the notebook back into his shirt pocket and took off toward the front of the mall.

It was forty minutes later when a shopper trying to escape the madness of Santa's arrival went out the back entrance of the mall. As she was walking toward her car, she spotted Tammy Aaron's car with the driver's door open. As she got closer, what caught her eye first was a puddle of dark fluid, like somebody's oil pan was leaking badly. Then she saw the ghastly sight of Tammy's blood-soaked body slumped near the driver's door. But something was out of place—where were her face and head?

The force of the blast of the shotgun at that close range had totally destroyed Tammy's face and head. All that was left were bone fragments, hair, and blood. The tall, attractive, dedicated naval wife and mother of two children lay there dead, killed instantly. The shopper who found her body still has nightmares from the horror of what she discovered and to this day sickens when she hears "We Wish You a Merry Christmas and a Happy New Year," which was roaring over the mall's public address system when she found Tammy's body.

The police were able to check the license tag number of Tammy's car and found that it was registered to Lt. Ronnie Aaron. They placed a call to the listing the radio dispatcher had found in the phone book for Ronnie Aaron, but there was no answer.

One of the police officers at the scene, who was in the Navy Reserves, suggested calling the sergeant at arms at the naval station in hopes of locating Lieutenant Aaron. It took several calls and two hours later to find out that Lieutenant Aaron was on an aircraft carrier steaming toward Charleston.

Lieutenant Aaron had been in the officer's mess having dinner when he was ordered to the captain's quarters. He almost fainted when the ship's captain and chaplain told him of his wife's tragic death. He sat there for several minutes unable to speak. When he finally did, he asked about his children. Had they been with their mother? Were they all right? He was told that personnel from the naval station were with the children and that they were fine. The captain told him they didn't have any more of the details, but they would have one of the jets from the carrier fly him ashore. Navy and police officials would meet him when they landed.

As the Navy jet roared off the deck of the aircraft carrier and started its climb, Lt. Ronnie Aaron looked out of the cockpit. Later he remembered that this would be his last take-off from the deck of a carrier. He had been gone so long and was so shell-shocked, he could not remember the last thing Tammy and he had done together.

With the help of the tag number written down by the maintenance man, the police were able to identify the owner of the car as Tony Nelson. A check of the police computer revealed Tony's criminal record, and an all-points bulletin was placed over the police radio. Less than one hour after the senseless killing of Tammy Aaron, an alert beat officer who heard the description of Tony Nelson's car spotted it in the parking lot of a bank.

The officer then spotted a black male dressed in a jogging suit standing in front of the ATM machine. The officer radioed for backup and walked within three feet of where Tony Nelson was standing, cussing and beating on the ATM machine because it had refused to give back one of Tammy's credit cards after he had repeatedly punched in the wrong PIN number while attempting to get cash from her account.

Tony Nelson was placed under arrest. His clothes were still soaked in blood. The crime lab later discovered fragments of Tammy's brain, blood, and hair on his jogging suit. The blood-soaked shotgun was lying in the back seat of his car.

Later at police headquarters, Tony Nelson confessed to the killing and robbery of Tammy Aaron. He also confessed to the other three assaults and robberies. He wrote in his confession that he kept going back to South Lake Mall because he never saw any security guards there and at night the lighting was bad.

Ronnie Aaron buried his wife on December 14, 1989, less than two weeks before Christmas. It would be months before he could deal with the details of what had happened in the parking lot of the shopping mall. Having been so close to their mother, the children needed professional counseling to help them deal with their loss. The airline company where Ronnie was to work held his job for six months while he cared for his wife's estate.

When talking with the police, Ronnie discovered that Tammy had not been the first shooting and robbery victim at South Lake Mall. In addition to the crimes committed by Tony Nelson, he learned that during the previous five years the mall had been the scene of hundreds of crimes, including rapes, robberies, assaults, and thefts. In talking with a local reporter who was covering the story, Ronnie found first that the mall manager had requested reports from the police departments not be released to the press; then he found the manager's quotations in the paper after Louise Collins' shooting. He was inflamed, and when he discussed his findings with the Naval Legal Office, they suggested he talk with a local attorney.

On May 9, 1990, Tony Nelson was found guilty of the murder and armed robbery of Tammy Aaron. He currently waits on death row for his execution date.

The South Lake Mall quickly and very quietly settled out of court with Ronnie Aaron in the lawsuit he brought against it for negligent security practices.

Ronnie Aaron today flies out of Atlanta for a major airline and hopes someday to put his life back together. Tim and Robin Aaron still have dreams in which they hear their mother's car pull into the driveway—of her getting out, swinging open the kitchen door, and asking, "How was the soccer game?"

What You Should Learn from This Crime

It is helpful to read the local newspaper and watch the local news in order to be familiar with crime trends in your community. Remember, a lone female makes an attractive target for a would-be assailant. It is highly recommended that if at all possible, go shopping with relatives or friends. Be ready to exit your car when you park, look around you, and exit with your keys in your hand. You can always take the time to freshen your lipstick and comb your hair once inside the mall or office building. Being alert and moving confidently can many times deter a would-be criminal.

■ ■ ■

CHAPTER FIVE

Home, Sweet Home

IN 1992, A YOUNG SINGLE WOMAN I'LL CALL JANE HAD JUST graduated from a small college in her hometown in central Georgia with a degree in education. She felt very fortunate that she had been accepted for a first-grade teaching position in the Atlanta school system. This would be her first stay away from home. Jane, a quiet, studious, devoutly religious woman was also relieved that she had ended her college relationship with a young man from her hometown whom she thought offered her no future but a humdrum life in the small town. Brent was a nice guy, she thought, but Atlanta should be *full* of nice, single men.

She was brimming with excitement when she came to the big city in search of an apartment. As she drove into Atlanta, the words of her father, who still thought of her as "Daddy's little girl," echoed in her ears. He had told her repeatedly that he was very concerned for her safety. "Be especially careful in selecting an apartment complex," he urged. He instructed her to ask the leasing agent or the manager about the apartment's environs and whether there had been any problems with crimes at the complex. She tried to assure her dad that she would be cautious in making her decision.

After several days of looking for her "first home," she found what appeared to be a very attractive apartment complex. It seemed to be in a nice section of town—winding, hilly streets full of modern apartments and condominiums—and reasonably close to her new teaching job in Atlanta's monied Dunwoody suburb. Jane felt she was very lucky to get a teaching position in that neighborhood rather than in one of the rougher sections with which Atlanta abounds. She felt good when she heard the school had a very diverse student population, knowing this would provide some reasonable but safe exposure to the "real world" which her sheltered upbringing hadn't provided.

At the leasing office of her apartment complex, she met a woman about her age named Sandy who identified herself as the leasing agent, and they hit it off immediately. Sandy introduced Jane to her manager, who also seemed like a very nice person.

The leasing agent showed Jane the model apartment, and the floor plan was just what Jane wanted. They then walked over to a building located at the rear of the complex. It backed up to a wooded area full of pines and oaks, and Jane fell in love with the setting. The only thing that bothered her was that the available unit was on the ground floor. She voiced some concern about the location, but the leasing agent sold her on the privacy it would afford her and the pretty view it offered. Her sliding glass door would be overlooking the wooded area behind her apartment.

Back at the leasing office, Jane questioned the leasing agent and the manager about any crime problems at the complex. They assured her that, to their knowledge, there had been none. They told her that there were many other single women living at the complex, and they had never received any complaints from them about their safety. They also told her they had full-time security on the premises, including a tenant/security guard who was a state trooper. In fact, Sandy fairly gushed, "He will be your neighbor in the next building." Jane knew that this knowledge would make her father happy.

She told them she would take the apartment and signed a one-year lease that same day. She couldn't wait to get back home later that night to tell her father and mother all about her new home. She was so excited she stayed up after midnight packing. Her parents were sad that their only child was leaving home, but at the same time they were very happy for her. They couldn't remember when they had seen her so excited. Had it been her high school senior prom?

On the first night in her new apartment, Jane noticed the lighting in the parking lot in front was fairly dim. Also, the only light in the rear of her apartment was a small porch light which didn't put out that much light. This worried her somewhat until she noticed a state police car parked outside of the building next to hers. She remembered about the apartment security officer who lived next door to her and decided she was being silly to worry.

On her second night in her new home, she called her parents and told them how happy she was with her new job and her new apartment. Her father, still being protective of his "little girl," again asked her about the area around the apartment and encouraged her to make sure she always kept her windows locked.

After going over classwork for the next day, Jane watched the late news on television before going to bed. She read for a few minutes until she fell asleep with the lamp on next to her bed.

The next thing she remembered was being suddenly awakened by the weight of a body on top of hers. In horror, she saw a man with a ski mask over his face sitting across her chest. He was wearing rubber gloves and holding a large hunting knife at her throat.

He placed his free hand over her mouth and rasped, "If you scream, I'll kill you." He stood up next to the bed with his hand still covering her mouth. He told her to take off her nightgown, which she did very slowly, thinking, "No, my God, no!" He then took the knife and cut her panties off.

She wished she could see his face, figuring if she could look him in the eye, maybe she could appeal to him to spare her. "Please . . ." she began.

His interruption was matter-of-fact: "If you don't scream or fight back, I won't harm you," he said.

She hardly felt relieved, as she saw him unzipping his pants. She felt utter terror. And, as she alternately cried and tried to scream, she was raped three times and was forced to commit oral sex on her assailant over the next three hours.

Before leaving, he cut the lamp cord and tied her hands and feet. He then placed a wash cloth in her mouth so she couldn't scream. He told her he had tied her loose enough that she would be able to work her way free after he left. As she looked at him helplessly through teary eyes, he threatened that if she called the police, he would come back later and kill her. He bragged, "I've raped other girls in this place. I can get back into your apartment any time I want." She could hear him exit the apartment by opening the front door.

She waited a few minutes to make sure her assailant was not coming back before working her way free of the lamp cord. Once free, she stumbled out of the apartment to that of the state trooper. All she was wearing were her panties, the only clothes she had the presence of mind to put on at that point. She knocked and knocked but no one was home. She thought she heard another door open and a pair of curious eyes surveying her before it closed. No one came out to help her and she ran back into her apartment, grasped the phone with shaking hands and called 911. The police operator kept her on the phone while she dispatched police units to the scene. The first police officer on the scene discovered the sliding glass door open and entered her apartment. He found her sitting in one corner of the bedroom holding the phone receiver tightly in one hand and clutching a stuffed teddy bear given to her by her father on her fourth birthday.

She was taken to Grady Hospital, Atlanta's largest public medical facility, which routinely treats the burgeoning number of rape victims. Although the police officers who took her were sympathetic at first, they asked over and over again how she could have taken a secluded apartment in that particular complex. "It was asking for trouble," one said. "We've had plenty of trouble there." Jane felt that they were victimizing her again. Meanwhile, the Grady Hospital Emergency Room was full of blood and gore—gunshot victims screaming to be treated, a woman whose arm had been severed at the elbow by a common-law husband wielding a butcher knife in a domestic argument that had gotten out of hand. The hubbub only intensified Jane's terror. Not only did she feel humiliated and mortified by the rape, but she was seeing a segment of society—at its worst—that she had never been exposed to in her hometown or at college.

Finally, they wheeled her in a wheelchair into the examining room. The doctor was young—almost as young as she, Jane thought—and very understanding, but when he tried to calm her down, she found she had nothing to say to him. Her feelings of disassociation from the entire scene were heightened when he took a semen specimen from her vagina. Although she realized he was trying to help her, his touching her private parts with a slide made her feel like another violation had occurred. Finally, *this* ordeal was over, and the police officers offered to take her home. "Home," she brightened, then she shuddered. She realized they meant her apartment. Finally, she allowed them to drive her over to a friend's house where she took her first shower since the rape and at least felt cleaner.

Meanwhile, the crime scene unit from the police department had concluded in a moment that the rapist had gained entry into her apartment by merely lifting the sliding-glass door off its track. This was accomplished fairly easily since the door had been installed improperly when the apartments were built five years earlier. The only locking device on the door was a flimsy sliding latch lock which is standard on patio-type doors.

During the course of my investigation on Jane's behalf, I discovered that there had been two other young, single girls raped in the apartment complex. They had all lived alone in ground-level apartments like hers, and the assailant had entered through the sliding-glass doors. I also found out that the apartment complex was all too aware of these rapes and the method of entry. In every case, police had supplied the leasing office with a description and sketch of the rapist and had encouraged the complex to distribute the sketch to all tenants. Police officers had also suggested that the complex not rent ground-level units to single females until the rapist was caught. All this had taken place just *weeks* before Jane signed her lease. The complex did not follow through on either suggestion.

Even as Jane moved back to her small town and in with her parents, I asked police if the apartments had ever had crime problems before the rapes. A computer check revealed more than fifty burglaries, two armed robberies, and several cars stolen from the parking lot of Jane's complex within the past twelve months.

The young schoolteacher who had such a bright future ahead of her was now a rape victim. She was faced with years of therapy and deep emotional scars that will, no doubt, be with her for the remainder of her life. Her parents tried to be as supportive as possible, and Brent tried to restart their relationship, but when he called at her house, she told her parents she didn't want to see him. How could she face him knowing that he had been her only lover prior to the rape? She felt guilty and dirty.

Her parents filed a $10 million lawsuit, still pending, on her behalf against the apartment complex. The suit alleged the complex was guilty of negligence by failing to warn her about the previous rapes and improper security measures, and breach of contract, due to the misrepresentation of the security services provided by the complex.

Continuing my investigation on Jane's behalf, I discovered the state trooper on the premises was being provided with a free apartment for his services as a "courtesy officer." He had received no instructions from the management of the apartments as to what was expected of him and, in fact, didn't even know the name of the new manager! He had lived there for more than a year at the time of Jane's rape. He also admitted to me that, due to his various assignments with the state police, he was gone from the complex for periods of up to two weeks. During these times he had not bothered to notify the leasing office that he would be gone. I was not surprised to hear all this. In previous cases, I had discovered that the use of off-duty officers for security was little more than a pretense of safety, even though more and more complexes were responding to the crime problem in this fashion.

I also found that the owners of the complex had been aware of the inadequate lighting and the improper installation of the patio doors. But instead of making the necessary repairs, they chose to invest in additional landscaping at the front entrance to provide more "curb appeal," albeit less security, to potential renters. The owners had also instructed their leasing agents not to warn potential or present tenants about the previous rapes and crimes committed on the premises. The reason: It might "scare them off."

The schoolteacher's case is still pending in court, but with the facts presently known, a victory for her is very likely. However, given her present emotional condition, it will be a Pyrrhic victory at best.

Hundreds of cases similar to this one are pending across the country against apartment owners. However, instead of reaching a courtroom where others may become aware of the dangers facing them when leasing or living in an apartment, this case will more than likely settle out of court—with the results sealed from public and media scrutiny. Potential renters at Jane's former complex will continue to fall in love with its woodsy property, totally unaware of the violent crimes committed there.

Recognizing the similarity between the hotel/motel and apartment industries, some courts have begun to impose a higher standard of responsibility on apartment owners. Perhaps this will force them to take reasonable measures to protect their tenants from criminal acts.

However, like the hotel/motel industry, most apartment owners would rather insure their risk against lawsuits than spend money on security and safety measures. It's a gamble apartment owners take, but the renter is at the greatest risk.

What You Should Learn from This Crime

When you are choosing an apartment, don't always trust the description a leasing agent gives of the complex's security and safety measures. Call the local police department and speak to the crime prevention officer. Tell the officer you are considering moving to a certain complex and ask what should you know about the past crime history of the complex. If you decide to move in, request that the crime prevention officer inspect your apartment and make recommendations concerning the door and window locks.

■ ■ ■

Dial 911 for Help in San Diego

IN THE SUMMER OF 1945 SPIRITS WERE HIGH THROUGHOUT THE country. Everyone was proud to be an American. The wars in Europe and the Pacific were coming to an end, and high hopes for the future abounded. Young servicemen by the millions were returning home to the families or sweethearts they had left behind. Marriage rates were at an all-time high, and the Baby Boom was underway.

John Taines, an Army Air Corps officer from Bakersfield, California, was one of the millions who returned home looking forward to a bright future. When the war broke out, John was finishing his senior year of college. He had experienced some rough times working his way through college. He had to work late at night and study well into the morning to keep up with his class work. With such a grinding schedule, John found little time to date or participate in other school activities.

Once overseas, John's buddies received letters from their wives or girlfriends back home, but John only received them from his mother and four sisters. This didn't bother John. If he were fortunate enough to make it through the war in one piece, he was confident that someday he would find the right girl, fall in love, and raise a family.

When the war in Europe ended, John returned home to his family and friends in Bakersfield. The people closest to John felt that he had changed. Maybe the difference came from the memories and scars of war, represented by the three rows of combat ribbons he wore across his chest. John had been assigned to one of the most hazardous duties during the conflict—flying combat missions over Germany. But after a few weeks at home with Mom's cooking and the companionship of good friends, John seemed more at ease. He was eager to get his discharge papers and get about the task of finding a job and a place of his own to live.

With four younger sisters at home, John had a built-in dating service. A night rarely went by without one of them encouraging John to meet a friend. John was convinced they had a contest going on among them to see who was going to introduce him to "Miss Right."

John had been home less than a month when his younger sister, Jill, approached him with what she felt would be the perfect place for him to meet somebody. A local civic group was sponsoring a beauty contest, and they wanted returning servicemen to act as judges. Jill had taken it upon herself to enter John's name. John's first reaction was anger that she would commit him to something like this without discussing it with him first. When John's scolding made Jill cry, he reluctantly agreed to accept, with a warning that she should never do anything like that again. Years later they would laugh together about how that evening would change John's life forever.

One of the requirements was that all judges wear their uniforms during the event. John's had been hanging in the closet since he returned home. When he took it from the hanger and tried it on, he was amazed at how snug it was around the waist. John tried to use that as an excuse to back out, but Jill assured him that he still looked dashing and handsome.

By the time they arrived at the assembly hall where the contest was to be held, John had made up his mind that this was going to be the most boring evening of his life. He took his place with the four other judges and received a short course in how to be a judge.

He was still feeling stupid and bored when the announcer introduced Contestant Number Five. As she walked out onto the stage, John sat up straight in his chair. All at once, he was glad he was there. Without a doubt, she was the most beautiful woman John had ever seen. For the remainder of the evening, his mind raced with thoughts of how he could get an introduction to her after the contest.

Terry Nash was indeed someone who would turn heads as she walked down the street. At 5' 5", 115 pounds, with luminous blue eyes and waist-length cornflower blond hair, she seemed the type of woman that both men and women admired. But there was a lot more to Terry than her good looks.

She was extremely intelligent and talented in many ways, and Jill later said that Terry's warm smile and effervescent personality made all who met her instantly fall in love with her. By then, John didn't argue.

Terry had recently graduated from college and had started to work at a life insurance company. A girlfriend at work had heard about the beauty contest and encouraged her to enter. She was reluctant at first, but after days of urging from her co-workers she agreed.

When it came time for voting, John had no trouble making up his mind. As the judges gathered to discuss the balloting, the leadership ability John had demonstrated in the military took over. It didn't take him long to convince the other judges that Contestant Number Five was the best choice. Terry won hands down.

As the ranking military officer among the judges, John was chosen to award Terry the prize money and trophy. After the presentation, John began talking with her and soon found himself asking her out. Much to his surprise, she accepted.

That night marked the beginning of a beautiful relationship that would result in their marriage just six months later—and their subsequent honeymoon at the idyllic Torres Villa Inn at La Jolla, four hours away. John treasured each moment of the honeymoon so much—it all seemed a dream after the horror of war—that he saved the room key as a keepsake.

Soon John passed his CPA examination and was hired by a large oil-well digging firm in Bakersfield. Over the next forty years, their marriage was everything John had ever hoped for and more. He and Terry shared the kind of special relationship found in very few marriages. They raised three children and were now starting to enjoy the pleasures of life as grandparents.

What with John's career and the responsibilities of raising a family, the couple had never had much time to travel. But now they decided to sell their home, buy a recreational vehicle, and travel the country as long as their health held out.

They spent weeks going over maps and plotting out routes they would enjoy traveling. Their children were delighted to see the excitement of their parents as they ran around making their plans. It reminded the kids of the first time Terry and John announced they were taking them to Disneyland.

During the preparation for their trip, John noticed that Terry was tiring easily. She had been complaining of a nagging back pain when she sat too long or bent over to pick up something. After several weeks of encouragement John finally convinced her to see a doctor. At first the doctor could not identify the source of her problems. He ordered extensive lab tests and x-rays, all the while reassuring John and Terry that it was probably nothing to worry about. Several weeks later, the doctor called them to a meeting in which he had terrible news: the results of all the tests had come back and the diagnosis was a very rare form of cancer called multiple myeloma. The cancer affects the marrow in the bone and weakens the spine. Eventually, even with treatment, patients become bedridden and totally dependent on others to care for them. The disease is usually fatal.

At first John and Terry were despondent and angry. But the same love and faith that had held their marriage together over the years finally prevailed. They had faced crises before, and they would confront this one together.

The Scripps Medical Center in La Jolla, California, is considered one of the finest cancer treatment hospitals in the world. John and Terry had no problem making the decision to use Scripps for Terry's treatment after her doctor in Bakersfield recommended it. It would mean making the four-hour drive at least once a month from Bakersfield to La Jolla.

La Jolla, California, is said by visitors to be one of the most beautiful locations in the United States. Its sun-washed beaches, cosmopolitan shopping centers, and quality restaurants are some of the best to be found anywhere. Its slow pace and calm lifestyle have a way of creating a unique euphoria. For those seeking a faster lifestyle, the great cosmopolitan area of San Diego is just minutes away. Looking at a snapshot view of La Jolla, one would find it difficult to believe the terror that awaited Terry, John, and their daughter in February 1987.

By then, Terry and John had grown accustomed to the monthly trips to Scripps for Terry's treatments. But this trip was to be a special occasion. Their oldest daughter, Nancy Taines Carlton, was going to come along with them. After Terry's treatments they would stay over for a couple days of sightseeing and shopping.

On their previous trips through the heart of La Jolla, they had driven by the picturesque Torres Villa Inn, the very place they had honeymooned forty years before. That was the place they wanted for their family holiday. "It will be like a second honeymoon," John said enthusiastically.

The Taineses and their daughter arrived at the Torres Villa Inn in La Jolla shortly after seven in the evening. They planned to get settled into their room and then go out for dinner.

The drive from Bakersfield had taken a toll on Terry. Instead of going out, John went to a nearby Kentucky Fried Chicken and picked up dinner for the three of them.

After eating, they talked about their plans for the next three days and watched television until around 10:00 p.m. With Terry's treatments planned for most of the next day, they decided to make an early evening of it. John and Terry took the bed closest to the windows. Before retiring for the night, Terry made John check the deadbolt on the door.

And then John had a surprise for her. He took out the room key from their honeymoon and related how he had kept it from her as his personal memento over the years. Feeling giddy with gratefulness for the many fine years of marriage Terry had given him, John tried the key in the lock. To his astonishment, it still worked!

Around 12:30 a.m., they were suddenly awakened by someone knocking loudly on the door. The knocking became more intense, and a male voice began yelling, "Hotel maintenance!" As the man bellowed, they heard what sounded like a key being inserted into their door and the jiggling of the door knob.

Nancy jumped out of bed and ran over to the curtains covering the window next to the door. As she pushed them back just enough to see out, she saw a Mexican-American man wearing what appeared to be work clothing standing at the door. When he saw her looking at him, he said in a more polite voice, "Hotel maintenance, let me in." Nancy told him they had not called for maintenance and to go away. He replied, "It's okay, it's okay, don't worry, let me in." Nancy again told him to go away or she would call the front desk to find out what the problem was. With this, the man turned and walked away.

Thinking this was a little strange, Nancy decided to call the front desk and report what had occurred. She dialed the office number and let the phone ring and ring, but there was no answer. Thinking she might not have dialed correctly, she hung up and dialed again. She let the phone ring for what seemed like ten minutes without an answer. John told her the desk must be really busy and that they would report the incident in the morning. They switched off the lights and went back to bed.

What they didn't know as they went back to sleep was that the man who had tried to enter their room was Antonio Robert Martinez, a former maintenance man of the Torres Villa Inn who had been fired several weeks earlier. Antonio Robert Martinez would be back.

He had already been on the hotel property for several hours that night and had tried to gain entry into other rooms by using the same guise. At room 211, he did manage to open the door by means of the master key he had stolen when he was fired. When the guest occupying the room, a visiting doctor at Scripps Medical Center, heard the sliding chain catch the door, he jumped up from bed and slammed the door in Martinez's face. Once he had re-engaged the deadbolt, he nervously asked who was there and what did they want.

Martinez told him that he was with hotel maintenance and he needed to check the room for water leaks. The doctor assured Martinez everything was fine in his room. Martinez insisted on gaining entry, but the doctor warned him to go away or he would file a complaint with the front desk.

The doctor listened as Martinez went down the stairway. He then walked over to the phone located between the beds and dialed the hotel operator. The phone rang between 15 and 20 times without an answer. Like the Taineses, the doctor figured the desk clerks were busy, so he hung up and went back to bed.

About thirty minutes had elapsed since Martinez had first tried to gain entry into the Taineses' room. In the meantime, the Taineses had gone back to bed and dismissed the first encounter with Martinez. The man had apparently gotten the room numbers mixed up, and they would say something to the manager about it the next morning.

John had just fallen back to sleep when a sound at the door and the turning of the door knob caused him to sit straight up in bed. His sudden movement awoke his wife and her hysterical scream, "What's wrong, John?" woke their daughter. John told both of them to be quiet, that he thought he had heard a noise at the door. The three of them sat staring at the door, fearful of what might happen next. The next sound they heard seemed like a cannon going off. A loud pounding began on the plate glass window nearest the door. This caused all three of them to jump to their feet.

John walked toward the windows, at which time the same pounding noise began on the second window and then the third. John, dressed only in his undershorts, slowly reached up with his left hand and moved the vertical blinds aside. It was extremely dark outside, but John could make out the outline of a man standing behind some tall bushes growing next to the window. John yelled, "Get away from here, fellow, or we are going to call the police."

Terry, her voice quivering and her entire body shaking in fear, told

Nancy to call the office and have them alert the police. Nancy picked up the phone and dialed "0" for the hotel operator. The phone rang and rang. No answer.

Nancy could not believe that no one was answering the front desk phone. Her hands were trembling, and she was crying. She turned to her mother and cried, "There's no one answering, there's no one to help us."

Martinez was pacing back and forth in front of the windows, which were about five feet high and twelve feet wide. As he paced, he muttered profanities and loudly demanded that John open the door to let him in. Martinez continued to insist that he was the hotel maintenance man and that he needed to check their room.

Terry told Nancy to hang up the phone and call 911. Before Terry could complete her sentence, the third window from the door came crashing in and glass flew all over. John, who had been standing near the window, was knocked back against the bed by the force of the breaking glass. A large fragment had entered John's right leg, and the blood was flowing freely. Panic and fear filled the room, and Terry and Nancy began to scream and cry. The horror and fear intensified when they saw a man's leg dangling through the broken window frame. John lifted himself off the bed and struggled back over to the window. Martinez had pulled his leg back and John leaned over closer to the broken window to see if the man had left. There were still fragments of glass hanging in the window pane so John carefully edged his face closer to the opening.

He was within inches of the window frame when an arm shot through the opening with a large bowie knife in its hand. Next, a leg appeared through the opening as Martinez attempted to climb into the room.

Nancy finally got a 911 operator on the line. The following is an account of the actual conversation between Nancy Taines and the San Diego 911 emergency operator:

Operator: San Diego Emergency.

Nancy: Hello (crying) — I called to get a police officer at the Torres Villa Inn. They just broke the glass out and they are trying to get into our room (crying) — please help.

Operator: Who just broke the glass?

Nancy: Someone from the outside. My father is cut and bleeding. Please send someone and hurry.

Operator: Okay, let me go ahead and transfer you to the paramedics. Hold the line, I will be right back.

Nancy: Thank you, but please hurry.

Operator: I'm back. We are sending a policeman right now.

Nancy: My father is bleeding. Is there an officer coming please? We are in room 110. Is there an officer coming?

Operator: Yes, please try and get control of yourself, talk to me. Who is trying to break into your room?

Nancy: A man, please help my father. He has a large knife.

Operator: Okay, we do have units on the way. They should be there shortly.

Nancy: Please hurry, help him, he's trying to kill him. He is still trying to get in.

Operator: We are en route.

Nancy: Okay, please hurry.

Operator: Your father is bleeding from where?

Nancy: He's been stabbed in the shoulder and I believe he has glass in his leg.

Operator: Okay, I want you to apply pressure to his wounds.

Nancy: I can't. He is fighting the man that is trying to come in the window.

Operator: Okay, we are going to be there in a few minutes.

Operator, to Police Unit: How fast is your unit going to be there?

Police: We have been responding for the past three minutes. We should be there any moment.

Operator: Okay, Miss, what I want you to do now is to compose yourself because you are going to have to help your father.

Nancy: Okay.

Operator: When the police arrive, I want you to get some towels from the bathroom and apply some pressure to that wound.

Nancy: All right.

Operator: Okay?

Nancy: Yes, the police are on their way?

Operator: Yes, the cops are on their way and we are going to get a medic there also.

Nancy: Would you please have the police turn their signals on?

Operator: They will. I am going to stay on the phone with you until they arrive.

Nancy: Okay.

Operator: Until someone gets there.

Nancy: We are on the bottom floor.

Operator: Are you in room 110?

Nancy: Yes, this is room 110.

Operator: We have the medics on the way now. The cops should be there any minute. Is this somebody trying to rob you or . . .

Nancy: I don't know. They have a long knife and he has been sticking it through the window. He has broken the glass trying to get in. My father is bleeding badly and there is glass and blood everywhere.

Operator: Okay, help will be there soon. Is your dad able to keep things . . . Are you two the only ones in the room?

Nancy: My mother and my father and I. We are here with my mother. She is getting treatment from Scripps Clinic.

Operator: I see. All right. We are going to be there and the cops will be there in a few minutes.

(Nancy hands phone to her mother in order to get her father some wet towels.)

Terry: Oh, dear God, is someone coming?

Operator: Oh, yes, honey, the police are on their way.

Police: We are en route.

Terry: Oh, thank you.

Operator: We are going to get a medic over to help your husband.

Terry talking to John: The police are on their way and the medics are, too.

Operator: Stand by, is the man still trying to break in?

Terry: No, he is not right now.

Operator: Okay, I am going to stay on the phone with you. The police unit is also patched into our line.

Police: Yes, our units are on the way.

Terry: Okay.

Police: You just stay on the phone with us.

Terry: Okay, I think there is someone at the front door. I hear him. Oh, I can't believe that no one shows up or no one helps.

Operator: Try to keep it together if you can. Is there a manager or anybody else around?

Terry: That I can't answer. We have been trying to call the front desk, but no one will answer.

Operator: They won't?

Terry: It looks like someone would say something or someone would come to help us.

Police: We have had another report on this. We have four units en route.

Terry: You have? Oh, good.

Police: Yes, that's right. So it's just a matter of moments now.

Operator: I know it seems like forever, but we are moments away.

Terry: Oh, it does.

Operator: I know it, but they will be there soon.

Terry: Especially since he broke the window out and no one has come from the hotel to help us. We have tried to call twice.

Operator: Okay, I will direct a unit to check on the welfare of the clerk.

Terry: Okay, I think the police are here. He says he is with the San Diego Police Department.

Operator: He is, I am going to have to drop off the line now. You can hang up the phone, the police are there.

Terry: Are you sure they are police officers?

Operator: Yes, they are police officers. Go open the door now.

Terry: I want to be sure. It has been so frightening.

Operator: Yes, I understand. They are police officers. I want you to hang up the phone and go open the door.

Terry: Oh, thank God . . . (phone goes dead).

While Terry and Nancy were on the line with the 911 operator, another 911 operator was having the following conversation with a Mr. Paul Briggs, another guest of the Torres Villa Inn in room 111.

Operator: San Diego Emergency.

Briggs: Yes, my name is Paul Briggs and I am a guest at the Torres Villa Inn and I am in room 111.

Operator: Yes, how can I help you?

Briggs: There is breaking glass and people screaming. It sounds like someone is getting killed.

Operator: The noise is coming from what room?

Briggs: I don't know where the noise is coming from . . . the south side of my room. There are women screaming. It's on the first level.

Operator: What is your name again, sir?

Briggs: It's Paul Briggs.

Operator: And what room are you in?

Briggs: Room 111.

Operator: And where is the noise coming from?

Briggs: It's outside of my room. There are people screaming and I hear someone running. I don't want to go outside my room.

Operator: Okay, stay in your room. We have received another call. There are police officers on the way.

Briggs: Thank you, good-bye. . . . (Phone is disconnected.)

As the frantic phone calls were being placed to the 911 operator, 72-year-old John Taines was fighting for his life against a much younger, much stronger man.

As Martinez stuck his leg through the window, he began waving the knife wildly through the air. John turned quickly to his daughter and shouted, "Nancy, hand me Mother's cane." Nancy leaped from the bed, almost pulling the phone out of the wall as she held tightly and tried to get the 911 operator. She managed to grab the cane which had been leaning against the night stand between the beds and handed it to her father.

John started fighting back, hitting Martinez as hard as he could with the cane. The blows caused Martinez to fall backwards and get tangled up in the window frame and broken glass. But each time, he would get up and come back again ever more determined, stabbing at John with the knife and screaming, "I'm gonna kill you."

This scene went on for what John would later describe as an eternity. All along John pounded Martinez with the cane around the face and wrist in an attempt to get him to drop the knife.

During the struggle with Martinez, John was stabbed several times in the shoulder and chest. John was losing strength and bleeding very badly. He knew he could not continue to fight much longer. But there was no way he was going to give up. He had to protect his wife and daughter, even if it meant his own death.

In one last attempt to stop Martinez, John threw down the cane and grabbed the hand wielding the knife with both of his own hands. Martinez fought back savagely and managed to cut John on both of his arms and hands. Still John hung on, twisting with all the strength he had left. But Martinez was much younger and much stronger.

John finally let go of Martinez's hands and turned back to grab the cane he had tossed on the bed nearest the window. As he turned to pick up the cane, Martinez thrust the knife into John's back. The pain was excruciating and John almost passed out. John kept telling himself, over and over, "I cannot pass out. I must protect my family." He kept on fighting. He grabbed the cane and again started hitting Martinez about the head and chest area.

John mustered all the strength left in his 72-year-old body as he lashed out fearlessly. He hit Martinez again and again until the attacker fell out of the window frame and into the bushes planted in front of the window.

As Martinez was falling, John could not believe his ears. In the distance he could hear the sirens of the approaching police cars. Help was on the way. The mere sound of the sirens gave John his second wind. With renewed strength, he continued to lash out at the figure of Martinez lying in the bushes.

Martinez heard the approaching police cars, as well. He was doing his best to get out of the way of the cane crashing down on him. He could not believe that such an old man was fighting so hard, even after being stabbed so many times. Martinez was finally able to roll out of the way of John's cane and get to his feet. He, too, was bleeding from cuts from the broken glass and from the blows of John's cane. He ran toward the back of the hotel property and down an embankment into a wooded area.

Four units of the San Diego Police Department arrived on the scene along with a K-9 unit. They tracked Martinez into the wooded area. When he refused to give himself up, they turned the dogs loose on him. Martinez tried to fight off the dogs by stabbing at them with his knife. In the end, the dogs won out and Martinez suffered several severe dog bites before surrendering to the police. Martinez's attorneys would later claim that releasing the dogs on their client was cruel treatment.

Martinez was charged with two attempted burglaries, assault with a deadly weapon and attempted murder. The police recovered a master key to the hotel from his jacket pocket which, when tested, fit all of the guest rooms' doors at the Torres Villa Inn.

During their investigation it was also discovered that Martinez was wanted in Texas for escaping from the state prison where he was serving a twenty-year term for assaulting a police officer.

Martinez was tried and convicted on all counts for the assault and attempted murder of John Taines. He received a sixty-year sentence, after which he will be transferred back to the state of Texas. There he will have to stand trial for his escape and complete his remaining Texas prison term. Martinez has seen his last days of freedom.

After the police had arrived at the Torres Villa Inn, one unit went to the front desk area in search of the clerk on duty. They found the front door locked and a phone number for the manager posted on the door which they radioed into their dispatcher. The dispatcher radioed them back, stating she had been unable to get anyone to answer that number.

When the paramedics arrived, they immediately set about tending to John's wounds. Still dressed in his undershorts, he was covered with blood from head to foot.

In obtaining medical history data from John, the medics learned that he was also suffering from a heart condition—angina. John was taken to a local hospital where he underwent surgery for the knife wounds. John recovered from his wounds in a remarkably short time and returned to his family. However, the nightmare was not over.

Terry's condition worsened after the attack at the Torres Villa Inn. Neither John or Terry could sleep at night without a .38 pistol at their bedside and a newly installed alarm system armed whenever they were in their house. When they would finally fall off to sleep, both would have nightmares about the awful night at the Torres Villa Inn and would awake shaking and crying. These conditions continued for months without improvement. They tried to handle the problem themselves, but finally realized they needed professional medical help if they were to overcome these emotional problems.

The Taineses first sought help from their family physician, who referred them to a specialist in dealing with psychological matters. In discussing their problems with family and friends, they were encouraged to seek legal counsel about help in paying for the additional medical treatment they required.

After meeting with a lawyer and explaining to him what had taken place, the lawyer suggested that the Taineses file a lawsuit against the Torres Villa Inn for inadequate security measures. Shortly afterwards I was retained as a security consultant. I was asked to evaluate the case and to determine if the Torres Villa Inn at the time of the Taineses' attack practiced reasonable security measures.

In reviewing the deposition of the manager of the Torres Villa Inn, I discovered that he had been employed only a short time prior to the Taineses' attack and had very little training and no prior hotel or motel management experience. His training had consisted of three or four days working at another hotel owned by the same owners before being assigned as the manager of the Torres Villa Inn.

He further reported that it was company policy to lock the lobby area at night. He lived on site and was responsible for answering any calls for assistance from guests. He had no explanation for why he did not answer his phone on the night of the Taineses' attack and denied hearing any noises which would have indicated a problem.

The manager was questioned about Martinez's employment at the hotel and what background checks, if any, were conducted prior to his employment. The manager stated that the only checks made were phone calls to previous employers. (Note: An examination of Martinez's application revealed that whoever called the previous employers listed did not get an answer at any of the numbers called.) Asked if he ever considered running background checks on employees through the police department, the manager replied that he was not aware he could do that. (Note: Martinez had, in fact, used his correct name and social security number when applying for the job, and a criminal history check through the police department would have revealed that he was wanted in Texas.)

When questioned about why Martinez was terminated from the Torres Villa Inn, the manager responded that he had been caught drinking on the job and sleeping in guest rooms after working hours on several occasions. He admitted that Martinez, in his position as the head maintenance man, had access to master keys and a key cutting machine.

He assumed that Martinez had turned all of his keys in when he was terminated, but admitted that an inventory was not conducted of the room keys or master keys after Martinez's termination. He also stated that no attempt was made to rekey or re-master the guest rooms.

We were well aware of that omission in good hotel management because the Taineses' forty-year-old souvenir key from their honeymoon still unlocked their room. The master locks had not been changed in forty years.

The manager testified that, to his knowledge, there had never been a crime committed on the premises of the Torres Villa Inn. A check with the San Diego Police Department, however, revealed that several burglaries and car thefts had been reported at the inn during the year prior to the Taineses' attack.

While in La Jolla, I located a former employee of the Torres Villa Inn named Janice Williams. An interview with Janice Williams went as follows:

Talley: How long were you employed at the Torres Villa Inn?

Williams: From May 1986 to February 1989.

Talley: What was your position at the inn?

Williams: Assistant manager and night auditor.

Talley: During your employment at the inn did you ever receive any training in guest security?

Williams: No.

Talley: Were there ever any discussions or concerns by the owners or manager of the inn about guest security?

Williams: No, never.

Talley: The general manager has said that, prior to the attack on the Taineses, there was a sign posted on the front door which notified the guests that there would be no one on duty at the front desk after 10:00 p.m. Do you recall such a sign?

Williams: Yes, but the sign was not put up until three or four months after the Taines incident.

Talley: Are you sure?

Williams: Yes, I am positive. If the manager says the sign was there before the Taines incident, then he is lying.

Talley: The Taineses have testified that they tried to call the front desk during the time the man was trying to break into their room and there was no answer. Was there supposed to be someone on call in case of emergencies?

Williams: Yes, the manager who lived on the premises, but I doubt it would have done any good.

Talley: Why is that?

Williams: The manager told me on many occasions that he hated to be bothered at night and he would turn his phone off.

Talley: Are you telling me that he would turn his phone off when there were guests in the hotel who might need help?

Williams: Yes, this happened all the time. You see, the manager had a drinking problem. There were many days when he would drink during the day and be out of it by the time night came.

Talley: During the time you worked there, was the property ever rekeyed?

Williams: No.

Talley: Are you aware of any keys missing to the guest rooms?

Williams: Yes, there would be two to three missing a week.

Talley: Were those rooms rekeyed?

Williams: Not to my knowledge.

Talley: Did you know Antonio Robert Martinez, the former maintenance man?

Williams: Yes, I interviewed him and had him fill out his employment application.

Talley: After he completed his application, did anyone do a background investigation or check his references prior to his being hired at the inn?

Williams: Not to my knowledge.

Talley: Who made the decision to hire him?

Williams: The manager.

Talley: Did you ever work at nights?

Williams: Yes.

Talley: How would you describe the lighting on the property?

Williams: It was very dark and sometimes it would be even darker because the manager would turn off some of the outside lights because he said they shined through his windows and he could not sleep.

Talley: Do you know why Martinez was fired?

Williams: Yes, he had been found sleeping in guest rooms on several occasions and you could almost always smell alcohol on his breath. Also, several of the maids had reported to the manager that Martinez had made a pass at them.

Talley: On the night that the Taineses were attacked by Martinez, do you feel there was any security at the Torres Villa Inn?

Williams: Only the locks on the doors, to which I understand Martinez had a master key, and whatever security the guests provided to themselves.

Talley: Knowing what you know about missing room and master keys at the Torres Villa Inn, would you spend the night there with your family?

Williams: No.

Janice Williams's testimony would later prove to be a smoking gun in the Taines case.

Upon completing my evaluation of this case, I rendered an opinion to the Taineses' attorney that the security at the Torres Villa Inn was grossly inadequate and was one of the worst examples of hotel/motel security programs I had ever seen. It was unbelievable that, in this day and time, a hotel would lock its doors at 10:00 p.m. and leave its guests to the mercy of people like Antonio Robert Martinez.

When the trial date approached, Terry Taines's health had deteriorated. Her doctors told John that there was no way she could survive that kind of an ordeal. Based upon the doctors' advice, John Taines instructed his attorney to settle the case. This decision was not a hard one for John to make. The possibility of getting a large jury award was never a consideration, given Terry's condition, even though John was informed a jury would be very generous to his family. He only hoped to recover the money it had cost them in medical bills. But most of all, he and Terry had hoped that, by bringing this lawsuit, they would force the owners and management of the Torres Villa Inn to take reasonable security measures to protect their guests in the future. John and Terry felt justice would be served if what they had undergone prevented anyone else from suffering the horror and pain they had suffered at the hands of Antonio Robert Martinez on the Torres Villa property.

Two days before the trial was to start, attorneys for the Taineses negotiated a settlement of $200,000. The Taineses were very pleased with the settlement, even after being told that a jury verdict might very well have been five to ten times that amount.

To my knowledge, John and Terry are still living in Bakersfield and continuing to fight the horrible disease from which Terry suffers. Hopefully, they are putting the memories of the night at the Torres Villa Inn—and their horrendous second honeymoon—behind them.

What You Should Learn from This Crime

When checking into a hotel or motel, ask if someone will be on duty at the front desk twenty-four hours a day. At the first sign of anything out of the ordinary, do not hesitate to call and report it to the hotel staff. If you don't get a response from them, call the police.

Train Ride to Death

ONE OF THE FONDEST MEMORIES I HAVE OF GROWING UP IN A
small East Tennessee town was sneaking off early from school and going
down to the center of attraction in our hometown—the railroad depot.
I was fascinated by the giant locomotives bringing in people and goods and
captivated most of all by the men who worked and rode on those trains.
They would call themselves, with a lot of conviction, "railroad men."

My richest memories involve the kindness and gentle nature of those
men. Those feelings came back to me years later while working as a security consultant when I was hired to evaluate a case involving such a "railroad man." But as I worked on the case of a "Train Ride to Death," I felt
an overwhelming sadness.

Randy Morris, a resident of a small town near Macon, Georgia, had just
turned forty years old. As he looked into the mirror, he could see the tell-
tale signs of age. He noticed more and more gray hair about his temples
and could see the etchings of wrinkles around his eyes. Instead of becoming depressed like most men faced with early middle age, Randy would
laugh it off and be thankful of how good life had been to him.

In the small south Georgia town where Randy Morris had lived his
whole life, one could not spend a lot of time worrying about growing
old. There were more important things—like making a living in a
region that had long been dependent on farming—to think about. It was
a never-ending struggle to make ends meet and, with luck, to have enough

money left over to buy your children new shoes for school.

When Randy was growing up, he had few options for his future. He could struggle like his father, plowing away at the earth, hoping that it would yield enough to make it to the next season. He could enter the military or work for the state highway department. He could also go to work for the railroad.

Randy had spent hours as a little boy hanging around the railroad station in the center of town. His father's brother had given up farming and, as he would say, "joined the railroad" after dropping out of school in the eighth grade. Randy's uncle would welcome the opportunity, whenever it presented itself, to gather a group of men and boys and spin tall tales about working the rails. One of Randy's favorite toys was an electric train set he had received on his tenth birthday. He would sit for hours watching as the train made circle after circle and dream about the days when he, too, would ride the rails like his uncle.

In all the years that passed, Randy never considered anything else but working for the railroad. Shortly after his graduation from high school, on which his father had insisted, he was hired, with his uncle's help, by the Southeastern Railroad. During his first years Randy worked every possible job the railroad had. He started in the yard, then worked as a brakeman, a fireman, and eventually an engineer—his real love.

Instilled with diligent, nose-to-the-grindstone work habits, Randy was admired by all of his co-workers and supervisors. He was soon known throughout the railroad as one of the best engineers in the company. When filling out a performance report, a supervisor described Randy as cheerful, honest, and good-natured in character, serious about his work, and always helpful to his co-workers. Frustrated, the supervisor finally wrote in the comment section, "Hell, there are not enough good adjectives to describe him."

Randy was singleminded in his dedication to his job. He worked extra hard the first couple of years he was with the railroad because he wanted to save money to marry his high school sweetheart. Indeed, on March 1, 1963, Randy realized another of his dreams. He married Betty Sue Grogan, a former high school cheerleader and his girlfriend since the sixth grade. Together they had seven children, each as special to them as the first, and they moved into the small but lovingly maintained red-brick house Randy had long dreamed of owning. Randy and Betty Sue were the ideal parents, making sure all the children took part in sports, scouting, school, and church events. It was a joke around their house that with two more children they could have started their own baseball team.

Neighbors and church members all said that Randy was a wonderful father and very well respected by his family. A young boy in the neighborhood would later say, "He was like a father to me." Randy found this amusing since he had so many children of his own. It truly seemed that Randy found the time for everybody. No one could ever remember his saying anything bad about anyone.

So, on the morning of February 13, 1982, Randy looked into the mirror, reflected on his life, and counted the many blessings it had bestowed upon him. He was getting ready to make a run to Cleveland, Tennessee, where he and other crew members would have to lay over for eight to ten hours. They would be staying at a hotel affiliated with a national chain located not far from the train yard. While at the hotel, he would have the opportunity to check on the reservations he'd made for his upcoming vacation. The whole family was looking forward to its first trip to Disney World in just three short weeks.

As he kissed his wife and children goodbye and boarded the cab of the locomotive, Randy never dreamed this would be his last train ride.

The city of Cleveland, Tennessee, has a population of approximately 27,000 people and is located northeast of Chattanooga on Interstate 75. It is mainly known as the home of Lee College, run by the Church of God. It is also one of the many destination points along the Southeastern Railway.

The train ride from Macon to Cleveland turned out to be an enjoyable one. Randy had drawn a crew he liked and had worked with many times in the past. The weather was excellent. It was only mid-February, but the smell of spring was in the air. Already, a small number of azalea blossoms were evident as Randy peeked out the window of the cab. As the train headed north, he could see that the leaves were already beginning to bud on the trees.

They left Macon early in the afternoon and made short stops in Atlanta and Chattanooga. They arrived in the Southeastern train yard in Cleveland a little after 4:00 a.m. on the morning of February 14, 1982. They secured the train and stopped to have a cup of coffee with the yard crew. It was around 5:00 a.m. when Randy finally called for the hotel shuttle bus to pick them up. None of them had any idea that, at that very moment, a chain of events was beginning to take place that would change their lives forever.

It was only a short distance to the Fiesta Inn-South from the Southeastern train yard. Steven Jones, the desk clerk on duty, had received the call from Randy. He then went into the lobby to shake awake Raymond Brown, the 59-year-old driver of the hotel's courtesy van. Steve laughed to himself as he stood there shaking old Raymond. He had grown up in Cleveland and he well knew Raymond's reputation as one of the town drunks. Raymond had worked almost everywhere in town, but mostly in janitorial or yard work.

The Fiesta Inn was part of a major chain, but the franchise was owned by a local doctor, who purchased the hotels years before as an investment. The owner had met Raymond through his church. Since then, he had used Raymond to clean up around his house. Feeling sorry for him, he instructed the general manager to hire Raymond as the night courtesy van driver and security person. Besides, the doctor told the general manager, hiring Raymond, who would be glad to work for a pittance, would save money. He could take the place of the contract security guard company they were paying $6.00 an hour.

As Steven Jones shook Raymond Brown awake, he thought to himself, "some security," but what did he know, he only worked there. He gave Raymond his instructions to pick up the railroad crew. As Raymond was leaving, Steven told him to make sure to tell the crew there would be a fresh pot of coffee when they arrived.

It would only take Raymond Brown about ten minutes to drive the short distance to the train yard. The cup of coffee Raymond had grabbed on his way out of the motel was strong. He started to throw it out the window, but decided it would help to wake him up. The skies were clear and the morning air was brisk. Between the strong coffee and the cool morning air rushing through the open van window, Raymond was almost awake as he approached the train yard. He pulled up in front of the dispatch office and saw that the four-man crew was already outside awaiting his arrival. Raymond recognized several of them, but especially the leader of the crew, Randy Morris. Raymond liked Randy because he was always cheerful, laughing, and making jokes.

About the time Raymond Brown was picking up Randy Morris and his crew, the county sheriff's department was receiving a call from a man stating that there was a disturbance in room 51 of the Fiesta Inn-North. The Fiesta Inn-North was owned and operated by the same people as the Fiesta Inn-South and was about six miles up the interstate from the southern location.

The county sheriff's department immediately dispatched one of its two on-duty patrols to the Fiesta Inn-North. The dispatcher did not know that the room numbers started at room 100. There was no Room 51. As the unidentified caller hung up the phone, he stepped out of the phone booth which was located in the parking lot of an Exxon Station near the foot of a hill, next to a driveway leading up to the Fiesta Inn-South. Waiting for him, in a car with the motor running, were the two friends with whom he had been out drinking and smoking marijuana.

They had met around 7:00 p.m. at a striptease joint in Chattanooga where they had remained until it closed at midnight. At 3:00 a.m., they found themselves at an after-hours club, where the booze flowed, but between them they had only a dollar left. They needed some money.

They left the club and drove around Chattanooga in a late-model Chevrolet that they had already stolen that night. They finished drinking some warm beer left over from the six-pack they had purchased earlier in the evening. When the beer ran out, they began smoking some marijuana, which Leroy Parker, the leader of pack, had been keeping to himself.

The conversation again turned to what they were going to do for money. Leroy Parker, by now feeling the effects of a night of drinking and drugs, pulled a Ruger .44 caliber pistol from under the seat and suggested they go steal some.

This was nothing new to 24-year-old Leroy, who had stolen plenty, even before this night. In fact, there was not much Leroy had *not* done. At the age of 13 he was arrested for a series of burglaries and sent to a reform school for three years. He had only been out of reform school a month when he was picked up by the police, this time for questioning in a burglary and rape. Leroy fit the description, but the victim could not identify him in a lineup.

Knowing he had beaten the rape and burglary charges, Leroy felt his foolhardiness grow. He wanted to advance to something more exciting. He found that excitement by buying a gun and robbing all-night service stations. Unfortunately for Leroy, the robberies were not that successful in terms of proceeds. The most he ever netted was $45.

During his seventh service-station robbery, Leroy was almost shot by a police stake-out team. The policemen testified that when they jumped out of the storage room where they were hiding, Leroy threw his gun down, and began crying and yelling, "Please don't shoot me!" Leroy's career as an armed robber was over, at least for a while. He was sentenced to twenty years in the Tennessee State Prison. Once in prison, Leroy had no problem playing the game. He became a model prisoner and was released on probation. He had served less than four years.

When Leroy suggested they go steal some money, his companions knew they were listening to an old pro. Besides, he had spent time in the "big house," a subject Leroy liked to brag about. The trio drove around for the next hour looking for a good target to rob. However, things had changed since Leroy had been away, and his old hunting grounds had dried up. Everywhere they went, the service stations he had robbed years ago were closed. The few they did find open were equipped with booths where you slipped your money through a slot. Robbing them would be next to impossible, and Leroy was cussing and complaining. How was a guy going to make any money this way?

The trio was about to give up when one of Leroy's partners spoke up. He knew an easy place to hit, he told them, a motel in Cleveland, Tennessee, where he had recently spent the night with a girlfriend. Unlike most of the motels on the interstate, there was no night check-in window. When he and his girlfriend had arrived at around 3:00 in the morning, the lobby was wide open. There was only one man on duty and he was sitting at the desk counting a lot of money. It was only a twenty- to thirty-minute drive to the hotel, and they could be back in Chattanooga in time for breakfast.

In order to make it appear that he was still in charge, Leroy had to ask several questions before making the decision to go and check this motel out. As they drove up Interstate 75, Leroy schooled his partners on the art of committing armed robbery. Sensing they were a little nervous, he told them not to worry. If anything went wrong, he would shoot their way out.

When they got off the first Cleveland exit, the young man who had come up with the idea of robbing the motel could not remember its name. He was sure it sat on a hilltop, but could not recall if it was to the right or left of the exit. He looked to the right and saw a Motel Six. He knew that was not it because Motel Six locked its lobbies at 10:00 p.m. and you had to use a night check-in window.

They turned left and saw an Exxon service station sitting at the foot of a hill and, atop the hill, the Fiesta Inn-South. Leroy's partner was sure this was the place because he remembered having to turn in next to a service station.

As they were turning into the driveway leading to the motel, Leroy noticed a police car sitting across the road at a Waffle House. They made a pass in front of the motel and could see clearly into the lobby by looking through the big plate-glass windows. He saw only one person sitting behind the front desk. No one else was in the lobby. At the rear of the motel office, he spotted a glass door leading into the lobby area. It all looked too good to be true. However, Leroy was still worried about the police car he had spotted at the Waffle House across the road from the motel.

Leroy told the driver to drive back down the hill to a phone booth Leroy had spotted as they drove in. Leroy got out of the Chevrolet, grabbed the phone book, and flipped to the yellow pages. He found the listings for the motels in the area and noticed there were two listings for Fiesta Inns in Cleveland. One was located on the north end of town and the second—the one they were going to rob—was on the south end. This gave him an idea. He reached into his pocket for a quarter, but realized that he did not have any change. He asked his two accomplices for a quarter, but between the three of them they only had a dollar bill.

Leroy noticed the card attached on the front of the phone which said that no money was necessary for emergency calls. He picked up the receiver and dialed 911. Within seconds the sheriff's department answered.

Leroy told the dispatcher he was calling from the Fiesta Inn-North. He reported that the people in room 51, next to his, sounded like they were killing each other. The dispatcher said she would send a car as soon as possible. However, she only had two units working. One of those was answering a call and the other was on his meal break. Leroy hung up the phone and smiled. He felt proud of himself, as he glanced across the road into the Waffle House. He saw the sheriff's deputy lift up his two-way radio as he answered the dispatcher's call. The deputy ran outside, jumped into his patrol car, and sped north on the interstate. Leroy's plan had worked perfectly.

Leroy got back into the car and told the driver to go back up the hill to the motel. As they went up the hill, Leroy laid out the plan. He would enter through the rear door while one of them went into the lobby and asked about renting a room. The driver would pull back around to the front and park near the front door. He was to keep the motor running so they could make a fast getaway. As Leroy was walking through the back door, he glanced down at his watch. It was 5:30 a.m.

Even while Leroy entered the back door, the motel's courtesy van carrying the railroad crew was approaching the underpass at Interstate 75. The crew was laughing and joking. Randy was kidding Raymond about what Raymond had bought his sweetheart for Valentine's Day. As Raymond turned into the driveway, Randy jokingly said that he hoped the coffee was better than the last time he had stayed at the hotel. Everyone was still laughing and having a good time as the van pulled to a stop in front of the motel.

The crew got out of the van and went around to the rear to retrieve their bags from the cargo bin. Sam Decker, Randy's brakeman, noticed a late-model Chevrolet sitting nearby with the motor running. Its driver was nervously moving around in his seat, as he constantly looked back and forth. When he spotted the van, it appeared that he wanted to say or do something. This made Sam Decker feel very uncomfortable, but he did not mention his feelings to the others. It was probably just someone checking out early to beat the early morning traffic. They gathered up their bags and proceeded into the lobby. Randy Morris, as usual, was leading the way.

Steven Jones would later testify that he had just finished the night audit and was counting the money, when he heard someone open the lobby door. He looked up and saw a "small, funky little black character" coming into the lobby. The man approached the front desk and acted a little nervous as he asked if there were any rooms available. There were, and Jones placed a registration card in front of the man to fill out. As he did so, Jones had a feeling that someone was behind him. He started to turn around to see when he felt a heavy blow to the side of his head. He fell to the floor and almost passed out. Lying there, he could hear the man he would later identify as Leroy Parker, yelling, "Don't try anything funny, or I'll blow your brains out."

Steven Jones did not pass out, but he was bleeding badly. The man who had been sent in to distract him had jumped across the desk. Leroy Parker was standing over Jones, with his foot on the base of his neck, pointing a gun at his head. Leroy's partner started cleaning out the cash register. Leroy repeatedly asked Jones if there was a safe. Jones told him there was one in the manager's office, but he did not have the combination to it. Besides, all the money was in the cash drawer, the victim said.

It felt like a lifetime to Steven Jones, but less than two minutes had expired. Jones began crying and begging Leroy not to kill him. He was relieved when he heard the front door opening.

He heard a voice call out, "I hope you have the coffee ready." Randy Morris saw the two men behind the front desk. What he could not see, and had no way of knowing, was that one of them had a gun pointed at Steven Jones's head.

Not recognizing either of them as the normal clerk, Randy said, "Hey, you must be new."

Sam Decker, Raymond Brown, and the other two crew members had just gotten inside the lobby. Randy Morris had barely finished his sentence when Leroy Parker pulled the gun from behind Jones's head and pointed it directly at him. Leroy yelled, "Put your hands up, motherfuckers, or I'll blow your heads off."

As Sam Decker later testified, Randy had a habit of talking with his hands. As Leroy yelled, Randy threw up his hands and said, "Hey, is this some kind of a joke?"

Leroy Parker didn't say a word. He simply pointed the gun at Randy Morris and pulled the trigger. The gun boomed like a cannon, as fire shot out of the barrel and cylinder.

The bullet struck Randy Morris squarely in the heart and exited out his back, leaving a massive exit wound. The force of the .44 caliber Ruger lifted him from his feet and threw him across a lobby sofa. Randy landed on the floor only inches from Sam Decker, who had dropped there when the shot rang out. Decker was splattered with blood as Randy's body hit the floor. One of the other crew members turned and fled out the front door. Raymond Brown and the fourth crew member stood motionless, shocked and stunned by what they had just witnessed.

Leroy Parker was yelling and screaming, "I'm going to kill all you sons of bitches." Leroy and his accomplice leaped across the desk and ran out the front door.

Sam Decker and the others would later say that, when Leroy leaped across the front desk, they were sure he was going to kill them all.

As the car sped off, they could hear Leroy Parker screaming, "I should have killed them all."

Leroy soon got over being upset. He was very pleased as he counted the money on the way back to Chattanooga. This had turned out to be his biggest haul yet—$1,200 in cash. He also had another reason to brag: He had killed his first man.

Once he felt it was safe to move, Sam Decker turned to his friend, Randy Morris. As Sam touched him, Randy made a gurgling sound as the last bit of life left his body. Spread about the floor near his body were Valentine cards for his wife and seven children. Sam's mind flashed back to the fun and laughter they had shared picking out the cards during their stop in Atlanta. What was he going to say to Randy's wife, Betty Sue?

Leroy Parker and his two accomplices were arrested several days later, after robbing another motel in Chattanooga. Due to the similar nature of that robbery, the Chattanooga police notified the Cleveland police of the arrests.

A lineup was held several days later with everyone present from the Fiesta Inn robbery. Everyone, with the exception of Raymond Brown, picked Leroy Parker as the man that had shot and killed Randy Morris.

Randy Morris's wife and seven children never missed a day of Leroy Parker's trial. They all cried when the witnesses described how he shot Randy for no reason at all and left him lying there to die. However, they showed no emotion when the jury found Leroy Parker guilty and sentenced him to die in the electric chair.

Randy Morris's estate, on behalf of his wife and seven children, filed a $10 million lawsuit against the Fiesta Inn. The suit alleged the inn should have foreseen this type of crime. The suit also alleged that the Fiesta Inn had no security measures which could have deterred or prevented Randy Morris's death.

Also sued was Fiesta Inns, the parent corporation. The suit alleged that the motel chain had a duty to insure that its franchisee had taken necessary security measures to protect its guests.

Naming the Fiesta Inns, the franchiser, in the suit was a smart move by the Morris attorney. During this time, Fiesta Inns had a respected loss prevention department, which was available to the Cleveland franchiser. This department could have assisted the Fiesta Inn-South in evaluating its security needs and offered recommendations to it. The parent corporation's position was that the Cleveland owners had to request their services. Under the licensing agreement they were not *required* to do so.

The attorneys representing the Morris estate hired a security expert to evaluate the measures in effect on the night of Randy Morris's death. In a deposition he gave in court, he cited several discrepancies in Fiesta Inn's security program. One, the motel should have followed sound security practices, making it unlikely for this type of crime to occur. Other national chains, such as Days Inns of America, used such measures, in particular the utilization of a night check-in window after 10:00 p.m.

At the time I was still employed by Days Inns as its vice president of risk management. The attorneys faced with defending the Fiesta Inn felt that since the plaintiff's expert was using Days Inns as the model, I was the best person to evaluate their case.

I received permission from my supervisor to assist the Fiesta Inn attorneys and set about doing so in July 1985. The first step, as in most cases, was to read the mounds of assembled depositions and discovery documents. After completing the initial review, I traveled to Cleveland, Tennessee, to conduct the on-site portion of the evaluation.

My first stop was a visit with the county sheriff's department. I needed to obtain records showing what type of criminal problems the county was experiencing during the time period of the suit. Second, I needed detailed information about crimes that had been reported by the Fiesta Inn or any of their guests. The Sheriff's Department indicated that, during the twelve-month period prior to the Morris incident, a rash of robberies and other crimes were reported among businesses located near the interstate.

Businesses located either at or near interstate highways have long been favorite targets for criminals. It affords the perpetrators several different options of escape after committing a crime. Law enforcement agencies have recognized this fact for years and have encouraged these businesses to take extra crime-prevention measures.

A review of serious crimes reported at the Fiesta Inn for a two-year period revealed ninety such incidents. Included were larcenies, burglaries, and one that would prove to be the most important to this case. On February 14, 1979, exactly three years before the Morris incident, the Fiesta Inn reported an armed robbery at the front desk. As in the Morris incident, the robbers had entered the lobby after 5:00 a.m. A large sum of money was also stolen. The desk clerk on duty was Bennie Simms, the present general manager.

In addition to the crimes reported at the Fiesta Inn, several other businesses at the interstate had experienced armed robberies, including the Exxon Station located at the foot of the hill near the Fiesta Inn-South. The owner told me he started closing at midnight six months prior to the Morris incident due to the increasing crime in the area and the fact that his station had been robbed twice in the early morning hours. He felt that if he had not made this decision, one of his employees might have been killed.

Bennie Simms, the general manager of the Fiesta Inn, was questioned about his knowledge of crimes upon the premises. He wasn't very cooperative and finally stated that he was aware of two or three hubcap thefts from guest cars in the parking lots, but no serious crimes to guests.

I asked Simms about the armed robbery at the front desk when he was a desk clerk, back in 1979. According to Simms, it was a little after 5:00 a.m. when two black males entered through the rear lobby door. They gained entry into the office located behind the front desk and sneaked up behind him. He stated that the robbers were armed with guns and had tied him up. They had rifled the cash drawer and had gotten away with a little more than $1,000.

I inquired about what, if anything, the hotel had done to increase security after that robbery. Simms said it had instituted a policy of locking the rear lobby and office doors at 10:00 p.m. For a time, the Fiesta had even hired off-duty police officers to work security after midnight. This continued for several months, but was discontinued due to the cost. Simms admitted that the policy of locking the back door had gone by the wayside several months later, simply because no one bothered to enforce it.

Simms related he had been through the training school at Fiesta Inn's corporate offices. He stated he "vaguely remembered" a portion of the training program directed at security measures. There were security manuals at one time at the motel, Simms stated, but they had been misplaced. Moreover, he had held no security-related training for his employees.

Simms said he was not aware of other armed robberies near the interstate exchange. I informed him about the two at the Exxon Station and the owner's decision to close after midnight. He responded by saying he thought they had closed because business had been bad. He was not aware that they had been robbed.

I asked about Raymond Brown's dual role as the van driver and night security person. Simms chuckled, saying, "That was the owner's idea; I never went along with that. Raymond was just a van driver."

Steven Jones no longer worked at the hotel and had moved out of state shortly after the armed robbery. I was able to contact him by phone, and the conversation turned out to be very revealing. Jones said he had asked the management of the hotel on several occasions to install a drop safe behind the front desk in order to secure the large sums of money that accumulated from one shift to the next. He also asked on several occasions why management did not use a night check-in window like the other motels along the interstate. He was told that, because of the design of the lobby, it would cost too much to install one. Besides, the general manager told him, "Nothing bad ever happens around here." I asked if he was aware that the hotel had a similar robbery exactly three years prior to that time. Jones said he'd asked the general manager, Simms, about any prior armed robberies and was told there had not been any.

Jones further stated he had attended several employee meetings, but the subject of security never came up. Jones said he was told Raymond Brown was the night security person. He felt this was a joke, but he had heard Raymond bragging to several guests that he was in charge of security. On a few occasions, Jones had seen Raymond with a gun, but never reported it to the manager. He said he always feared being robbed, especially since he was forced to keep such large sums of money at night.

If he were asked in court, Steven Jones said, he would say that the lack of a night check-in window and the policy of keeping large sums of money contributed to the armed robbery and death of Randy Morris. Jones also stated that if he had been made aware of the other armed robberies in the area, he would have quit.

The attorneys for Randy Morris's estate hired their own security consultant a few months after the incident. The consultant wrote a report about his observations at the motel during a two-day stay five months after Randy Morris's death. While none of the conditions he observed might be relevant to the night of Morris's death, they could show the motel's overall attitude toward security. The following are excerpts from his report.

> I arrived at the Fiesta Inn around 9 p.m. I found the front lobby doors opened. I then walked down the hallway leading from the front desk and found the rear door unlocked. As I was walking back toward the front desk I noticed the door leading behind the front desk. I saw no one was watching, so I tried to open it. To my surprise it was unlocked and I could see it led to the area behind the front desk.
>
> As I walked back around in front of the desk, I noticed only one person on duty there. However, I did notice a Cleveland police officer sitting in a lounge chair. His shoes were untied, shirt unbuttoned and his feet were resting on a table as he watched television. I asked the desk clerk why a policeman was there, and he said the officer was off-duty but working security for the motel. I asked if they had problems with crime on the premises. The desk clerk said, "None other than some hubcaps being stolen, but that's why we hire security." I also noticed anoth-

er middle-aged man sitting with the police officer reading a paper. He was identified to me as the night van driver. I later overheard the police officer call him Raymond.

After checking in and putting my baggage away, I walked around the premises. I counted a total of six lights burnt out, which caused dark areas on the premises.

I walked back into the lobby and went back to the front desk in hopes of striking up a conversation with the desk clerk. I asked for change. I noticed three closed circuit television monitors sitting on a table behind the desk. I casually asked the desk clerk what those were. He said at one time they had cameras in the parking areas for security. However, they had quit working about three to four years ago. The owners had made the decision not to repair the cameras, due to the cost involved. The desk clerk told me they kept the housings up and the monitors behind the front desk in hopes of making people think they had security cameras.

I went back to my room, but kept a watch on the parking lot from my room window until 3 a.m. During this time, I never saw the off-duty police officer patrol the grounds. Around 5 a.m. I walked back around to the lobby, where I found the police officer and the van driver asleep. The front and rear doors were open and the desk clerk was counting money behind the front desk.

In the materials I had been provided was the sworn statement of Danny Benson, the brakeman on Randy Morris's railroad crew on the night of Morris's death.

The following are excerpts from Benson's statement:

I was about three feet behind Randy when we entered the lobby. I saw the two black men standing behind the front desk. I felt uneasy, because I did not recognize them.

I had known Raymond Brown since I started staying at the motel. I always thought he was the security officer. He always told us that he was in charge of security and we always joked with him about it. On the night of Randy's death, Raymond had come to the train yard to pick us up. He got out of the van and was showing us a new gun that he had bought. We kidded him by saying, "No one would think of messing with the Fiesta Inn now." He put the gun into his back pocket. During the robbery and Randy's shooting, I worried about Raymond pulling the gun. I was afraid he was going to pull the gun and try something stupid and get us all killed. However, Raymond dropped to the floor like the rest of us. I thank God he did not make any attempts to do anything.

After completing my review, I rendered the following opinions in the case of *The Estate of Randy Morris v. Fiesta Inn*:

> A: The armed robbery of the motel was a foreseeable event. This opinion was based upon the prior armed robbery to the motel and the recent armed robberies to area businesses.
>
> B: Due to the foreseeability of the armed robbery, the Fiesta Inn should have taken some security measures to deter or prevent robberies to its premises. Its failure to take these necessary measures contributed to the death of Randy Morris.
>
> C: The Fiesta Inn was negligent in failing to abide by the security policies and manuals provided by the Fiesta Inn Corporation.
>
> D: The Fiesta Inn was negligent in not providing any security training for its employees.
>
> E: The Fiesta Inn was negligent in creating a "false sense of security" by implying that Raymond Brown was a security officer there to provide protection for its guests and employees.
>
> F: The Fiesta Inn violated reasonable security measures by keeping large sums of money in the cash drawer. This practice created a target for potential robbers.
>
> G: The totality of the security violations by the Fiesta Inn may prove to be gross negligence, therefore opening the Fiesta Inn up to possible punitive damages.

The lawsuit was settled with Randy Morris's estate within weeks of the presentation of my opinion.

The court, at the request of the defendants, ordered the terms of the settlement sealed, so no one outside the case will ever know its amount. However, I am informed it was substantial—given the extent of the Fiesta's proven negligence and the size of Randy's family.

Incidentally, many hotels/motels where serious crimes have occurred prefer sealed settlements even if it means paying out more money than if the settlement were public. They don't want news of a heinous crime—and tremendous pay-out to the victim's family—to reach the traveling public, which might not frequent the facility if it knew the truth. So travelers remain unaware that staying in hotels like the Fiesta Inn-South means taking one's life into one's hands. This is extremely unfortunate, and, I believe, a flaw in our tort system.

There is no way to determine if Randy Morris would be alive today had the Fiesta Inn taken reasonable security measures. However, the facts indicate that a high probability exists that he would still be riding the rails.

There is a railroad crossing less than a block from the Morris's red-brick home where Randy's wife and children still live and try to somehow justify the untimely death of a good man. A Southeastern Railroad train passes four times a day. As it disappears into the distance, you can hear its whistle blowing one last time as if in memory of Randy Morris.

What You Should Learn from This Crime

If you should walk into a situation that appears to be out of the ordinary, do not take any unnecessary risks. If you should be a victim of a robbery, always do exactly as the robber requests. Don't make any sudden moves or attempt to question the robber. Remember, in most cases the robber will be just as, if not more, scared than you and will want to complete the crime and escape. Any provocation could result in injuries to you or other victims.

■ ■ ■

CHAPTER EIGHT

Rape in the Heart of Jackson

IN EARLY DECEMBER, 1985, PATTY RUGGS FELT LONELY AND depressed as she went about her daily routine of cleaning house and picking up after her four-year-old daughter.

James, her husband, had been out of town working for the past several months, and now it did not appear that he would be able to spend Christmas at home. This would be very difficult for her to cope with, but would be extremely hard on their daughter, Maggie.

Maggie was at the age when she needed the love and affection of both parents. Not a day would go by that Maggie didn't ask when her daddy was coming home and would he be home in time for Santa Claus. It was not unusual for Maggie to cry herself to sleep at night wanting her daddy to come home.

James Ruggs was born in the small south Georgia coastal town of Brunswick. Like many such towns, Brunswick depended heavily on the fishing industry and, in its case, the local military bases. The economy in the mid-1980s had taken its toll on the Brunswick area, and James, like many of his friends, had found himself in the unemployment lines. With his benefits only two weeks away from expiring, James found a job with Southeastern Bell. The only drawback was that his new job would require him to be away from home months at a time. But, he had to care for his family. It was a little easier for James to deal with his separation problems when he reflected on how fortunate he was compared to some of his friends who were still in the unemployment lines and who faced losing everything they had worked for their own entire lives. James only hoped that he could be home for Christmas.

Patty's prayers and James's hopes finally paid off. Around the 10th of December, James's boss called the whole line crew together after work for a meeting. He started off by saying, "I have some good news for you and some bad news. The good news is we will be finishing our present assignment on the 19th of December and we will all be home for Christmas with our families. The bad news is we have to report to our new assignment, in Jackson, Mississippi, the day after Christmas. But the company has arranged for all of the married crew members to take their families with them if desired."

As soon as the meeting was over, James ran to the nearest pay phone to call Patty and share the news with her. James's boss told the crew that the company would be making the motel arrangements for them and their families and that these would be within walking distance of where they would be working in downtown Jackson. Everybody would be expected to check in by 7:00 p.m. on December 26, and there would be a short meeting of the crew members at 8:00 p.m.

Christmas that year for James, Patty, and Maggie was a special one. For the first time in months they were together as a family, and they looked forward to being able to remain together after the holidays. The time passed by quickly as they visited family members and made their plans for their trip to Jackson.

They arrived in Jackson just as it was turning dark on the evening of December 26, 1985. The trip had been a long one, and, like a typical four-year-old, Maggie became cranky toward the end. They followed the directions to the motel that the company had mailed to them over the Christmas holidays and had no problem locating it. As they pulled into the driveway they were pleased with its outer appearance. The grounds appeared to be well maintained, and the parking lot and walkways were brightly lit.

James pulled the car up near the entrance to the registration desk and parked in the space marked "guest check-ins only." It had been several hours since they had stopped, so Patty and Maggie got out of the car to stretch their legs while James went inside to register.

As James walked into the lobby, the first things that caught his attention were a camera pointing at him from behind the front desk and a video monitor, projecting his image, sitting on the counter. In all of his travels this was the first time that he had ever seen such a set-up. He gave his name to the attractive young lady behind the front desk, and she immediately handed him a guest registration card and informed him that several other members of his company had already checked in.

The presence of the camera and monitor somewhat concerned James, and he wondered if there were a possibility that the motel may have been experiencing security problems.

As he was filling out the guest registration card, he casually asked the clerk if the motel were located in a safe area of town. Before he could finish his question and before the desk clerk could respond, a man stepped out of a doorway with a beaded curtain. It was almost as if he had been standing there listening to their conversation. He immediately identified himself as Mr. Patel, the manager and owner of the motel.

Mr. Patel first welcomed James and his family to his motel and them set about reassuring James that the motel was located in a very safe area of town. He said that there had never been any security problems at the motel. Mr. Patel stated that the camera and monitor were installed as part of his security plan for his guests and attributed the lack of security problems to these high-tech devices. James commented that this was comforting since his wife and daughter would be there alone during the day. Mr. Patel replied by saying that everyone at the hotel was part of one big happy family and to let him know if the Ruggses needed anything at all during their stay.

After James finished filling out the registration form, Mr. Patel offered to show them to their room. He directed them where to park and commented that their room was visible from the office. Mr. Patel helped James unload the car and pointed out where the ice and vending machines were. James and Patty both thanked Mr. Patel for his kindness. As he was departing, he told them that he also lived on the premises and if they needed anything at all, just call. They watched as Mr. Patel walked back through the parking lot towards the office and agreed that he seemed to be such a nice man.

James and Patty had no way of knowing that this was their second major false impression of the night. The first: that the Heart of Jackson Motel appeared to be a safe place.

Patty began unpacking their bags and set about getting settled into what was going to be their home for the next couple of months. James, in the meantime, called his boss to let him know that they had arrived and their room number. Tired from the trip, Maggie had climbed up on one of the double beds and had fallen asleep. Instead of waking her up, James and Patty decided to order a pizza from a local delivery service that advertised in the room. As promised, the pizza was promptly delivered in less than thirty minutes. As James was hurrying to answer the knock of the pizza delivery man, he noticed that the room door was equipped with a sliding bolt lock in addition to the knob lock, but it had no safety chain. He assumed the knob lock operated like its counterparts at all the other motels in which he had stayed—automatically locking when you closed the door. James paid for the pizza and closed the door behind him, making sure that he also engaged the sliding bolt lock.

While eating dinner they watched television, and it wasn't long before Maggie fell asleep. James and Patty watched the late-night news and talked about how great it was to be together. Before they went to bed, James walked over to the door to make a final check and cautioned Patty about keeping it locked while she and Maggie were alone during the day.

The next two mornings James left around 7:00 a.m. and walked the short distance to the local telephone company building where he would be working for the next several months. He planned to get off work normally between 6:00 p.m. and 7:00 p.m. Patty and Maggie would be waiting on him to go to dinner and to tell him how they had spent their day. James thought how nice it was to be able to share this extra time with his family. He hoped that some day he would be able to find a job where he could enjoy this lifestyle every day.

On the second day, December 28, Maggie was especially excited and could not wait for her daddy to arrive back at the motel. Earlier in the day, her mother had taken her to a nearby air force base where she had seen planes, troops marching, and large military trucks everywhere.

As soon as James knocked on the door, Patty had barely gotten it open when Maggie rushed into James's arms and began telling him about her big day at the air force base. The remainder of the evening was spent pretty much like the previous two. They went out for dinner, drove around town for awhile, came back to their room, put Maggie to bed, and watched television until it was time to go to sleep. As customary at this time, Maggie said her prayers and ended them by telling God how happy she was to have both her mommy and daddy at home with her.

That night it was Patty's turn to make sure the door was locked and to turn off the lights. She walked over to the door and turned the latch into what she thought was the locked position. She then shut off the lights in the main part of the room, but left the bathroom light on with the door partially closed in case Maggie had to get up in the middle of the night to use the bathroom. The room had two double beds, and James had chosen the one nearest the door. Patty ran over, jumped in the bed beside James, and kissed him good night. It didn't take long for both of them to fall sound asleep.

Around 2:00 a.m., Patty was abruptly awakened by a noise. Drowsily, she thought it must be outside. She closed her eyes and fell back asleep. She had no way of gauging how much time had gone by when she heard the noise again. But this time it sounded as if someone had bumped into a piece of furniture.

Again, half asleep, she thought it must be Maggie going to the bathroom; on her way she must have bumped into the dresser. Patty opened her eyes and looked in the direction of the noise. Patty immediately saw a silhouette of a man cast on the wall from the light she had left on in the bathroom earlier. At first she felt it had to be James checking on Maggie, but she broke out in a cold sweat and got a sick feeling in her stomach when she reached over and touched James, who was still lying in the bed next to her.

Patty tried to scream but nothing came out of her mouth. She tried to move her arms to wake James, but they felt as if they weighed a ton. She could not lift them. She finally managed to sit straight up in the bed and let out a gagging sound as if she were gasping for her breath; James awoke.

James was attempting to gain his senses and was in the process of asking Patty what was wrong when she finally screamed, "James, there is someone in the room."

This was enough to wake James completely. He glanced around the room and saw the figure of a man standing near Maggie's bed. James jumped up and ran toward the figure, but before he could reach him, the intruder jumped on the bed with Maggie, grabbing her and placing a knife at her throat.

The intruder, later identified as Eugene Sams, was an ex-convict with a long history of burglaries, robberies, assaults, and rape. He was well known to the local police. His last big crime spree ended in 1979 when he rode up to a local 7/11 store on his bicycle to commit an armed robbery. He failed to notice that there were two police cars parked just outside the door and that two police officers were taking their morning coffee break inside. Sams parked his bike, dismounted, walked inside, pointed a gun at the store clerk and announced, "This is a hold-up." The store clerk, thinking the robber was surely crazy or hyped up on drugs, calmly placed the $67.20 that was in the cash register in a brown paper bag and handed it over to him. Feeling proud of himself, Sams then demanded a pack of Kool's, and the store clerk immediately complied. Sams turned to walk out of the store only to find himself facing two police officers aiming 9 mm automatic pistols at him.

The officers, who had been standing near the coffee machine when Sams had entered the store, had done all they could to not burst out laughing during the "robbery." The situation seemed so ludicrous. The robber had missed the two police cars sitting right in front of the store, he was going to attempt his getaway on this battered bike, and his clothes consisted of an old pair of army fatigue pants, a bright orange shirt with parrots on it, and an old World War II pilot's skull cap pulled down over his ears. He certainly seemed dressed to blend in with the crowd during his getaway!

Sams received five years to serve for his infamous 7/11 robbery, and the only question he had for the judge was whether his bicycle would still be there when he got out of prison.

A few days before the Ruggses checked into the Heart of Jackson Motel, Mr. Patel noticed a worn-out bicycle propped up against the wall near room 103 around ten o'clock in the morning. He went back to the office and checked his records to see if room 103 had been rented the night before. It hadn't been, and he proceeded to the room and opened it with his pass key. Lying crosswise on one of the beds was one Eugene Sams passed out, but still holding a bottle of Mogan David wine in one hand. It took several minutes for Mr. Patel to wake up Sams, and, in a verbal combination of broken English and East Indian, to banish Sams from the premises. Mr. Patel never bothered to call the police or question Sams about how he had been able to enter one of the secured motel rooms.

Now, Sams yelled at James to stop or he would cut Maggie's throat. Maggie by now was awake and screamed for her mommy, as Sams placed his hand over her mouth and told her to "shut the fuck up." James pleaded with Sams not to hurt Maggie, and the burglar responded by yelling, "Shut up or I'll kill all of you." Sams then ordered James to sit down on the bed with Patty.

Sams demanded, "If you don't tell me where the money is, I will kill this little bitch." James told him all the money they had was in his wallet on the dresser. Still holding Maggie tightly in his arms, Sams stood up and walked over to the dresser. He fumbled around searching for the wallet, mumbling and cursing because he was having difficulty finding it. James finally told him that it was in the pocket of his pants which were lying atop the dresser.

Sams finally located the pants and removed the wallet from the rear pocket. He then walked over to the entrance to the bathroom and pushed open the door, allowing more light to enter the room. Sams was having trouble removing the money from the wallet and holding Maggie at the same time, so he threw her onto the bathroom floor, causing her head to strike the side of the bathtub with a bang.

This brought both James and Patty to their feet. Sams reacted by waving the knife in their direction and demanding that they sit down or he would kill their daughter. James and Patty obeyed Sams's command at once.

James pleaded, "You have what you came for, please leave." Apparently taking this as an order, Sams angrily shouted back, "Don't tell me what to do, motherfucker. Get up and get over here."

James stood up and walked slowly toward Sams. As James got close, Sams grabbed him by the arm and thrust the knife toward him. Sams worked his way into a position where he was now holding the knife against James's throat from the rear, and he snarled, "Try and be a hero and you will never live to see your wife and daughter again." Sams then shoved James into the bathroom along with Maggie.

James again pleaded with Sams not to harm them and to leave since he had gotten what he had came for. This only seemed to provoke Sams even more. Sams shouted back, "I told you to keep your mouth shut, and besides you don't know what I came for." As he said this, Sams turned toward Patty, who was still sitting on the bed.

James knew without a doubt what was on Sams's mind. He made an attempt to rush Sams, but the streetwise robber merely sidestepped and struck James on the back of his head with the butt of the heavy knife. James fell forward stiffly, bouncing off the wall and landing on the floor. The force of hitting the wall combined with the wound to the back of his head almost caused him to pass out. James struggled to keep conscious, fearing that if he passed out he would never see Patty and Maggie again.

Sams stood, straddled James, and yelled, "Stay put, you cracker son of a bitch, or you'll make me kill all of you."

At the same time, he detected movement from the corner of his eye. He looked in the direction of Patty and saw that she had moved toward the end of the bed and was grabbing at a robe. For the first time, Sams could tell that Patty had been sleeping nude. He yelled at her to lie back down, and she complied, grabbing at the bed covers in an attempt to cover herself up.

Sams then turned his attention back to James, who by now realized that he was bleeding severely from the wound on the back of his head. Sams ordered James to crawl back into the bathroom. As James positioned himself between the toilet and the bathtub, Sams reached down, grabbed Maggie by the front of her nightshirt, and yanked her into his arms. James tried to react, but the strength was completely gone from his body. The only thing he could do was to weep uncontrollably.

Feeling that he now had total control of the situation, Sams told James, "Shut up, you pussy, or I'll kill both of these bitches when I'm through with them." He told James that if he stuck his head out of the bathroom they would all die.

Still holding Maggie in one of his arms, Sams walked over to the bed where Patty was lying, grabbed the bed covers with the hand in which he was holding the knife, and tossed them aside, exposing Patty's nude body. He lay Maggie down at the foot of the bed and told her to lie still if she didn't want her mommy hurt. Sams then turned his unswerving attention to Patty.

Sams reached over and stroked the inside of Patty's thigh and said in a hoarse voice, "My, my, what do we have here—a little extra bonus?" Patty reacted by jerking away from his reach. Her whole body began to shake, and she could not control the crying. Patty pleaded with Sams not to hurt her and to please just take whatever he wanted and leave. Sams replied, "That's just what I intend on doing—take what I want and leave." He then drew nearer and slapped her across the face, causing her lip to burst and start bleeding. Sams sat down on the side of the bed and began taking his shoes and pants off.

For the first time, Patty could smell the strong odor of alcohol and body odor coming from Sams, and this made her sick to her stomach. Patty pleaded over and over again, "Please don't rape me, please don't rape me," but Sams responded by grabbing Maggie and pulling her up beside her mother. Sams then placed the knife against Maggie's throat and pulled it just enough to cause a little scratch from which trickled some blood. "You want this little bitch to die?" Sams screamed at Patty.

Patty begged, "No, no please don't hurt my baby. I will do anything you want—just don't hurt my baby any more."

Still lying on the bathroom floor, James could hear what was going on in the other room. He managed to pick himself up off the floor and stagger to the door. He peered around the door frame and could plainly see Sams stroking the inside of Patty's legs. James yelled for Sams to stop. Sams responded by again grabbing Maggie, but this time by her hair, causing her to scream with pain, and again pointed his knife at her throat. Sams stated, "You crackers are unbelievable, you don't believe I'm in control here." Sams ordered James back into the bathroom and screamed at Patty and him, "This is my last warning. If I hear one more word out of either of you, I will kill this little bitch [Maggie] in front of both of you." James retreated from the doorway and sat down on the toilet seat, feeling totally helpless to defend his family. Not knowing what else he could possibly do, he silently began to pray.

Sams again turned his attention back to Patty. He laid the knife down on the night stand and reached over and grabbed her left breast, squeezing her nipple hard between his dirty fingers until she yelled out in pain. He responded by slapping her across the face, this time breaking her nose and splattering blood about the bed.

This obnoxious deed seemed to exhilarate Sams even more. He mounted Patty, reached down and spread her legs apart, and entered her forcefully. For what seemed like a lifetime, Sams moved up and down, moaning and growling. He licked her with his tongue about the face and repeated, "Baby, baby, I know you like this, I know it's good for you."

Reeling from the blood flowing down her face, the weight of Sams's body atop her and the dreadful smell of his body, Patty did all she could do not to throw up. When he could not ejaculate, he rolled off her, grabbed her by the hair, forced her head down on his penis, and ordered her to fellate him. Patty did as she was told, fearful that if she didn't he would surely kill Maggie. After a few minutes, this didn't seem to please him either. He yanked her back, rolled her over on her stomach, entered her from the rear, and almost instantly ejaculated.

Sams lay atop of her back for a few minutes, and in one last sign of arrogance and defiance, rolled off, lay down next to her, reached into his shirt pocket, removed a cigarette from a pack, lit it, and smoked it.

Finishing his cigarette, Sams sat up in the bed, reached across Patty to where Maggie was lying, and began to stroke the child's arm.

All kinds of horrible thoughts ran through Patty's mind. Sams must have sensed her anxiety, because he looked at her and said, "Don't worry, bitch, I've had enough." He then stopped, got up off the bed and began putting his pants and shoes back on.

When he finished dressing he walked over toward the door, stopping briefly to pick up Patty's panties which had been lying atop the dresser and stuffing them in his pocket as a souvenir. He opened the door slightly, then turned toward Patty, who was still lying on the bed tightly holding Maggie in her arms, and said, "Maybe this will teach you to lock your door at night."

He then left, shutting the door behind him.

Patty just lay there holding Maggie. It was quiet except for the humming of the Coke machine and the falling of ice as it was being made in the ice machine outside of their room. Patty just lay there praying that her ordeal must have been a bad dream. She hoped against hope that any minute she would wake up and James would be there lying next to her sleeping and Maggie would be in the bed next to them peacefully sound asleep as well.

However, the pain in her face and the blood dripping into her mouth brought the reality of what had occurred back to her; it had not been a dream but a true-to-life nightmare.

Patty managed to pull herself up off the bed, still holding Maggie firmly in her arms, and stagger toward the bathroom, where James had been held hostage. It took all the strength she had left in her body to make the short walk. She slowly pushed open the bathroom door. At first her eyes had trouble adjusting to the brightness of the light shining in her eyes. She did not immediately see James, and she thought this was strange. She opened and closed her eyes quickly several times. Then she heard a whimpering sound coming from the direction of the toilet.

In a total state of shock, James had wedged his body between the toilet and bathtub. He was curled up in a fetal position, making it difficult for Patty to see him. Patty called out to him, but he did not move. She called his name a second time and said, "James, Maggie and I are all right. He's gone." James just lay there. Patty kneeled down next to him and laid her hand ever so gently against his face. At first he reacted by jerking away from her touch as if someone was trying to harm him. Patty again laid her hand on his cheek and said, "James, it's all right. He's gone, and he won't hurt us any more."

James finally looked up at her and sobbed, "Patty, I'm so sorry I let you and Maggie down, I love you, I love you." Patty helped James stagger to his feet and took him into her arms. They both cried uncontrollably while Patty tried to reassure James there was nothing more he could have done.

After a few minutes, they stood up and cautiously walked back out into the room where Patty's assault had taken place. Then Patty realized that she had not checked to make sure the room door was locked after their assailant had left. Fear and panic once again swept over her. She ran to the door, leaned her weight against it, and turned the sliding latch lock.

That's when she realized how Sams could have entered even when the door was locked.

James in the meantime ran over to the nightstand and grabbed at the phone. He dialed "0" for the hotel operator, and the phone rang and rang for what must have been twenty or thirty rings. A sleepy-sounding desk clerk finally answered. James screamed into the phone, "My wife has just been raped and we have been robbed—call the police!"

While waiting for them, James began to think a little more clearly. He wondered why the clerk on duty at the front desk had not seen someone trying to enter their room, especially since there was a perfect view of their room door from where the clerk was supposed to have been working. But that was a question the police could answer, and besides, the camera system would have recorded the break-in and the tape would help police to catch this animal.

In a mere matter of minutes, several patrol units from the Jackson Police Department arrived. Patty gave a quick description of the assailant to one of the police officers who immediately put out a bulletin over his hand-held radio. Then the motel desk clerk walked over and identified himself to police officers as the one who had called 911. Upon hearing Patty's description of the assailant he immediately told one of the police officers that a few minutes before James called the front desk he had seen a man fitting that description. The suspect had walked through the parking lot and retrieved a bicycle which had been leaning up against the Coke machine. The clerk added that the suspect then rode off down Main Street, heading north toward one of the low-rent housing projects in the area.

Upon hearing this, two of the officers ran from the room, jumped into their patrol cars, and sped off in the direction given by the desk clerk. It didn't take long for them to locate the "master criminal." They found him less than a mile away from the motel, lying beneath an underpass sound asleep. His bike lay close by. It took the police a few minutes to shake Sams awake, because between the time that he left the motel and when the police located him he had stopped at an all-night liquor store. He had purchased a cheap bottle of wine with the money he had stolen from the Ruggses and had consumed it. This, along with what he had already drunk earlier in the evening, had made him sleepy, so he decided to stop and sleep for awhile. Thus another one of his great escapes came to an end. Patty's underwear was still hanging from his pocket.

The Ruggses were transported to a local hospital for treatment. At the hospital, the doctors performed the standard rape test on Patty in hopes of collecting useful evidence for the police to use in their investigation. The doctors informed Patty that they had found a significant amount of semen and that they were concerned that she might become pregnant as a result of the rape. Almost hysterical, Patty asked what could be done to prevent this and was told of a medication she could take which might prevent pregnancy. However, there was no foolproof guarantee. Nevertheless, Patty decided to take the medication and pray that it worked. If it didn't, she told the doctors grimly, she would have an abortion.

What really scared her, however, was the possibility of contracting AIDS. She was told there was a chance, but that it might take months or years for the AIDS virus to show up if she had been exposed to it. One of the doctors treating her suggested that if the police arrested her assailant, she demand through the courts that he be tested for the AIDS virus. They set her nose and stitched her lip, and she was ready to be released.

James received sixteen stitches to the back of his head, and Maggie was given a quick examination to make sure she had not been injured.

While James had been waiting to be treated, one of the police officers who had accompanied them asked him why in the world would he have ever stayed at the Heart of Jackson Motel. James explained how he had been sent to Jackson by his company to work and that it had chosen the motel for his crew to stay in. James asked the officer why he had asked such a question, and the officer replied that the Heart of Jackson Motel was notorious for drug deals and prostitution and more. It had been the site of everything from burglaries of guest rooms to murders, rapes, assaults, and armed robberies. James related to the police officer what Mr. Patel had told him about the motel's safety when they checked in, and the officer sort of laughed and said, "Old man Patel would tell people anything to get them to stay there." Already angry about the assaults, James was further infuriated by this statement.

As they were getting ready to leave the hospital with the police officer, he received a call over his walkie-talkie which requested that he call the station at once. The officer excused himself and went to one of the nurses' stations in the emergency room and called in. The officer was informed a suspect had been arrested. He was asked to transport the Ruggses to police headquarters for a line-up. The officer found the Ruggses sitting in the hospital waiting room. For both Patty and James, the news of the capture evoked a mixture of emotions. The awful memories of what they had experienced only hours before were still fresh, and, to make matters worse, now they had to face their attacker again.

Upon arriving at the police station, they were taken upstairs to the detectives' office and introduced to two detectives who had been assigned their case. The detectives explained what the lineup would involve and assured them that the men in the lineup would not be able to see them through the one-way mirror.

Patty and James were led into a small viewing room. The lights were off, but they surmised that was intentional so that it took away any possibilities that the suspects on the other side might see in.

Patty and James stood holding hands as they peered through the glass, waiting on the suspects to be brought into the room. As the doorway to the room opened, Patty squeezed James's hand ever so tightly. Even before the suspects were ordered to turn to face them, Patty spotted her assailant. Once the police had the suspects go through the routine of facing them, then turning to each side, both Patty and James exclaimed that suspect 3 was without a doubt the man.

Suspect 3 was none other than Eugene Sams.

The next several hours were spent being interviewed and going over and over the same story. Then Patty and James were separated and required to give written statements. It was around 10:00 a.m. when they were finally finished. They were both exhausted. It had been over seven hours since this nightmare had begun.

James asked if someone would please take them back to the hotel to freshen up. One of the detectives volunteered, adding that he would wait for them if they wished to pack and check out. The detective suggested another local motel, which he assured them did not share the same reputation as Mr. Patel's Heart of Jackson.

As they sat next to each other in the back seat of the detective's car, James held Patty's hand and began to cry. He told her over and over again how sorry he was that he had been unable to protect her and Maggie. He felt "terrible" because he had let them down. James could hear her response— that everything would be all right—but the tone of her voice and the new way she seemed to look at him told him something very different.

The motel was only a mile or so away from the police department, and the traffic was very light at that time of the morning. The detective pulled up in front of their room, got out of the car, and opened the rear door for the Ruggses. James was carrying Maggie, who had long ago fallen asleep on a small sofa in the detective's office, and Patty was walking at his rear. They approached the room slowly, and James reached into his pocket to remove his room key. However, before he could, the police detective reached out and grabbed the door knob, turned it, and it popped open. James looked at the officer in dismay. How could the officer had opened the door without a key?

Before James could ask him the question, the police detective stated, "That's one of the problems with the motel and the reason so many of the rooms are broken into. It's equipped with standard residential type locks which don't lock automatically when you close the door."

As they entered the room, the detective pointed out another major problem with the door locks—the slide bolt. He showed James how the lock turned in both directions, making it very easy for a person to believe that he had locked the door, when in fact he had only turned a sign on the outside of the door indicating that he wanted room service. That would be a dead giveaway to someone like Sams that the room was occupied and unlocked. The detective also pointed out to them that there were no written notices on the rear of the door warning about how the locks operated. In addition, he said that Mr. Patel had been warned about the dangers of the locks many times by various police officers, but that he had elected not to do anything about it.

The police detective volunteered to drive over to a nearby fast-food restaurant and pick up some breakfast for them. Would they be all right in his absence? They assured him that they would lock the door while he was gone. Little did they know that they were about to be assaulted for the second time within twenty-four hours.

The motel room was a wreck. Their clothes and personal belongings were scattered throughout the room. Residue from where the police had dusted for fingerprints was everywhere, and backings from the instant film the police had used to take photographs were lying about the floor.

Patty had just begun to pick up their clothes when a series of loud knocks commenced at the door. Patty thought that could not be the police detective back so soon—he had just left—and she was right.

Standing outside the door pacing back and forth was Mr. Patel, the owner of the Heart of Jackson Motel, who had been so nice to them when they had checked into the motel. Patel was getting angrier by the moment as he awaited an answer to his repeated knocks. He reached out again, banging on the door, yelling this time, "I know you are in there. I just saw the police drop you off. Open the damn door—now!"

James walked over to the door and unlatched the sliding bolt lock; before he could reach for the knob handle lock he heard a key being inserted into the door handle. The door was pushed open, striking him in the chest. There, standing at the doorway with key in hand was Mr. Patel himself.

Mr. Patel immediately burst into the room and began shouting at them and waving his hands and arms in the air like a mad man. He was completely out of control, screaming at the top of his lungs in broken English, "What have you caused to happen at my motel? Look at this room, who's going to pay for this mess?"

Patty and James could not believe what was happening. Here they had been assaulted, raped, and robbed, and this idiot was in their midst, raving about who was going to pay for the mess in the room. James tried to explain to Mr. Patel what had happened, but Patel rudely cut him off, demanding that he shut up.

Patel was pacing back and forth, still waving his arms and hands around as he talked. He told them, "You have caused the police to come to my motel. I run a good place here, for to make money for my family. You try and destroy my good name and ruin my motel."

Patel added, his voice carrying throughout the motel, "You must pay me for damage to my motel room and leave at once."

Then Patel started into his next rage. "I guess you think you are going to sue me, but I tell you what, if you even think about it I will get the man out of jail and give him your name and address."

James had heard enough. He grabbed Patel by the arm and forced him out of the door.

The stunned Patel shouted, "You attack me. I will have you arrested. This is my hotel, you leave right now."

James slammed the room door shut and relocked it with Patel still standing in the middle of the parking lot screaming.

A few minutes later, there was another knock at the door. James yanked it open viciously, expecting to find Mr. Patel, but it was the police detective with the food. James explained about Patel's conduct, and the officer replied that it did not surprise him. It sounded like the Patel he knew. The Ruggses shouldn't worry about the threats.

The victims sat down and took a few minutes to try and eat, but neither of them could force the food down. They finished packing and left the Heart of Jackson Motel with the police detective. He drove them across town, pointing out that while the particular street on which the Heart of Jackson Motel was located appeared to be a nice, the surrounding neighborhood was made up of housing projects, liquor stores, and porno shops.

The detective helped them settle into their new motel room and pointed out the difference in the locks on this room door compared to the ones at the Heart of Jackson Motel. He told them he would be back later that afternoon to pick them up in order to finish up some paperwork at the police department.

They both showered, and Patty lay down on the bed after taking some of the pain medicine given to her by the doctor. She wanted to sleep, but couldn't. Few words were spoken between Patty and James for the remainder of the afternoon. Their interaction was rather cold. Neither knew then that this was only the beginning of the problems between them which lay ahead as a result of Eugene Sams's intrusion into their lives.

When they arrived back at the police department later in the afternoon, they were surprised to find the night desk clerk there giving a statement. James got a cup of coffee and asked one of the detectives if he could speak with the desk clerk for a few minutes. The detective agreed and excused himself.

In the ensuing conversation, James learned many new things about how Patel ran his motel and its previous crime problems. The clerk told James that people complained all of the time about the locks on the doors. Worse, numerous people had reported waking up to find an intruder in their room.

The clerk also stated that most people thought, like James and Patty, that there were security cameras throughout the property. He said Mr. Patel certainly wanted people to think that, but there were no other cameras on the premises. Patel had installed the one in the lobby only after the front desk had been robbed. The clerk said Patel had exclaimed after he had installed the camera, "This won't happen again, stealing my money. I catch them with my camera."

The clerk also told James how Mr. Patel would threaten guests when they reported a crime to him and that all of the employees had been instructed to lie if they were asked if the motel were safe.

The clerk said he was sorry that Patty had been raped. He admitted that he only continued to work there because jobs were hard to come by—a statement James could relate to.

James was furious after talking with the clerk. Not only had Patel lied to them when they checked in, but he had threatened them like common criminals after the attack.

After learning what happened to James and his family, the telephone company immediately made arrangements for him to be transferred back home. He was given a job which required no travel, an action for which he was thankful. In the meantime, the phone company canceled the lodging agreement with Mr. Patel and moved the remaining crew members to another motel.

The next several months were pure hell for James and Patty. Their physical wounds healed quickly, but the emotional ones worsened. With his newly acquired quick mood changes and fits of anger, James made it almost impossible for Patty and Maggie to live with him. Patty wasn't much better—she was short with Maggie and James and would go days without speaking to James.

During the day when James was away, Patty would keep all the doors and windows locked, and a newly purchased gun lay nearby at all times. Once a delivery man knocked repeatedly on the door—only to see the door thrown open and to face Patty standing there with a gun pointed at his head. At night she didn't sleep well; the least bit of noise would wake her up. When this happened, she would sit up and reach for her gun. She would scream for James to wake up and would make him search the house before lying back down.

Patty would never go out of the house by herself, and James now found himself doing all of the grocery shopping on his way home from work. They never showed any affection toward each other, and lovemaking was out of the question. Patty blamed James for this, claiming he was afraid of catching AIDS (even though the tests conducted on Sams and herself had come back negative).

Patty and James realized that they could not go on living like this and finally sought the advice of a divorce attorney. He immediately concluded that they still loved each other and recommended additional professional counseling for them before they made such a devastating decision. After hearing the unbelievable story of their attack, he also recommended that they seek the advice of a personal injury attorney.

They hired one to represent them in a civil action against Mr. Patel. I was hired as the security expert in the case. With the help of my testimony, the Ruggses settled their case for several million dollars and were able to afford the long-term counseling they both needed to put their lives back in order.

Maggie is now 12 years old, and has a new one-year-old baby brother to play with and help care for. Patty's and James's love for one another has never been stronger, but occasionally the horror of their stay at the Heart of Jackson Motel still looms in the night.

Eugene Sams sits staring at the four walls of his prison cell, hopefully never to ruin other people's lives again.

What You Should Learn from This Crime

If your company is making arrangements for you at a hotel or motel, ask the person making the arrangements if he or she knows about the security at the premises. A call to the local police department may give you the information you need in making a reasonable decision about staying there. After checking into a hotel or motel, always familiarize yourself with the proper operations of the locking devices on your room door. If the room is not equipped with a self-locking lock and deadbolt, you should consider staying elsewhere.

■ ■ ■

It's Safe at the Sunrise Inn

OVER THE PAST FEW YEARS, LITERALLY MILLIONS OF WOMEN have begun traveling for work. This brings them into the previously predominantly male traveler's world of airports, rental cars, and hotels/motels. Increasingly, some of them are also coming into harm's way, as a growing number of traveling women are discovering something many of their male counterparts have known for some time: Traveling can be a dangerous activity, particularly in unsecured motels and hotels.

Indeed, traveling women are particularly vulnerable to attacks and assaults. Instead of going out of their way to assure these women are protected, however, many hotels/motels do all they can to attract them—without providing for their security. The result can be a safety disaster, as it was for Deborah Johnson, a 40-year-old woman from Palm Beach, Florida.

In early August 1991, Deborah was in a very upbeat mood. She had an enviable marriage to her husband, Fred, a salesman. They had experienced some money problems in the recession, and he had lost some of his most reliable clients. However, they still owned a spacious, split-level home in West Palm Beach, each had new cars, and the future looked bright—so bright that for the first time the Johnsons were committed to having children before their biological clocks ticked too far. They began trying to get pregnant late in 1990, and when it eventually appeared they could not succeed, they made an appointment with a fertility specialist at a local hospital. It would take place when Deborah returned from her pending business trip.

Meanwhile, Deborah's career was taking off. A graduate in public relations from the University of Miami, she had worked in a public relations agency in Boca Raton in her twenties, first as an administrative assistant, then as a junior account executive. Then she married Fred, and his income was so large at the time that she quit the agency and devoted herself to being a full-time housekeeper. In 1985, though, she did some copywriting for her old agency, and she found that she had missed it. Eventually, she began to handle small accounts in Palm Beach and Boca Raton, and her business flourished.

She incorporated herself, hired several account executives, and began seeking even more ambitious and lucrative accounts. In early July 1991, she was thrilled to hear that the Tourism Department of the State of Florida was considering her bid for a state contract. She made an appointment with a state official in Gainesville for an official presentation on July 16, 1991. She planned to travel to Gainesville on the 15th, spend the night, and meet with the state official first thing in the morning.

Deborah's mood was jaunty as she kissed her husband good-bye on the morning of the 15th. She promised to call him that night as soon as she reached a hotel in Gainesville. They parted with her winking at him and saying that she didn't care who was to blame for their inability to conceive; they would get it all straightened out when they visited the fertility specialist.

Her six-hour drive to Gainesville went smoothly, but she was tired and looking forward to a quiet night in her hotel room to prepare for her meeting the next day. Humming to herself, she pulled into the parking lot of the Sunrise Inn located right off the interstate highway. Her good spirits would have dissipated had she known that, in her rush to leave Palm Beach and drive to Gainesville, she had made a terrible mistake: this high-powered executive who would never leave any business details hanging had failed to check with a travel agent to find a safe hotel/motel in a good neighborhood of Gainesville.

She had thought about her safety. She had read in the Palm Beach newspaper about the recent brutal murders of college students in Gainesville-area apartments. She had become concerned enough to refuse a friend's offer to stay in her apartment while there. But she quite foolhardily had neglected to make a motel reservation.

Instead, here she was arriving after dark in a city that she didn't know. The situation was brimming with the ominous potential of her choosing a hotel/motel that could not guarantee her safety. However, she had seen numerous billboards advertising the Sunrise Inn. She felt better, knowing it was part of a national chain, which she believed would guarantee security.

As she entered the off-ramp from the interstate, she noticed that the interchange was very heavily populated with a variety of businesses and several motels. The overall area appeared to be well maintained, and to Deborah it seemed to be in a middle- to upper-class area of town. But looks can be deceiving. The area in which the Sunrise Inn was located had been the scene of hundreds of crimes, many violent, over the preceding two years. The local police department considered the neighborhood one of the most dangerous in Gainesville. Anyone who knew Gainesville would have advised her not to stay there—particularly because of the newspaper reports of the robbery of one tourist family and the rape of a woman tourist in the presence of her husband there only a few weeks before. But, like many women who had recently begun to travel alone, Deborah's mind was on her business and career—not her safety.

She drove the short distance from the off-ramp, pulled up under the covered canopy of the Sunrise Inn, and parked in the area designated for "registering guest only." She got out of the car and, in keeping with habit, locked her car doors before walking into the lobby. As she entered, Deborah thought to herself how nicely decorated and spacious it was. The check-in counter was to her left, and a large lounge area with a wide-screen television was located to her right. She looked around the lobby and noticed a man who looked like a college student sitting in the lounge area watching the news on CNN.

To the rear of the lobby were several racks of literature advertising local attractions. Standing there was a man whom Deborah took for a tourist because of the way he was dressed. He had on a brightly colored shirt with tropical flowers covering it, baggy over-the-knee shorts, and tennis shoes with black dress socks. Around his neck was a 35mm camera, and sitting atop his head was a straw hat which was at least two sizes too small. Yes, he was a tourist—or so she thought.

The young man behind the front desk was busy studying a textbook when she walked up and stood there for a minute or so until she got his attention. When the desk clerk finally noticed her, he jumped to his feet and apologized for his inattention. He started to explain that he had mid-term exams the next morning, but Deborah cut him short and said that she, too, had once been a college student. She understood what it was like to have to work and go to school at the same time.

Deborah told him that she did not have a reservation, but wondered if he might have a room available. He told her that would be no problem and asked if she needed a room for one or more persons. Deborah explained that she was alone, traveling on business, and inquired about a business rate. The young man quoted her a nightly rate of $49.50, which was acceptable to her. She then asked about the area in which the motel was located. The clerk quickly replied that there was a major shopping center located at the rear of the motel and there were many nice restaurants within walking distance. Deborah thanked him for that information, but explained to him that she was more concerned for her safety after reading about the murders of the college students in the newspaper.

She believed the desk clerk when he informed her that because of the student murders there was a climate of fear in Gainesville; however, the motel was extremely safe. He said he couldn't remember the last time there had been problems at the Sunrise Inn. She was further reassured when the desk clerk told her that there was one particularly safe room—room 211—that he usually gave to women traveling alone. She could stay there, and if there were any problems at all she could call the front desk. Almost as an afterthought, she asked the clerk the distance to the nearest Hyatt or other well-known hotel. He told her such hotels were six or seven miles away, and it would be completely dark by the time she arrived there. Besides, it was safe at the Sunrise.

So Deborah made her decision to stay at the Sunrise Inn. She had even seen some goofy weatherman on national television advertising how great a place the inns were to stay. She filled out the guest registration card and gave her credit card to the clerk for payment. The young man then handed her the key, announcing she would be in room 211. As he was handing her the key, he leaned over the desk and pointed to the rear of the motel, indicating the best place to park. Deborah had no way of knowing that the weirdly dressed tourist pretending to be looking at the information rack was also paying particular attention to the directions given her by the helpful young desk clerk.

Deborah didn't think twice about her decision to stay at the Sunrise. She bade the desk clerk good-night, and she exited the lobby. The "tourist" also left but through a side door which led to room 211.

Deborah drove around to the side of the motel building. It was dark now and she was have difficulty locating her room. She knew it was on the second floor because of the number, but the parking lot lights were not on. She drove completely around the motel building before realizing she had passed by her room. She finally located it on the second floor right behind the office. She was able to find a parking space about two spaces from the stairway which led up to the second floor walkway.

Deborah parked her car and began unloading her baggage. Like most women, she had overpacked. She needed to make more than one trip to the room. As she carried one bag up the stairs, she spotted the weirdly dressed man she had seen a few minutes before in the lobby. He was standing at the top of the stairs, leaning over the handrail and looking out into the parking lot as if he were just passing the time. They ignored each other, and she went to her room, which, she was pleased to see, was the nearest to the stairwell.

She set the first load of baggage down and retrieved her room key from her purse where she had placed it. She inserted the key, opened the door, reached inside, and found the light switch. Deborah was pleased with the size and condition of the room. She reached down and grabbed one of her bags and used it as a door prop as she carried the rest of that load inside. Then she returned to her car, retrieved the rest of her baggage, and climbed up the stairs again. Again, she passed by the strangely dressed tourist. She looked at him quizzically, and he seemed to turn and move away. She walked on toward her room.

The man, who Deborah had wrongly assumed was a tourist and fellow guest, was actually one Jeffrey Lee Webster—and he wasn't a tourist or a guest. Jeffrey Lee, 26, had been born and raised in a small town about fifty miles north of Gainesville. He came from a divorced family and was raised by his mother, who in her drunken rages would abuse him for hours on end. Jeffrey Lee dropped out of school in the seventh grade and had quickly turned to a life of crime when he found out it was easier than working for a living. He had tried to have meaningful relationships with women, but they would quickly end when the women found out the only way he could realize any sexual satisfaction was through abusing them. Besides, Jeffrey Lee wasn't sure what his sexual preferences were. He had engaged in homosexual sex in prison during most of the last ten years when he served time for a variety of charges ranging from rape and assault to armed robbery.

In Jeffrey Lee's mind, he was surely a bad man, and he could not understand why society didn't keep people like him locked up. He had been released from prison about four months previous to seeing Deborah, and he had been a very busy man. He had been traveling up and down the interstate highway from Florida to Virginia and had terrified, robbed, and raped numerous motel guests. In many of these crimes, Jeffrey Lee bound his victims with duct tape and handcuffed them with plastic ties; he would terrify them for hours on end by waving a gun about and blaming them for the way he was.

As Jeffrey Lee Webster stood watching Deborah unload her car, he thought to himself what easy pickings most motels made. Not only were there plenty of unsuspecting victims from whom to choose, but most hotels had little or no security. Some, like the Sunrise Inn, will even give out guests' room numbers to strangers. Jeffrey Lee's Gainesville trip had been especially successful in the past two weeks; he had robbed and raped two women, one at the same Sunrise Inn and the other at the motel across the street. As a bonus he had netted over $700 in cash, a handgun, and the camera which he now had around his neck.

Yes, life was good, and he had targeted his next victim.

Deborah reached her room and for the second time inserted her room key into the lock, opening the door. Suddenly, she sensed the presence of someone behind her. Jeffrey Lee Webster was making his move. He placed a gun at her temple and pushed her into the room.

"Don't scream or I'll shoot you," Jeffrey Lee ordered, as he secured the door and reached to pull the drapes shut.

"Oh my God," said Deborah. "I can't believe this is happening."

"Shut the fuck up," Jeffrey Lee said, as he pushed her toward the bed and ordered her to sit down.

"How much money do you have?" he asked her matter-of-factly, tightening his grip on the gun at her temple. For the first time she noticed that he was carrying a small black bag.

"About $50," lied Deborah, starting to cry. Actually she had about $150. "You've chosen the wrong person. I'm here on business. I have mostly credit cards," she pleaded softly.

"Shut up," he screamed. "I don't want to hear your shit. Stand up and take your clothes off." Deborah began pleading with him not to rape her. He could have all her money and credit cards and the keys to her car, as long as he didn't rape her. Deborah had no way of knowing that her fears only fueled Jeffrey Lee's sexual ardor.

Sensing what was coming, Deborah summoned up her courage and looked him in the eye and said, "I feel sorry for you that you're doing this to me."

This made Jeffrey Lee laugh out loud. "Lady, don't feel sorry for me, feel sorry for yourself because of what I'm going to do to you."

When she heard this, Deborah began sobbing loudly. This only excited Jeffrey Lee more. He reached over and ripped her blouse off and pushed her back down on the bed. He again ordered her to take her clothes off. Deborah slowly began to remove her clothes, first her shoes, then her pantyhose. Sensing that she was stalling, Jeffrey Lee decided that he had to take more control of this situation. He leaned over her and struck her across the cheek with the barrel of his pistol. This caused a cut about four inches long on the side of her face, and the blood began to seep out.

"Now bitch, do as you are told or I'll kill you—then fuck you," Jeffrey barked as he moved even closer and licked the blood dripping down her cheek. "Now finish taking your clothes off."

As she removed her skirt, he ordered her to stop. He reached into the black bag, placed the gun inside and removed a large hunting knife. Jeffrey Lee then climbed on the bed and straddled Deborah. He took the knife and very carefully cut off her bra, exposing her breasts, and buried his head between them. He kissed and licked all about her breasts. He then started biting them. Unable to stand the pain, Deborah let out a scream.

"You stupid bitch, what are you trying to do, scream for help? There is no helping you now," he said as he slapped her several times across the face and then leaned forward and took a bite out of one of her breasts and spit the blood into her face. Jeffrey then got off the bed and opened up his black bag once again. This time he removed a roll of duct tape and a set of plastic handcuffs, like the police sometimes use. Jeffrey Lee knew this type of cuffs was very effective because they had been used on him many times.

"What are you doing?" Deborah cried out.

"What do you think I'm doing? I'm going to shut you up." He tore a large piece of duct tape from the roll and placed it firmly over her mouth. At first Deborah had trouble breathing, and she thought she would suffocate. But she soon realized that she could breath through her nose, and she was determined that she was going to do whatever it took to live through this ordeal.

He began removing her jewelry, first her wedding band, then her anniversary ring, a tiny rope bracelet, and finally her prized possession, a Rolex watch.

He rolled her over on her stomach, pulled her arms across her back and placed the plastic cuffs tightly around her wrists. He then slapped her across the rear and told her to stay put until he returned.

Then he systematically began going through all her luggage, looking for her wallet. He couldn't find it and became even angrier. He walked back over to the bed, started poking her with the gun and demanded, "Where is the goddamn wallet?"

Deborah kept trying to reply but her mouth was taped. Finally, he realized this and jerked her over so that she was face up on the bed. He ripped off the tape, poked her with the gun, and screamed, "If you know what's good for you, you'll tell me where your wallet is."

"It's in the car," she sobbed.

"Goddamn it, I don't have time to go search your car," he bellowed.

Then, his mouth tight, he flipped her over again. He took his knife and cut away her panties. He sat on the bed, reached down, and picked up his black bag off the floor and placed it on the bed next to him. He opened the bag and removed a pair of surgical gloves and put them on. He then removed a jar of Vaseline. He dipped his fingers into the Vaseline and smeared it in and out of her rectum. He took his time as if he were preparing to perform major surgery. After finishing his preparation, he began to slowly move his fingers in and out of her rectum. The force and pain of this caused Deborah's body to shudder, and this served to excite Jeffrey Lee even more. The more her body reacted, the more pleasure he received. Sweat began to drip off his forehead and fall onto her back. At first Jeffrey Lee moaned ever so slightly, but the more he moved his fingers in and out and the more her body shuddered, the louder his moans became. To Deborah, the assault seemed to last a lifetime. The pain was unendurable. Jeffrey Lee finally worked himself into such a frenzy that he climaxed in his pants.

He then rolled her over on her back and began committing sodomy on her. Deborah tried to scream, but to no avail—the duct tape muffled any sounds she was able to make. Why, God, is this happening to me, she thought. While he was between her legs she tried to raise her head to get a better look at him. If she lived through this nightmare she damn well was going to be able to identify this bastard later.

He caught her looking at him and he stopped for a moment, stuck the knife against her throat and said, "If you look at me again, I'm going to cut your throat out."

He went back to what he had been doing for a few minutes more. When he had satisfied himself he stood up and walked into the bathroom to clean himself.

Hopefully, her prayers had been answered. He was through and would be leaving soon. He walked out of the bathroom and sat down on the side of the bed next to her. Only the worst thoughts were running through Deborah's mind—now he was going to kill her. Instead, he sat there and began to weep and asked, "Why do you all make me do these terrible things?" This frightened her even more. This creep is crazy as hell, she thought. Then he reached out and rubbed her on the stomach and said, "You are a nice woman, I'm sorry."

He stood up and packed his black bag. He then reached down and pulled the phone cord from the wall. Jeffrey Lee walked over to the door and opened it slightly. He looked down the hallway, first to the left and then the right toward the stairs. Seeing that no one was out there, he exited the door and shut it behind him.

Deborah lay there and breathed a sigh of relief. She knew that the motel room door had locked behind him and that the key was lying on the nightstand. She felt somewhat safe at last.

She began to wiggle her mouth against the duct tape and was finally able to catch the corner of it against the bed. By moving from side to side she was able to work it off. She then rolled off the bed and kicked the nightstand away from the wall where she could get to the telephone jack. She scooted about the floor until she found the telephone and grabbed it with her hands, which were still tied behind her back. It seemed like it took forever, but she was finally able to work the plug back into the wall jack. She rolled over and with her feet was able to replace the receiver back in its cradle, so that she could then remove it and get a dial tone. With her feet she managed to dial "O" for the office and leaned over and placed her ear and mouth near the handset. To this day she can't tell if it was a man or woman who answered on the other end. All she remembers is screaming into the phone, "For God's sake, please call the police, I've been raped."

Before passing out from physical and emotional exhaustion Deborah managed to look at the clock on the front of the television set and saw that it read 9:15. Her attack had lasted over two hours.

The next thing she remembered was waking up and seeing a room full of men in uniforms. One man, apparently a paramedic, was kneeling over her, covering her with a blanket and reassuring her she was going to be all right. She recalls being whisked away in an ambulance and the bright lights of the examining room at the hospital. She recalls one of the nurses or doctors telling her that her husband had been notified and was on his way. She would not totally regain her senses until several days later.

As she was recovering in the hospital, the hunt went on for her assailant. The police immediately suspected it was the same man who had committed the similar crimes along the interstate.

Back in Palm Beach, Deborah's life was hell while her attacker was still at large. She became so scared of being alone that some days she cried until Fred agreed to stay home from work with her. She herself was unable to work, and soon she was forced to lay off all her employees and close the business. At night she didn't sleep and when she did manage to doze off, she would wake up screaming, "No, no, get away from me." Deborah's and Fred's once active life together was at the brink of total disaster.

Finally, Jeffrey Lee Webster was captured. The TV show "America's Most Wanted" aired a reenactment of one of Jeffrey Lee's crimes, and it led to an anonymous tip which resulted in his arrest in Charleston, South Carolina. Next, numerous law enforcement agencies began working together to piece together the trail of terror that Jeffrey Lee Webster had canvassed throughout the Southeast. Several of Webster's victims picked him out of line-ups, and he was charged with armed robbery, rape, burglary, and car theft in five different states. Since he had been arrested in South Carolina, that state put him on trial first. In February 1992, after a two-week trial, Jeffrey Lee Webster was convicted of five counts of armed robbery, three rapes, five burglaries, and auto theft. In sentencing him, the trial judge said that he only wished he could impose the death sentence on his tormented soul, but that the law would not allow him. However, the judge stated, "I can see to it that you will never spend another day without looking through bars." Jeffrey Lee was sentenced to five life terms without parole.

Deborah's condition improved slightly after Webster's arrest and conviction. While she still had trouble sleeping, often awakening to scream, she became less dependent on Fred's presence during the day. Knowing she probably needed professional help, she and Fred consulted their family doctor who recommended a psychiatrist whom she started to see. Meanwhile, another friend recommended another psychiatrist who specialized in helping victims of crime suffering from trauma. For a while, Deborah saw both of them at almost the same time. Eventually she realized that the simultaneous treatments might be confusing her more than helping her. And the cost was tremendous. She settled on the specialist in trauma, who diagnosed her as suffering from Post Traumatic Stress Syndrome, a malady often associated with shell-shocked combat veterans of the Vietnam War.

Meanwhile, her relations with family and friends continued to deteriorate. Deborah felt that they didn't fully appreciate what she'd been through, and she began pulling back from them. Worse, problems arose in her relationship with Fred. She found that, try as she might, she couldn't give herself to him sexually. It was as if the attack had driven a wedge between them.

The bills for her counseling kept adding up, and with her not working, the financial stress on Fred was becoming unbearable, causing ever more problems with their day-to-day relationship. At dinner one night with friends someone mentioned that they had read an article about a woman having been raped in an apartment complex and how she had suffered not only the physical attack, but severe mental problems afterwards. The woman had filed a lawsuit against the apartment complex, alleging it had not provided adequate security, and won the suit. The next day the Johnsons visited a local attorney and related their story. The attorney advised to proceed with a lawsuit against the Sunrise Inn's owners.

I was hired by Deborah's family as part of their suit against the motel. My investigation revealed that on June 23, 1991, a gunman had accosted a couple checking into room 157 of the Sunrise Inn, robbed them of $300, and sexually assaulted the woman while her husband was forced to watch. The gunman was later identified as Jeffrey Lee Webster, who terrorized Deborah some two weeks later. And two years earlier other guests were robbed, indicating that the desk clerk's claims of safety were lies. My investigation also revealed a terrible pattern of crime in the area around the hotel. Despite the overwhelming number of attacks in the area, the Sunrise Inn owners in an attempt to save money had elected not to hire any security for the premises. This was doubly unfortunate because the man who fit the description of the suspect in nineteen similar crimes along the interstate was spotted at the motel several times prior to Deborah's assault. The motel throughout the lawsuit continued to deny any liability and vowed to fight the suit.

During the discovery stages of the lawsuit, several of the motel's employees and owner were deposed, a process by which Deborah's attorney had the opportunity to question them about the security of the premises prior to her checking in. The desk clerk, who signed Deborah Johnson into the motel, gave some particularly damning testimony during his deposition. He stated:

- When he was hired, no one had ever given him any security and safety training.

- On most occasions he worked alone and the manager had demanded that during those times he walk the premises and pick up trash and report any lights out.

- It was not uncommon for lights to be burned out for weeks at a time without being fixed. He would report these findings to the manager and owner, whose only reaction would be pride at saving money on the electrical bill.

- The night that Deborah Johnson checked in, all the lights on the side of the motel where her room was located were burned out and had been for the prior two weeks.

- He recalled Deborah's checking in and her asking if it was a safe area; he had told her that she didn't have anything to worry about, knowing that it was a lie.

- That he had been instructed by the owner and manager of the motel never to tell guests that any crimes had occurred there or they would fire him.

- He had been on duty the night the other couple had been robbed and the woman sexually assaulted and that he knew now that the weirdly dressed man who had been hanging around in the lobby thirty minutes before Deborah Johnson arrived had fit the description given to him by the police after the first incident. However, he had been too busy studying to pay too much attention to the man.

The manager of the Sunrise Inn, when questioned, gave the following responses:

- If we told potential patrons about our crime problem, they would never stay with us.

- It's not our job to keep people safe, it's the police department's job. That's what we pay taxes for.

After completing my review of the facts in this case, it wasn't hard to render opinions concerning the negligence of the Sunrise Inn.

Indeed, in March 1993, after a week-long civil trial, a jury agreed by deciding Deborah and Fred needed compensation for the motel's negligence. It awarded her $3 million.

While the money is nice, today Fred and Deborah would give it back for the peace of mind that has escaped them since her brutal attack. She still has trouble sleeping at night—on occasion waking with a scream—and a family for now is out of the question.

Hopefully Deborah's case will stand as a warning to traveling businesswomen that hotels and motels may be more interested in their business than their safety.

What You Should Learn from This Crime

If you are a female traveling alone, always make reservations before departing. Try to arrive at your destination before dark, and if you have any concerns for your security, ask that you be escorted to your room. Remember, just because the establishment is part of a national hotel or motel chain does not always guarantee your security. When registering, if anything causes you concern, you will be better served to leave and find a better situation, no matter how tired you are.

CHAPTER TEN

▪▪▪

Terror at Inner Harbor Baltimore

TYPICALLY FOR A LATE FRIDAY AFTERNOON, THE BALTIMORE-Washington Parkway was bumper to bumper. It didn't help matters any that it was the first week of December, and the season's first snow was falling. The snow was light—not enough to cause any real road hazards—but enough to slow traffic down even more than usual.

The rhythmic movement of the wipers pushing the gingerly falling snow off the windshield, combined with the slow-moving traffic, was enough to make Vickie Caldwell drowsy. She reached over and opened the driver's door window slightly to let in some fresh air and turned up the volume on the radio. Vickie looked at her watch—it was 6:30 p.m. The teacher's conference in Baltimore started with a cocktail party and reception at 8:00.

Vickie Caldwell grew up in a family of teachers in Richmond, Virginia. Her mother had been one, and so had her mother's mother. From the time Vickie was a little girl, all she talked about was that when she grew up she wanted to be a teacher just like Mommy and Granny. Vickie had excelled in grammar and high school and won a scholarship to a teaching college. She graduated with honors and had no trouble finding a job in the Richmond school system after graduation. Vickie's second year of teaching was marked with yet another achievement when she was chosen Teacher of the Year. She took great pride in marching across the stage to accept the award with her mother and grandmother in the audience. It was the proudest moment in her life.

This was the third year in a row that she had attended the National Teacher's Conference. Each year, it was in different places, and the site of this year's conference was Baltimore. While Vickie still enjoyed teaching, she was looking forward to a break from the classroom, as well as touring the Inner Harbor area of Baltimore. Some friends of hers had visited there several months ago and commented on the nice restaurants and shops lining the harbor. Vickie only hoped she wouldn't be late for the reception.

In 1965, Baltimore undertook a massive project called the Inner Harbor program which took until the early 1980s to complete. The purpose of the program was to help revive the failing inner-city area by boosting tourist and convention trade to the area. In addition to fine restaurants and shops, many new plush hotels and office buildings began to spring up with the help of industrial revenue bonds. One such hotel was the Inner-Harbor Inn, which was part of a national chain and the 1990 site of the National Teacher's Conference.

The alarm clock on the clock radio sounded at 6:30 a.m. on Friday, December 7, 1990, as it did every weekday, and Bobby Cook reached over as he did every morning and hit the "snooze button" for fifteen minutes of extra sleep. The alarm went off a second time, and Bobby Cook reluctantly pushed the covers off and rolled out of bed. He sat there for a few minutes trying to wake up. The announcer on the radio was reading off the upcoming events for the weekend, one being the start of the National Teacher's Conference at the Inner-Harbor Inn.

"While on the subject of teachers," the announcer said, "Do you know what today is? Give up? Fifty-one years ago today, the Japanese bombed Pearl Harbor." Bobby rubbed his eyes and flashed a small grin. How fitting, he thought. The Japanese planned a sneak attack on a harbor, and he, too, had chosen a harbor area as the scene for his sneak attacks.

Bobby Cook was born and raised in an upper-middle-income family in Baltimore, and he, too, graduated with honors and went on to college. He graduated from the University of Maryland with a degree in finance. Within days of finishing college, Bobby was hired as a loan processor at one of Baltimore's largest banks and placed in its management training program. His office was located downtown, and often he walked the short distance to enjoy lunch at one of the many restaurants at the Inner Harbor area.

On the job, Bobby was well liked, and because of his personality, dedication, and hard work, he was on a fast track for advancement and promotion.

However, Bobby had a dark side to him that would shock his co-workers.

As a child Bobby grew up in a home with abusive parents, both of whom were alcoholics. He would be beaten and battered about for no apparent reason other than that he was just there. He sought comfort in his uncle, who ended up sexually abusing him and introduced him at a very young age to pornography.

By the time he was in high school, Bobby had sexually assaulted two grammar school girls, but hadn't been caught. His history of sexual assaults continued while a student in college, but again he was never discovered or even suspected in a series of rapes on the campus. By now, rape had become a game for Bobby, and he thought that due to his superior intelligence, he would never be apprehended.

Bobby jumped into the shower, shaved and dressed. He was a meticulous dresser and spent more money than he should on his clothes. When he stepped outside of his apartment, he would certainly pass for a "yuppie" business executive. He would go to work during the day and excel at whatever task was assigned to him. After work his second life would begin.

He would start his evenings by going to four or five different sleazy strip joints located along Howard, Eutaw, and Baltimore streets downtown. He would sit for hours on end drinking scotch and water while watching the dancers remove their clothes. Bobby became well known in the various bars, and the doormen and dancers would all joke among themselves—here comes the banker.

After watching the girls strip away their clothes down to their G-strings for several hours, Bobby would end up in a "peep show" where he would watch hard-core pornography for a couple of hours. That would arouse him even more. By then it would be around 11:00 p.m., and he would head off to the hotels around the Inner Harbor looking for a woman to rape.

Bobby's favorite hunting ground had become the Inner-Harbor Inn. It was apparent to anyone that the security was pretty lax there. The hotel had multiple entrances, and at two of them, Bobby noticed on careful inspection, the boxes mounted to hold security cameras actually had no cameras but only loose wires hanging down where the cameras had once been. The hotel had security guards, but they spent most of their time hanging around the lobby area talking with the female desk clerks.

Bobby used the same tactics on each of his visits to the Inner-Harbor Inn. He would walk into the main lobby, wave hello at the security guard, and walk straight to the lobby lounge. Once inside the lounge, he would sit at the bar, order a drink, and strike up a conversation with the bartender, who after several months had come to know him by sight. After a couple of scotch-and-waters, he would walk out into the lobby area, purchase a newspaper, and sit watching the activity around him. When he was sure the security guard was paying him no attention, he would get up and casually walk over to the bank of guest elevators and ride up to a guest floor.

Upon arriving on one of the guest floors, Bobby would walk up and down the hallway looking for signs that a particular room was occupied, like a room service tray not collected or linens sitting outside the door where some lazy housekeeping employee had laid them instead of placing them inside of the guest's room.

Once he spotted a potential target, he would walk over to a house phone conveniently installed on each floor (unlike most hotels where they are located only in the lobby areas) and dial the room number of his targeted victim. The hotel was even accommodating enough to place instructions on the phone to dial "7" first, then the room number you wished to call.

If he couldn't reach anyone on that floor, he would just move on to the next floor and try again until someone answered the phone. If a male answered, Bobby would immediately hang up. If it was a female, he would give the woman some story about being on the hotel staff. He would first ask how many people were in the room. If she answered two or more, he would just excuse himself and hang up. If she answered just one, he would proceed with his plan.

He would tell the woman that he had received a signal at the front desk that something was wrong with her smoke detector. He would ask her to look at the smoke detector and tell him if the red light was blinking. It didn't matter what the answer was; he would say it was broken. He would then ask her if she would like for someone to come up and check it before she retired for the night. In most cases, the woman said, "Sure," and he would proceed to her room.

Once inside, Bobby would size up the situation, and if the occupant of the room appealed to him he would rape her. Bobby was very picky about his victims, and on several occasions had changed his mind about attacking them. To avoid suspicion in those cases, he would stand up on the desk chair, remove the cover of the smoke detector and act as if he were adjusting something inside. After a few minutes, he would place the cover back on and apologize for any inconvenience he may have caused.

From the middle of June 1990 to the first week in December 1990, Bobby

Cook had used this cunning method to gain entry into eight guest rooms at the Inner-Harbor Inn. He raped three women. During this same time period, the Inner-Harbor Inn failed to increase its security, did nothing to scrutinize its security needs, and failed to warn other guests of the ploy used by the rapist.

Vickie Caldwell looked at her wrist watch as she pulled in front of the Inner-Harbor Inn; it was exactly 7:30 p.m. If she hurried, she could make the start of the reception.

The valet and the bellman ran over to her car to meet her. They welcomed her to Baltimore and the Inner-Harbor Inn and asked if she was there to attend the teacher's conference. The bellman escorted her into the lobby and walked her up to the front desk. He announced that she was there for the teacher's conference, and the desk clerk asked her for her name. Vickie's name was located in the computer, and they handed her a pre-registration package which she was told contained her room key.

Vickie opened the package and removed the room key and her conference identification badge. She gave the bellman her room key and pinned the badge on her dress. The bellman motioned her toward the guest elevators, and they rode up to the tenth floor. They exited the elevator and walked a short distance down the hallway to her room—number 1010.

The bellman opened the door and held it while she entered. The room was very spacious and had a king-size bed. The bellman hung her hanging bag in the closet and placed her suitcase on the luggage stand at the foot of the bed. He offered to get her a bucket of ice, but she declined, telling him that she was in a hurry to make the start of the reception.

She took a dollar bill from her purse and tipped him. He thanked her and told her that if she needed anything at all during her stay, not to hesitate to call the front desk. The bellman then left the room and closed the door behind him.

Vickie quickly opened her suitcase and removed her overnight pouch with her makeup and toothbrush. She raced to the bathroom to brush her teeth, wash her face, and put on some fresh makeup before going downstairs to the reception. She looked around the bathroom for a wash cloth and hand towel but found that the maid had only left one full-size bath towel. "Oh well," she thought, "this will just have to do for now." She would stop by the front desk when she went downstairs to the reception and request more towels and wash cloths. She finished applying her makeup, straightened up her clothes, and left her room.

She went by the front desk and informed the clerk that she needed more towels. The clerk apologized, asked for her room number, and assured her that he would take care of it immediately.

At the reception, Vickie saw and visited with many friends whom she had met at past meetings. She had a couple of glasses of wine and ate hors d'oeuvres while chatting with her friends. But she soon began to feel tired, she guessed from the drive and the tranquilizing effects of the wine. What she needed was a good hot shower and then a restful night's sleep. She told the people with whom she had been sitting good-night and left the reception.

As Vickie walked through the lobby, she noticed a nicely dressed man sitting and reading a newspaper. She couldn't see his face clearly because the newspaper partially covered it. However, from the way he was dressed he appeared possibly to be a hotel staff employee taking a break. She walked past him and rode the guest elevator up to the tenth floor.

She entered her room, sat her purse down, kicked her shoes off, and started taking her clothes off. She removed a robe and a nightgown from her suitcase and laid them across the foot of the bed for when she got out of the shower.

Vickie turned the shower on and stuck her hand out to test the water. "Ah, just right," she thought. She started to step into the shower and suddenly noticed that the hotel had failed to send additional towels and wash clothes up to her room as she had requested. She reached over, wrapped the same bath towel she had used earlier around her, and went to the phone.

She dialed "O" for the hotel operator and asked to be connected to the front desk. She informed the person answering that she had requested additional towels and that she had yet to receive them. This clerk also apologized and stated someone would be right up with the towels.

Vickie grabbed the remote control and flipped on the television while waiting for the towels to arrive. She caught the last of the local news, and "The Tonight Show" started to come on. She switched off the television and decided to go ahead and get in the shower. She would worry about the towels in the morning.

Meanwhile, the night maid slowly made her way down the hallway with a handful of towels and wash clothes. She had been told to deliver them several hours ago but had got busy and forgot. The night manager had yelled at her, and she assured him she would take care of it immediately.

The maid knocked on the door to room 1010 several times, but no one responded. She placed her passkey in the door, but the door would not open because Vickie had engaged the safety chain before getting into the shower. With the door cracked open, the maid could hear the shower running, so she shut the door. She decided to just leave the towels and wash cloths in front of the door.

The maid wasn't the only one interested in the occupant of room 1010. Bobby Cook had noticed Vickie when she walked through the lobby and entered the elevator. He watched the indicator light on the elevator go from the lobby floor to the tenth floor. This would be easier than he had thought. He pushed the button for an elevator and awaited its arrival.

Bobby entered the elevator, and before the door closed three or four people attending the teacher's conference also rushed on. "Damn it," he said under his breath; now he would not be able to see which room she had entered.

Much to Bobby's dismay, every person pushed a different floor number. He quickly surveyed his fellow passengers, but just as quickly decided that none of them appealed to him. By the time Bobby reached the tenth floor, no one was in the hallway. He walked down the hall and noticed that a room service tray was sitting outside room 1009, but it had enough plates and glasses on it for two people. Scratch that one. Discouraged, Bobby entered the stairwell and walked down to the ninth floor. Maybe the pickings will be better there, he thought.

As Bobby exited the stairwell on the ninth floor, he saw the night maid opening a hallway storage closet and removing some towels and wash cloths. He walked by her and said, "Hello." The maid failed to acknowledge his presence. He continued to walk down the hallway toward the elevators and watched over his shoulder as the maid entered the same stairwell that he had just exited.

He would play a hunch: he entered the elevator and pushed the button for the tenth floor. It only took a second for the elevator to reach the tenth floor. The door opened, and Bobby got out and stuck his head around the corner, just in time to see the maid lay the towels down in front of room 1010, turn, and reenter the stairwell.

He waited a few minutes to see if the occupant of the room would open the door to claim the towels. About ten minutes passed, but no one came to the door. A situation made to order for Bobby Cook.

Bobby walked down the hallway and looked back toward the elevators to see if anyone else might be coming. The coast was clear, and he bent over and picked up the towels, knocked on the door, and very professionally announced: "Housekeeping, with your towels."

Vickie had just finished putting her nightgown on and wrapping the only towel she had around her wet hair. She had reached inside her suitcase and had just removed her hairdryer when the knock came.

Vickie put her robe over her nightgown and walked over to the door. She looked out of the peephole and saw a man dressed in a suit and tie holding an arm full of towels. She slid the chain off the door and opened the door slightly.

"You requested extra towels," Bobby said with a commanding voice. He was delighted to see that it was the same attractive woman he had noticed in the lobby.

"Yes, well not extra towels, the maid forgot to put them in the room when she cleaned it," Vickie responded.

"Well, we will have to speak to housekeeping about that," Bobby said as he tried to look into the room to see if there was anybody else inside. However, she was blocking his view.

"Are you sure this will be enough for your party?" Bobby said, hopeful to get a response from her that would indicate how many people were in the room. But it didn't work.

Vickie only responded by saying, "I'm sure this will be plenty." With that, she reached out and took the towels from his hands, thanked him, and closed the door.

Bobby stood there, disgusted, as he heard her place the chain back on the door and lock the deadbolt.

"Damn it to hell," he cussed as he kicked at an imaginary object. "That was her, and I'll find a way," he mumbled to himself.

Bobby walked back to the elevator, pushed the down button, and when it arrived rode it down to the lobby. He strode back into the bar where the bartender recognized him and asked, "Do you want the usual?" The bartender poured a scotch-and-water and placed it on the bar in front of him.

Bobby took a long drink of the scotch and began to think of his next step.

Vickie put the towels and wash cloths in the bathroom and then blow-dried her hair. Then she sat down on the side of the bed and removed some of the conference materials from the package she had been given earlier at the front desk. She thumbed through the listing of various workshops and circled the ones that she was interested in attending. She glanced over at the clock on the nightstand and saw that it was 12:15 a.m. She put the papers up that she had been reviewing and reached over and turned off the lamp next to her bed.

Just as Vickie was laying her head down, the phone rang.

The sound of the phone at that time of the night made her jump. "Who would be calling me now?" she wondered.

"Hello," Vickie answered.

"Yes, this is the front desk. We are awfully sorry to bother you this time of night, but we have just received an indication on our fire alarm panel that your smoke detector has gone off," a male voice said.

"It must be a mistake, my smoke detector has not gone off," Vickie responded.

"Well, it may be an indication that the battery is low. Would you please look up at the smoke detector and let me know if there is a red light on?" Bobby Cook said from the house phone only twenty feet from Vickie's room door.

"Yes, the red light is on," Vickie said.

"Well, I know what the problem is, the batteries are low which causes the detector to send a signal to the front desk. For your safety we need to send someone up to change the batteries," Bobby said.

"Do you have to do that tonight?" Vickie asked.

"It's for your own safety, it will only take a second," Bobby answered.

"Oh, okay, if it will only take a second. I was already in bed."

"I promise. Someone will be right up." Bobby smiled and hung up the phone.

Bobby waited about five minutes before making the short trip down to Vickie's room. The room service tray was still sitting outside the room next to Vickie's and he reached down and took a steak knife from the tray. He thought this might come in handy and slipped it inside of his belt under his suit jacket.

He walked over and stood in front of Vickie's door and knocked. "Hotel staff here to check your smoke detector," he announced.

Vickie had already put her robe back on and had turned the lights on in the room. She walked over to the door, slipped the security chain off, unlocked the deadbolt, and opened the door.

Bobby said, "Sorry again to bother you at this time of night, but this is for your safety in the event of a fire."

"It's all right. Better safe than sorry," Vickie said.

Bobby walked over to the small desk in the room and pulled the chair out and placed it against the wall directly underneath the smoke detector. He stood up on the chair, removed the cover of the smoke detector and took out the battery. He then replaced the cover and pointed out to Vickie that the red light was now off. He situated the chair back under the desk and turned toward Vickie.

"It's fixed. As we suspected, the battery was low. Sorry for the inconvenience. I hope you have a good night." With that, Bobby turned as if he were leaving the room and walked over toward the door. Vickie was close behind him to re-lock the door once he left.

Bobby got to the door, reached up and placed the chain on the door, and flipped the deadbolt into the lock position. He reached inside of his suit jacket and grabbed the knife which he had lifted off the room service tray and sprung around toward Vickie.

"What are you doing?" Vickie demanded. Then she let out a scream when she saw the knife.

Bobby placed his hand over her mouth and thrust the knife against her throat.

"Just shut up, and I won't hurt you," he ordered.

Bobby pushed her toward the bed and threw her down across it. Vickie began to cry and to plead for her life.

"I'm not going to kill you or hurt you as long as you cooperate, I just want to have sex with you and then I will leave," Bobby told her.

Bobby ordered her to take all her clothes off and to lie on the bed. Bobby stood there silently for a few minutes admiring her firm nude body. He then began to take off his clothes and very carefully hung them across the back of the desk chair. Bobby then sat down on the bed next to her and began rubbing her thighs. He slowly worked his hands along her body until he reached her breasts. He rubbed them and rolled her nipples between his fingers, applying a little more pressure with each roll until Vickie let out a scream from the pain.

"Just calm down, I'm not going to hurt you. This can be good for both of us if you will just relax a little," Bobby told Vickie.

"But I don't want to make love to you," Vickie blurted out.

"Well, I don't see that you have much choice in the matter, do you?" Bobby said.

Bobby leaned down and kissed her breast. He then grabbed her hand and forced her to hold his erect penis. He started kissing her stomach and running his tongue across her body until he worked his way down between her legs.

After committing sodomy on Vickie, Bobby mounted her and forcibly had sex with her until he ejaculated. Having finished, he stood up, walked over to the bathroom, washed himself off and dried himself with one of the towels he had handed Vickie earlier at the door. He then walked back into the room and put his clothes back on.

Bobby stood there in front of the mirror and tied his tie while Vickie lay motionless on the bed sobbing. He turned toward her with the knife in his hand, and Vickie reacted by curling up on the bed.

"Please don't kill me," she pleaded. "You said you would not hurt me."

Bobby told her that he was not going to hurt her or kill her. He reached out and picked up the phone from the nightstand next to the bed and cut the wire.

"I just don't want you calling for help until I have time to get away," Bobby told her.

He then cut the phone cord into smaller pieces and tied her hands and feet. He covered her up with the sheets and bedspread.

"Please, don't try and get loose until I have had time to get out of the hotel," Bobby said, almost politely.

Bobby turned all the lights off in the room and left. He walked down the hallway, got on the elevator, and rode back down to the lobby. He exited the elevator and nonchalantly walked through the lobby, waving at the security guard standing near the front desk who tipped his hand in acknowledgment.

Bobby Cook walked across the street to a phone booth. He pulled out the yellow pages from the holder and looked up the number for the Inner-Harbor Inn. He dialed the number and waited for an answer.

"Inner-Harbor Inn. How may we help you?" a friendly female voice answered.

"You can't help me, but you can help the lady in room 1010. She has just been raped," Bobby said in a gentlemanly voice and hung up the phone.

Thinking it was a quack call, the switchboard operator hung up and waited more than twenty minutes before saying anything to the night manager. When she finally mentioned it, he told her to ring the room and see if someone would answer the phone. In the meantime, he pulled the information up on the computer screen and saw that the room was rented to a single person, Vickie Caldwell, from Richmond, Virginia.

When the switchboard operator received no answer, the night manager and the security guard went upstairs to room 1010 and knocked on the door. Again, no answer. They used the night manager's passkey and entered the room. They found Vickie curled up in a fetal position, still bound about the feet and hands. She had managed to kick the covers off, but she only lay there, naked and not moving. The night manager spoke to her, but she did not respond. She only stared at him. The hotel security guard radioed back to the front desk and told them to call the police and an ambulance.

Vickie was transported to a local hospital, where she was treated for shock and examined for the rape. She would not respond to questions asked of her by the doctors and nurses, and preferred to lay curled up in a fetal position on the stretcher. She was admitted and for the next several days lay in her hospital bed without saying a word. Her only sign of emotion was a single tear flowing down her cheek when her mother and grandmother walked into her room.

On the fourth day, Vickie spoke her first words. She looked at her mother and asked, "How was the conference?" and again went back into the solitude of her silent world.

On the seventh day, Vickie started speaking—first saying things that did not make much sense and then becoming more coherent. She was finally able to talk with the police, doctors, and her family and tell them what had happened in her hotel room. Vickie was released from the hospital two days later and was taken home by her mother and grandmother, who had remained by her side throughout her recovery.

Vickie was not able to work for the next two years. Most days, when not going to counseling, she would sit and stare out the bay window of her mother's house, where she had moved after the rape.

On behalf of Vickie, her mother sought the advice of a local attorney. After hearing the story, the attorney advised that they retain a lawyer in Maryland and start legal action against the hotel for negligent security. Vickie's mother spoke to her about that, and she agreed to follow the advice of the attorney.

One month after Vickie Caldwell was raped at the Inner-Harbor Inn, Bobby Cook was back at the hotel looking for another victim. Using the same ploy that had been so successful for him in the past, he gained entry into another female guest's room. Bobby forced her back onto the bed with the same knife he had stolen off the room service tray the night he had raped Vickie Caldwell. But he finally made a mistake. He had failed to look in the bathroom, where the 6' 3", 225-pound husband of his latest victim had been using the toilet. The irate husband grabbed Bobby from behind and almost choked and beat him to death. When the police and security people finally arrived, Bobby was begging to be taken away from this crazy man.

Six months later, Bobby Cook pleaded guilty to four counts of rape and one count of attempted rape. As he stood in front of the judge to receive his sentence, he reached up and rubbed his neck which was still sore from where he had almost been choked to death.

Bobby was sentenced to four life terms plus twenty years for the rapes of Vickie and others. He is presently sitting in a prison cell in Maryland without any hope for parole.

Vickie Caldwell started teaching again at the beginning of the 1993 school year. She has moved back to her own apartment and still attends weekly counseling sessions. She settled her lawsuit against the Inner-Harbor Inn and is very active in crime victims' rights groups.

The Inner-Harbor Inn in January 1993 was the site of yet another brutal attack and armed robbery of a female attending a conference. On the night of the attack the security guard was still standing at the front desk, and the boxes for the cameras were still empty.

What You Should Learn from This Crime

If you receive a call from the front desk requesting that they send someone to your room to check out something, ask for the name of the person who will be coming to your room. Once the caller hangs up, call back and speak to the manager on duty. Inform him or her of the nature of the phone call and verify all of the information. Remember, it is unusual in most hotels for maintenance personnel to be working past the usual eight-hour day schedule. Never admit anyone to your room without first positively identifying him or her.

■ ■ ■

A Shopping Trip in the Suburbs

DONNA GLENN HAD JUST TURNED OVER, GRABBED HER PILLOW, scooted closer to her husband, and was preparing for what she was sure was her last hour or two of sleep when the clock radio went off. While this was the same routine each morning, it always startled her. She scrambled to hit the "snooze alarm" for just ten more minutes of sleep. She reached out, groping for the clock radio, and, typically, almost knocked it off the nightstand before she found the right button. After hitting it, her arm slid off the nightstand and bounced off the side of the bed. She was out like a light.

At 5:30 a.m., those extra ten minutes of snooze time could either feel like hours or seconds. For Donna this morning, it felt like she had never hit the snooze button.

The radio station helicopter pilot, who must have flown helicopters in Vietnam, was screaming, "Good Morning, Los Angeles, it's another smog-filled day, and the traffic on most major freeways is already bumper to bumper." Donna had a notion that someday someone was going to get sick of the chopper jock's "Good Morning, Los Angeles" routine and shoot him down. She said to herself, "Now, that's not nice"—but at 5:30 in the morning, who's nice?

Donna sat up on the side of the bed and slid her feet, one at a time, into her house shoes, stretched, and for a fleeting second thought about lying back down. However, she knew that was not possible since she had a husband to get off to work and two children to get to school. The newest addition to the family, an 18-month-old baby boy, would be waking up any minute screaming to watch "Barney." Besides, this was one day of the week she really looked forward to—Mother's Day Out. She would get everyone off, get the baby ready for nursery school, and have the rest of the day to herself.

That particular day she had several errands to run, and then she was going to meet her best friend, Janet Simpson, at Westport Mall in Burbank for lunch and some shopping. Donna often told her friends that whoever invented the concept of Mother's Day Out should run for president because he or she had to be brilliant.

Once she got started in the morning, Donna was like a whirlwind. Within about forty-five minutes, she fixed breakfast, awakened her husband, got the two older kids up, helped them get dressed for school, snatched little Jimmy from his crib, changed his diaper, dressed him, and sat him down in the den with a fresh bottle and his first "Barney" tape of the day. While Donna's life would seem hectic by anyone else's standards, she would not trade it for the world.

As Donna put the finishing touches on breakfast, she turned on the television in the kitchen. The news of late had been consumed with the Rodney King affair, along with the battle between Chief of Police Daryl Gates and Mayor Tom Bradley and the speculation as to which official would win. The next story dealt with another drive-by shooting between rival gangs in east Los Angeles. Finally, a group of black ministers in Watts was meeting with Mayor Bradley later in the day to seek more assistance in the aftermath of the riots that occurred after the LAPD officers were acquitted. The ministers demanded that Chief Gates resign or be fired. While listening to the news accounts, Donna understood what they were saying, but, like most of us, could not connect these events to her everyday life. The social problems with crime, drugs, violence, gang killings, and carjackings were something that happened to other people in other places—not in her life. Little did she know that tomorrow she would be part of the morning news headlines.

Westport Mall in Burbank was built in 1980, and, like most malls, its developers had spent millions of dollars trying to create an atmosphere that would attract shoppers. They emphasized perfect landscaping and a mall interior decorated with flowing fountains and expensive light fixtures. In such an atmosphere, while most people might expect an occasional act of shoplifting to occur, they would never dream that assaults, rapes, robberies, and kidnappings from mall parking lots—which some security experts refer to as "no man's land"—are occurring daily in malls across the country.

Since many malls are located in highly populated suburban areas and near major freeway systems, they have become the favorite stalking grounds for inner-city criminals who commit crimes and then escape back into the ghettos and barrios. In addition, many youth gangs will try and establish a mall as their "territory" and have even developed a sport called "mall-mauling."

In the twelve years since Westport Mall was built, it had experienced more than its share of criminal activity, and the surrounding neighborhood, once characterized by upscale apartments, was now surrounded by iron fences, access-controlled gates, and armed guards walking the premises at night to control the drug dealing and nightly violence. But to the average patron of the mall the area still seemed okay, and like most businesses, those at the mall were not going to advertise to the contrary.

As the manager of the Westport Mall had stated in a recent employee meeting, "We are in the retail business, not the security business. It's the police's problem, not ours, that they cannot control the crime in the area." Whenever the mall's security director would ask for more manpower, lighting in the parking lot, or security cameras, he would always be given the same answer—maybe next year.

In 1985, Westport Mall hired 30-year-old Jerry Long to be its director of security. From the time he was a teenager, Jerry longed to be a police officer, but bad eyesight had caused him to be rejected from the LAPD and the police departments of four surrounding communities. He had to settle for what he felt was the next best thing—working as a contract security guard. Over the years Jerry Long had attended every possible training course he could on security and police procedures. Each of his supervisors would always rate him outstanding, and he quickly rose in the ranks of private security. When Jerry applied and was selected to be the director of security for the Westport Mall, he was overjoyed and made a pact with himself that he would run the best security program to be found in the industry. However, it didn't take long for him to become disillusioned; request after request was turned down by the mall management. While attending criminal justice classes at a community college taught by a police captain from the LAPD, he learned that, no matter what, you should always document your actions. So Jerry Long would do just that. He would document his data about crime trends at the mall and his recommendations for additional security—and then it would be up to management if it responded or not. At least he would be doing his job.

As Skip Glenn, Donna's husband, finished his last cup of coffee before leaving for work, she ran into the bedroom, pulled a pair of jeans on, and slipped a sweatshirt over her head. She hurriedly brushed her hair and put a pair of tennis shoes on so that she could drive the two older children to school and drop off the baby at the day-care center. As Skip was walking out the door, he turned, kissed her on the cheek, and like always said, "I love you; be careful." Typically, she replied, "I have to be careful; who would take care of this wild bunch if something happened to me?" Donna then rushed the children into the mini-van, and off they went.

Donna pulled up in front of the school and stopped in the area designated for parents to drop their children off. The school crossing guard waved and said good morning to Donna as Tommy, the oldest of the two children, opened the front passenger's side door and jumped out. He started to run off in the direction of some of his friends who were standing nearby when Donna ordered him back to the car. "I know you are 11 years old, but you are not too old to give your mother a hug and a kiss," she said.

Tommy responded like most kids his age who are embarrassed in front of their friends. Worried that this might not be the manly thing to do, he hugged his mother's neck ever so slightly and stood at the curb while his sister Ashley got out of the rear of the car. Ashley leaned across the front passenger's seat and gave her mother a kiss and a hug.

"One last check, guys: Do you have your lunch money? And don't forget, Mrs. Jackson will pick you up after school," Donna said. Tommy and Ashley both acknowledged that, yes, they had their lunch money and that they knew Mrs. Jackson would pick them up.

"I love you, guys, see you around 6:00. Be good!" Donna said as Tommy closed the van doors and she pulled away from the curb. She waved at them and had no way of knowing that would be the last time she would see them. The 18-month-old started crying and screaming that he, too, wanted to go to school and Donna assured him that he was going to his own school.

After dropping the baby off at the day-care center, Donna drove to the drive-in window of the bank and deposited Skip's paycheck before the checks she had mailed the day before could bounce. She then ran into the supermarket to get some snack food for Tommy and Janet when they got home from school that afternoon. She then drove back home.

Donna looked at her watch. It was already 10:00 a.m., and she had promised to meet her friend Janet at 11:00 a.m. for some quick shopping before they had lunch. She jumped in the shower and halfway blow-dried her hair. Since it was such a nice spring day, she put on a sundress and sandals. Before leaving the house, she called Skip at the office to see how his day was going; as usual he couldn't talk right now because he was late for a meeting. She quickly reminded him that she would be out for the rest of the day and that she would see him tonight at home. She hung up the phone, grabbed her purse, and out the door she ran.

Donna looked at her watch as she pulled into the parking lot of Westport Mall. It was ten past eleven, and she knew that Janet would be pacing back and forth, dying to descend on their first store. As she pulled into the main entrance of the shopping mall, Donna saw a police car in the middle of a group of people. "Must have been a wreck," she thought. Actually, what she was seeing was a police officer taking a report of a lady who had been mugged as she walked back to her car—a crime that was becoming almost an everyday affair at the mall.

Donna had to circle the lot near the main entrance of the mall several times before she found a parking space that another shopper had just vacated. By the time she parked her Dodge mini-van, it was almost 11:20, and she prepared herself for the lecture she would get from Janet about how she was always late. Donna's typical reply was that if Janet, who was only recently married, had three kids, then she would be late, too. As it turned out, Janet was not the only one pacing back and forth that morning. Jerry Long, the mall's director of security, had been fit to be tied. "Another damn customer robbed! When is this going to stop and when is the mall management going to pay attention to me?" Jerry shouted out loud to the security officer who had come to fill out an incident report on the latest crime victim at Westport.

Six months before, Jerry had written a detailed memorandum to the mall manager outlining the crimes during the past year and his recommendations. The memo read:

> During the past year Westport Mall has seen a dramatic
> increase in criminal activity. During the past year customers have
> experienced the following types of crimes:
>
> 1   Abduction

3 Rapes
49 Armed Robberies
44 Purse Snatchings
17 Aggravated Assaults
198 Thefts from Vehicles
52 Thefts of Vehicles

Also, for your information, the following are crimes that have been committed within a one-mile radius of the mall:

24 Murders
81 Rapes
825 Armed Robberies
89 Aggravated Assaults
782 Auto Thefts

As you know, we have repeatedly requested more police patrols, but the zone commander has stated that they are doing all they can and recommend that we hire more security. In addition to the crimes I have outlined above, there are several youth gangs that are now trying to establish the mall as part of their "turf." This poses an even greater danger to our patrons. Also, the type of criminals we are now seeing are supporting drug habits and are usually armed. The area in which the mall is now located is considered one of the highest crime areas of the city.

We presently have a staff of fourteen (14) security officers to cover all three shifts; I recommend that we double that number, increase lighting in the parking lot, and install surveillance cameras in the parking lot. I also recommend that we send a letter to all the stores in the mall notifying them of the seriousness of the crime problem here.

Please reply as soon as possible so that we can make Westport Mall once again a safe place to shop.

For years Jerry Long had begged for increases in security, and now he believed that once the mall manager read this memorandum, management would respond favorably to his request. He again would be proven wrong.

After writing the memo, Jerry attended the weekly staff meeting where mostly marketing plans and mall events were discussed, but the topic of Jerry's memo never came up. Another week and another meeting and still no discussion of his memo. On Tuesday of the third week, Jerry received a routing envelope from the mall manager. Inside was the original copy of his memo to the mall manager with a hand-written note, in red, which read:

> Jerry: Good memo, great ideas, thanks for the good job you and your staff are doing. Keep up the good work and bring this back to my attention in six months or so.
>
> Thanks—FWR

Thus Jerry realized once and for all that he was fighting a losing battle. He immediately began preparing his résumé and started looking for another job. That would solve his own problem, but what about the patrons who shopped at the mall daily and did not know of the crimes? Someone was going to get killed, Jerry thought to himself as he typed his résumé one finger at a time.

Janet soon got over her displeasure with Donna for being late, and they enjoyed an hour of shopping before deciding to eat lunch. They selected a "theme" restaurant located inside the mall and had a good time catching up on events in each other's life. After lunch they again hit the stores. Donna had an appointment to get her hair and fingernails done at 3:00 p.m., but the salon was also located in the mall so they could shop right up to the time of her appointment. Janet walked Donna to the entrance of the hair salon and said good-bye, giving Donna a tight hug before she left.

Donna thoroughly enjoyed her day out. While getting her hair and nails done, she could relax after several hours of shopping and make mental notes of what she needed to do during the coming week. Of course the customary gossip of the shop attendants was always something to look forward to as well.

At approximately 5:00 p.m., Donna left the hair salon. As she walked through the mall, she stopped at a pay phone and called to check on the children. The babysitter answered and assured her that everything was all right and the children were fine. The babysitter reported that the two older children had completed their homework and were out in the backyard playing. The baby was in the den watching the afternoon session of—what else?—"Barney." Donna told the sitter that she had one more stop to make and that she should be home no later than her planned 6:00 p.m.

The sales clerk in the toy store wrapped a "Barney's Blanket" in tissue paper and placed it in the shopping bag. He rang it into the register—$49.95 plus tax—and Donna handed him her MasterCard as payment for the "Barney Blanket," which she had promised the baby. Forty-nine dollars for a blanket with a big purple dinosaur on it? Why couldn't she have been the mother who thought this one up? Donna thought.

If the mall had installed the surveillance cameras in the parking lot or increased the security patrols, maybe someone would have noticed the late-model black Oldsmobile with three Chicano males that pulled into the parking lot around 4:30 p.m. and began circling slowly, driving up and down each row of parked cars. At one point a lady shopper was walking toward her car, and the black Oldsmobile pulled alongside of her and almost came to a stop. However, her companion exited the mall and yelled for the woman to stop so he could catch up. The Oldsmobile sped away. The lady shopper thought that it was just someone waiting to see where she had parked so they could get her parking space.

The lady shopper would never know how lucky she had been. The occupants of the Oldsmobile were looking for something all right—but it wasn't a parking space. They were like predators looking for prey.

Donna gathered her shopping bags after having paid for the blanket and started toward the entrance of the mall. She glanced at her watch. It was 5:15 p.m. "Good," she thought. "I should be home at six, just in time to start dinner.

She exited the main entrance to the mall and started walking down the rows of parked cars towards her Dodge mini-van. As Donna was halfway down the row in which her van was parked, the black Oldsmobile with its three predators pulled into that row. Donna had her back to the Oldsmobile so she didn't even notice or sense their presence.

The driver of the Oldsmobile had spotted the attractive woman in the sundress, her arms full of packages, when she first exited the mall. He watched as she began walking toward her car and announced to his two friends in the car with him that maybe this was the one. He slowed down and, while watching Donna with a keen eye, glanced up in the rearview mirror to make sure she was by herself. He told his buddies to get ready—this appeared to be it.

Donna reached her van and had to set her shopping bags next to the sliding door in order to get her keys from her purse. She reached in, removed the keys, inserted them into the door, opened it, and reached inside to push the automatic door locks. They made a clicking sound as they opened, and Donna threw her purse in the passengers seat and opened the sliding door to store her packages.

The black Oldsmobile stopped right in front of Donna's van. The front and rear passenger's door swung open at the same time as if the two men who jumped from the car had practiced this a hundred times before. The man who had been sitting in the front passenger's seat removed a pistol from the waistband of his pants and held it down by the side of his leg as the two of them quickly ran around to the side of the van.

A witness later told the police that he was getting out of his car about two rows over when he saw an older black Oldsmobile stop in front of a blue mini-van and two Hispanic males jump out. One of the men appeared to be holding what looked like a gun down by his side.

The witness stated, "I could see a lady at the side door of the van and it looked like she was putting shopping bags into the van.

"I saw the two men run up behind her, and the one who had been holding a gun struck her on the top of the head.

"The lady let out a scream and fell forward into the van. The man who hit her then picked her up and threw her into the van like a sack of potatoes, and then he jumped into the van behind her.

"The other man ran over to the front door, opened it, and got in. The driver of the black Oldsmobile leaned over and shouted, "'Let's get out of here' as he was pulling the two passenger's doors shut," said the witness. "The Oldsmobile then sped away with the mini-van close behind."

The witness ran into the mall and dashed into the first store he came to. He ran up to the cashier and, almost out of breath, began yelling out what he had seen in the parking lot. The man asked where the mall security office was and the clerk stated that she didn't know. He then asked if she could call the security office and the clerk stated that no one had ever given her the number, but that they could look it up. It took her around five minutes to find the phone directory and another minute or two to find the mall's main number in the book.

The store clerk called the main number and got a recording stating that the mall's business office was open from 9:00 a.m. to 5:00 p.m. and if you knew your party's extension, please dial it now. "If not, thank you for calling and please try back in the morning."

The clerk told the now very frustrated witness about the recording, and he ran from the store looking for someone who looked like a security officer. Instead of calling the police, the store clerk went back to work ringing up sales.

The man who had witnessed Donna's abduction desperately looked for a security officer. After about ten minutes he saw a hallway where a door read, "Mall Employees Only." He swung open the door and ran down the long hallway until he came to what appeared to be a break room. Inside of the room sat a grossly overweight man eating a sandwich and watching a small television. The man eating the sandwich, startled by the appearance of the half-crazed witness, announced that he was a mall security officer. (It was later discovered that he was the only mall employee on duty at the time and had been in the break room for more than forty-five minutes.) With food spilling out of his mouth, he demanded to know what the witness was doing in an "off-limits" place.

The witness by this time was in a state of panic. He tried to explain to the mall security officer what he had seen. Instead of calling the police, however, the officer immediately pulled out a notebook from his pocket and started taking notes on what the man was trying to tell him.

"Did you get the tag number of the van or the car? Can you give me a description of the assailants?" barked the security officer. This line of questioning went on for close to twenty minutes with the same questions being asked and the same answers being given over and over.

The witness had not been able to get the tag numbers of either vehicle. The mall security officer finally told the man that would be enough for now and that he would notify the police. The security officer thanked the man and told him he could go and that they would be in touch with him later if they needed him. There was only one slight problem: With that statement, the witness walked down the hallway, exited through the door, and disappeared into the mall never to be seen again. The security officer between bites of his sandwich and asking questions forgot to obtain the man's name or phone number.

The mall security officer also had never asked for the exact location where the incident took place, and that detail might never have been known had not one of Donna's shopping bags fallen from the van as her assailant was pushing her inside. It contained the credit card receipt for the Barney's blanket purchase with her name on it.

After the unidentified witness had left the breakroom, the mall security officer went back to eating his cheeseburger and French fries. He reached over and turned the volume up on the portable television and finished watching the evening news. He never called the police.

At 7:30 p.m. Skip Glenn pulled into the driveway of his house. He reached up and pushed the button on the garage door opener. "That's strange," he thought as the garage door began to open. Donna's mini-van was not in the garage. He remembered that this was Mother's Day Out, but she was always home and had dinner on the table when he arrived. Skip pulled into the garage and parked his car. He grabbed his briefcase and hurried into the house.

Skip was met at the door by his two oldest children. "Hi, Dad," they shouted. "Is Mom with you?"

"No, she's not with me," Skip replied. "Why do you ask?"

"Well, Mom's not at home and the babysitter said she called sometime ago and said she was on the way home. When she didn't get here by her normal time, we thought she might have met you or something," Tommy answered his father.

Skip felt a sense of panic rush through his body as he ran through the kitchen and into the den where Mrs. Jackson, the babysitter, was with the baby. Not realizing he was shouting, he scared the baby when he loudly and almost rudely demanded to know about his wife's earlier phone call.

Mrs. Jackson explained to him what time Donna had called and what she had said during the brief conversation. "Have you heard from her since?" Skip demanded.

"No," Mrs. Jackson replied. "Is something wrong?"

"I am sorry, Mrs. Jackson, I am probably just overreacting, but Donna has never been this late before, and I'm worried," Skip answered.

He picked up the telephone and called Janet Simpson.

"Hi, Janet, this is Skip. Nothing is wrong, but what time was it when you last saw Donna?"

"I left her at the mall around three or so and she was going to get her hair done and come home. Why, Skip, what's wrong?"

"Nothing I hope; it's just that she's not home yet and she hasn't called," Skip answered.

"Maybe she had some more shopping to do and she has just let the time get away from her. You know how women are," Janet offered.

"Yes, but this is not like her, Janet. Well, maybe you're right. Sorry I bothered you."

"Oh, don't be silly, Skip. You haven't bothered me, I'm sure everything is fine. Have Donna call me when she gets home."

After hanging up with Janet, Skip called information and asked for the phone number of Westport Mall. He hoped he could get the security office and find out if Donna might have reported that she was having car trouble or something. Still, it was unlike her not to call. He dialed the number the operator had given him for the mall and got the same recording as the store clerk who had attempted to call security. Skip slammed down the receiver in disgust.

Skip asked Mrs. Jackson if she would mind watching the children for a while longer while he drove down to the mall to see if it was possible Donna had experienced car trouble.

He drove the route that he felt she would take and looked along the way for her mini-van. He kept praying that he would find her merely stranded along the side of the road. He knew that it was very unlikely that she had forgotten what time it was and continued shopping. She would never do that. Something was wrong and he had to find out what.

Skip didn't see any sign of Donna on the way to the mall. He drove around the massive parking lot in hopes of spotting her mini-van. He remarked to himself how poor the lighting was in the lot. Not finding her van, he parked his car in the same general area where Donna had parked hours earlier. He entered the mall, and, ironically, walked into the same store that the witness to Donna's abduction had rushed into more than two hours earlier seeking help in locating the security personnel.

Skip walked up to the cashier and asked where the mall security office was located. As before, the clerk answered she didn't know and anticipated his next question by stating that she did not have a phone number either. Skip started to turn and walk away when the girl behind the register said, "Gee, this must be a busy night—you are the second person tonight looking for security."

Skip turned around and looked her directly in the eye and asked what did she mean by that. The clerk told him about the man who had earlier run into the store, yelling that he had seen a woman being assaulted and kidnapped from the parking lot.

"What else did the man say?" Skip shot back. "Did he say anything about what kind of a car the woman was in?"

The clerk said, "Yeah, it was an Oldsmobile mini-van or something like that."

When he heard the word "mini-van," Skip felt sick to his stomach, and it was all he could do to fight back the tears. But he had to remain calm. "What did you do, did you call security or the police?" Skip demanded. The clerk explained to him about trying to call the mall office and getting the recording and that the man had then run from the store searching for the mall security office.

Dashing out of the store, Skip ran toward the center of the mall hoping to spot a security officer. After running up and down the halls of the mall, he finally spotted an overweight man in a security uniform standing in front of the mall theaters talking with the ticket-taker.

Skip identified himself and related the story which the store clerk had told him. The security officer admitted that an unknown man had disturbed his supper break with a story of how he had witnessed a woman being hit over the head and kidnapped, but the man could not give a description of the woman, the assailants, or tag numbers of the vehicles involved.

"Did he tell you what kind of vehicles were involved?" Skip asked.

The security officer removed a tattered notebook from his pocket and began flipping through page after page.

"Let's see—here it is. He said it was a Dodge mini-van and an old black Oldsmobile with two or three Chicanos," the security officer replied.

It was all Skip could do to fight back the nausea. He knew that his worst fears were coming true—something horrible had happened to Donna.

"What did you do, did you call the police, what the hell did you do?" Skip screamed at the security officer.

"No, wait a damn minute here, you need to calm down, mister. I looked around but couldn't find anything, and besides, we get kooks like that all the time reporting they saw something when it's just their imagination running away with them," the security officer shouted back at Skip.

"Well, this is not a kook this time. My wife is missing and she was driving a Dodge mini-van," Skip shouted in return.

Hearing the verbal confrontation between the security officer and Skip, the theater manager walked over and suggested that they go to his office and call the police.

The police arrived within ten minutes and began taking what limited information the security officer and Skip had. The patrol officer called over his radio and requested some additional units and detectives. The officer then put out a look-out for Donna's mini-van and a limited description of the black Oldsmobile.

The other police units arrived and after searching the parking lot they discovered the shopping bag dropped from Donna's van. The police officers began stopping anyone leaving the mall and asking what time they had arrived and if they had seen anything suspicious. No one had.

The detectives arrived and asked Skip to accompany them down to the police station to wait for any word on his wife's whereabouts.

At approximately 10:00 p.m., while sitting in the detectives' office, Skip and the detectives overheard a firetruck being dispatched to a deserted area about five miles from the mall. Someone had reported what appeared to be a vehicle on fire. One of the detectives called the fire dispatcher and asked if there were any additional information and was told no. The detective requested that when the responding units arrived at the scene they notify him with any possible identification of the vehicle.

The phone rang in the detective office about ten minutes later. It was the fire department's dispatcher. The detective grabbed a note pad and began taking notes. The seasoned detective hung up the phone and turned toward Skip, who by this time had jumped from his chair and was standing.

The detective had done this a hundred times, but it never got any easier; if anything, it got worse. He asked Skip to sit back down, but Skip pleaded with the detective to tell him what he knew. The detective told him that the vehicle on fire had been identified as Donna's.

"How about my wife, is she all right?" Skip asked.

"I'm sorry, Mr. Glenn, your wife was found lying about ten feet from the van and she had been shot and killed," the detective said.

Everything that came afterwards seemed to be in slow motion—the identification of her body, the funeral arrangements, family members and friends coming to comfort Skip and the children, and finally the church service and burial.

A local newspaper reporter had followed the story from the time the body was discovered and had written a detailed account of Donna's abduction and murder—an account which Skip could not bring himself to read until months later. When he did get around to reading the article, Skip was incensed with the account of all the other crimes that had been committed at the mall. He also read how the mall security director had resigned in total disgust the day after Donna's abduction and murder and how he had pleaded for more security measures at the mall. The former security director was also quoted as saying, "I knew that it was just a matter of time before something like this was going to happen."

The police detectives had described the crime scene to Skip. Donna's body had been found nude, and she had been repeatedly sexually assaulted, beaten, then shot through the head twice with a large caliber pistol after which the assailants covered her face with the Barney blanket she had purchased for the baby. The force of the bullets had been so brutal that the positive identification had to be made by her fingerprints and dental records. Apparently, after raping and killing her, her assailants had set her van on fire to destroy any possible evidence they might have left behind.

A lawsuit was filed on behalf of Skip and the children a year after Donna's death. With no defense, the mall agreed to a large settlement shortly after the suit was filed.

One would hope that such a tragic incident would cause the mall to improve its security measures. However, it is sad to report that another woman at Westport Mall was abducted, robbed, and raped a little over a year and a half after Donna's death.

The security policies and measures remained the same as they did on the day Donna was abducted, and Donna's abductors have gone unidentified.

What's it going to take?

What You Should Learn from This Crime

Always park as close to the entrance of a mall as possible. If valet parking is available, use it. Go shopping with others, not alone. Remember, if you are confronted by an assailant in an open parking lot, faking a fainting spell may scare off your would-be assailant. Always be cautious and heed your own best alarm—your common sense.

■ ■ ■

Car-jacking

IN THE LAST EIGHTEEN MONTHS OR SO, A NEW CRIME PHE-
nomenon has erupted across the country—one so heinous and frightening that it has garnered headlines throughout the world. The crime is car-
jacking.

In one ten-day period in September 1993:

- The father of basketball superstar Michael Jordan was shot
in the head when he stopped to grab a nap at a North Carolina rest stop. His flashy sports car was stolen, and his body was
dumped in a river in South Carolina.

- A German tourist leaving Miami International Airport in a
rental car was almost immediately bumped from behind by a
potential car-jacker. (This is a favorite car-jacking tactic. When
the driver of the bumped car gets out to inspect the damage,
the car-jackers pull a pistol on him.) When the driver in this
incident tried to avoid stopping, the second car pulled up
alongside of him, and he was shot to death.

- Another tourist couple, this time from England, was attacked
in their car at a north Florida rest stop. The man was shot to
death, and the woman was wounded.

While all crimes that I describe in this book are frightening, car-jacking is among the most disturbing because it occurs totally at random. Anyone in a car can be a victim at any time. And car-jacking, by its very nature, is an extremely violent crime. The best a victim can hope for is that a gun will be pointed at him and he will be ordered to abandon his car—and that is all.

But many, if not most, car-jackings are accompanied by further violence: Victims are thrown from their cars onto the street—or they are shot and wounded or killed as their cars are taken. In one particularly brutal incident in suburban Maryland, a young mother was car-jacked as she was taking her little daughter to her first day of preschool. The car-jackers tried to throw the woman out of the car, but she became entangled in her safety belt and shoulder harness and ended up hanging out of the car. The assailants drove the car alongside a fence to dislodge her body, leaving a trail of blood a mile long behind the car.

Further, there are no typical victims. While women are much more likely than men to be raped, car-jackings claim victims of both sexes, all ages, and all socio-economic groups. Even a drug enforcement agent, armed with a gun, was car-jacked, shot and killed in Birmingham, Alabama.

Tourists have been particularly singled out, especially in the Miami area. Unsure of the highways, riding in rental cars with bumper stickers and license plates that are dead giveaways that the car is leased and they may be tourists, a number of foreigners were attacked in the Miami area in 1993.

In response, rental car agencies there began distributing detailed maps and anti-car-jacking instructions to tourists and removed telltale stickers from their cars. Still, the carnage continued, and Florida governor Lawton Chiles was forced to appeal to President Clinton for help. In addition, Governor Chiles ordered state license tags—which indicated which vehicles were rental cars—removed, and increased police patrols at rest stops and inner-city areas frequented by tourists.

However, abiding by the following tips, plus those in the chapter on safety while traveling, can reduce your chances of being car-jacked.

- First and foremost, do not stop in a dangerous or doubtful neighborhood to use a pay phone or look at a map. This is how an incredibly high percentage of car-jackings begin. Ask for directions before leaving the car rental agency and make sure you understand them before leaving the lot.

- Keep all doors and windows in your car locked at all times.

- Always ensure that you are driving with plenty of gas. It's amazing how many car-jackings occur because someone forgot to fill up.

- If you are visiting a strange town, do not rent a car with bumper stickers that indicate it is rented. If you can, avoid renting one with a telltale license plate.

- To avoid being "bumped," always leave enough space between your car and the car in front of you while stopping. This will allow you enough room to drive out in the event a quick escape is necessary.

- If your car should break down, turn on the emergency flasher, raise the hood, tie something white to the driver's door, get back into your car, and lock the doors. When someone stops to help, roll down the window slightly and ask the person to call the police.

- Pick well-lit areas if you should stop for gas or to eat.

- If you should be confronted by a car-jacker and are unable to get away, try and remain as calm as possible and follow instructions completely. Do not provoke the car-jacker!

- Do not stop for flashing white lights. Emergency vehicles in the United States always use red or blue flashing lights.

- Do not pick up hitchhikers under any circumstances.

- If you are a foreign tourist and arriving late, you may want to catch a shuttle bus to your hotel or motel and have the rental car agency deliver a car to you the next morning. This helps eliminate the chances of your getting lost in a strange city at night.

The Federal government has passed a law that makes car-jacking a federal crime. This new legislation plus better awareness of the crime among potential victims may eventually help curb the trend. But until car-jacking ends completely, many Americans will be wondering, "If I can't be safe in my own car, where and when can I be safe?"

■ ■ ■

Security and Safety Tips for Traveling

MILLIONS OF PEOPLE TRAVEL ANNUALLY ON BUSINESS OR FOR pleasure. Increasingly these trips are becoming nightmares as more and more travelers are falling victim to crimes. The following personal safety tips may prevent you from becoming the next victim of a crime while traveling or staying in a hotel or motel.

- Always let family members or co-workers know the name and address of the hotel or motel where you are staying.

- If possible, inform them of your plans during your evening hours and what time you expect to be back in your room.

- If you use name tags on your briefcase and luggage, *do not* use visible ones. They allow a would-be criminal to obtain your name, business or home address, and phone numbers—and use this information to obtain further information on you, such as your hotel and room number. Luggage tags can be useful, but use the concealed type. Female travelers should consider using initials instead of their first name.

- If you are driving to your destination, make sure you start your trip with a full tank of gasoline and *do not* wait until you are near empty to stop and purchase another tank.

- A car phone is an excellent security measure in today's society. In the event of an emergency, it allows you to call for help no matter where you are, without leaving the safety of your car.

- Never leave luggage in the backseat or garment bags hanging in the window. These are welcome mats to a would-be criminal.

- While traveling in your car, keep all the doors and windows locked at all times. This security measure is especially important in inner-city areas where incidents of car-jacking are becoming common.

- Pick well-lit areas if you should stop for gas or to eat.

- If possible avoid using rest stops along interstate highways. Most are isolated and are not frequently patrolled by law enforcement personnel. A well-lit truck stop parking lot may be a better choice.

- Remember always to lock your car when parking. Upon reentering, always check the backseat and floorboard for "unwanted traveling companions." As you approach your car, always have your keys in your hand ready to open the door. Keys also make an excellent weapon against a would-be assailant. You can scrape them across the eyes and face.

- If you are driving in a strange city, do not stop in unfamiliar areas and ask for directions. Look for a mail carrier, fire station, or police officer to ask for directions.

- *Do not* pull over in unfamiliar areas of a city to read street maps. You have no way of knowing the crime history of that part of town, so do not take the chance.

- Do not get out of your car to use a pay phone in a deserted area of a city. Look for well-lit areas and places with some activity around them.

- If your car should break down, turn on the emergency flasher, raise the hood, tie something white to the driver's door, get back into your car, and lock the doors. When someone stops to help, roll down the window slightly and ask the person to call the police. If you are a female traveling alone, tell the person that your husband or boyfriend has gone for help. However, ask them to notify the police of your whereabouts. If a passing motorist tries to signal for you to pull over, *do not* pull over. Turn on your emergency flashers and keep driving to the nearest open business where other people are present. Remember, you can also look for a fire station or police officer to flag down. Another ploy used by car-jackers is to bump you from behind. If you feel the least bit suspicious, do not get out of your car. Motion for the driver to follow you to the nearest police station or fire station.

■ If you feel someone is following you, try and remain calm. Drive to the nearest open business or look for a police or fire station. If possible, try and obtain a good description of the car and driver. Write the tag number and descriptions down to turn over to authorities later.

■ Never pick up a hitchhiker no matter how "innocent" he or she may look. It's better not to take any chances, and remember that no one knows what a criminal really looks like. If you are flying to your destination, do not become overfriendly with people in the airport or the person seated next to you on the airplane. Try to avoid giving out your name and where you are staying.

■ Think about your personal appearance. Expensive clothing, flashy jewelry, and large sums of money may draw unwanted attention.

■ Do not develop a "Disneyland Mentality" when traveling, and be alert for what is going on around you. If you practice the same reasonable security measures that you do at home, then you dramatically decrease the chances of being a victim of a crime while away from home.

■ If you should rent a car, ask the rental agent to remove any obvious bumper stickers. This is an advertisement to would-be assailants that you are most likely from out of town.

- Remember: As with your own car, never leave luggage in the backseat or garment bags hanging in the windows of your rental car. This is another advertisement that you are from out of town.

- If you are staying at a hotel, drive to the front entrance and allow a bell person to assist you with your luggage and use the valet parking service if available.

- If you arrive at night and you observe the parking lot area is not well lit, you may decide you do not want to stay there. Lighting is a very effective security measure, and the absence of good lighting may be an example of the hotel or motel's attitude toward security.

- If you are staying in a motel, always ask if they have ground-floor rooms available. If so, park as near as possible to your room.

- If you are staying in a motel, never leave your room door open while unloading or loading your luggage.

- If you are a female traveling alone and you are staying in a motel or hotel, do not hesitate to ask for an escort to or from your room if you feel the least uncomfortable with your surroundings. Always ask for an escort if you are returning from a late meeting or dinner. Have the person escorting you check the closet, bathroom, and other hiding places in the room before they depart. Remember, most *motels* will not have personnel available to escort you to your room.

- Beware if the desk clerk calls out your name or room number when checking into a hotel or motel. This may be a good indication that the hotel or motel has provided little or no training to its employees on guest security measures. If you should decide to stay there, ask the desk clerk to assign you to another room and this time to *not* call out your room number.

- If you are a female traveling alone, you should always use your initials, not your first name, when filling out the guest registration card.

- When checking into a hotel or motel, the type of room key

you receive may be another indication of the concern placed on your safety. As a rule, the newer "card access" locks provide the best key control and guest-room security. This is not to suggest that a hotel or motel that uses brass keys and hotel/motel function locks—which automatically lock when you close the door—is not a safe place to stay. However, all hotel or motel rooms should be equipped with a dead-bolt lock and latching U-bolt or chain lock. No key device should display the address or number of your room.

- As you are going to your room, be observant and make a mental note of the surroundings.

- Always have your room key out and in your hand when entering or exiting your room. Remember: like your car keys, a room key or plastic card key can make an excellent weapon against a would-be assailant.

- When entering your room, make sure your door shuts securely and observe what type of locks have been provided for your safety.

- While in your room, always use all of the locking devices which have been provided for your safety.

- After entering your room, walk over to the telephone and make sure you have a dial tone. Hotel and motel phones should have emergency phone procedures on them. If yours does not, call the front desk and ask what number you should dial in the case of an emergency. This is very important since all communities do not have "911" service and your phone may be restricted from calling an outside operator direct. Remember, in the case of an emergency, the room phone is your best means for summoning help.

- Familiarize yourself with the positions of all light switches in your room. If you have a lamp next to your bed, make a mental note of how to turn it on. This way, if you are awakened in the middle of the night and sense a problem, you will not fumble for the light switch.

- Always check any windows or sliding glass doors that may be in your room to insure they are locked. Windows and sliding glass doors should have at least two locking devices. Never stay in a ground-floor room or other floors which may be easily accessible from the ground if they do not have secondary locks.

- If your room has a connecting door, check to see if it is secured and locked. It should also have two locking devices on it.

- Always inspect all windows and doors before retiring at night. Windows and doors should always remain closed and locked whether you are in the room or away from it.

- All hotel or motel doors should be equipped with a peephole viewer. Always use the peephole to aid in identifying anyone knocking on your door. Never answer your room door without first verifying who it is. If the person claims to be an employee, call the front desk and ask if they have sent anyone to your room and for what purpose.

- If you should receive a call from someone who claims to be a hotel employee and wants to gain access to your room, do not automatically invite him or her to your room. Ask for the person's name, department, and for what purpose he or she wishes to enter your room. You may want to ask questions such as, "What address do you show for me on my guest registration card?" "What date do you have that I checked in?" etc.—information which only a hotel employee should have access to. If you still feel uncomfortable, hang up, call the front desk, and ask to speak to the manager on duty. Inform the manager of the call and ask him or her to verify the nature of the call. Placing such calls to guest rooms has been a very effective way for would-be criminals to gain access into rooms to commit their crimes.

- When leaving your room, always be observant of your surroundings and make sure that your room door has shut securely behind you. If you observe anything which you feel is suspicious in the hallway or walkway, immediately reenter your room and call the front desk.

- Try to avoid any clues that your room is empty. Never leave a "Please Clean My Room" sign on the door. If you want your room cleaned while you are away, call the housekeeping department and request it.

- You may want to leave a television or radio playing while you are away. This would give the appearance to a would-be criminal that your room is occupied.

- For the security of your valuables, use in-room safes or safe-deposit boxes provided by the hotel or motel. Never leave valuables in your room.

- Never prop your room door open for any reason and never leave sliding-glass doors or windows open.

- If you are a female traveling alone, consider using room service for ordering drinks or ice instead of venturing out of your room at night to find the vending or ice machine.

- If you have ordered room service and someone knocks at your door wanting to pick up your tray, make sure that you look out of the peephole and identify that the person is with the hotel staff. If you have any doubts, *do not* open the door. Go to the phone and call the room service number to verify that they have indeed sent someone for your tray.

- While away from your room, do not needlessly display your room keys or carelessly leave them at the swimming pool, health club, restaurant, or other places where they can be easily stolen.

- Never invite strangers to your room. If you have children traveling with you, never send them to the room or to run errands in other parts of the hotel or motel without parental supervision. There are no age or maturity exceptions to this safe practice.

- If portable travel alarms and locks made for hotels or motels make you feel comfortable, by all means use them. A very effective and very inexpensive personal door lock can be purchased at your local hardware store for under a dollar—a rubber doorstop. It does not take up much room in a briefcase, purse, or piece of luggage, and by merely placing it securely under your room door at night you will add extra protection.

■ Never hesitate to call the police or hotel management if you should ever feel threatened in any way. Always trust your instincts: they are usually your best guide. It is always better to be embarrassed than to be sorry later.

■ If you are a female traveling alone and you are attacked outside your hotel or motel room or in the parking lot, faking fainting is a very effective self-defense measure. There is nothing that creates more panic in would-be criminals than a woman's fainting. If you do scream, yelling "fire" may get more attention and results than yelling "help."

■ Remember: Using good common sense and practicing reasonable safety measures are the best protections for avoiding becoming a victim of a crime while traveling.

...

Security and Safety Tips for Renters

APARTMENT RENTERS ARE EASY TARGETS IN TODAY'S HIGH-crime, tight-budget climate. Apartment owners are often apt to spend their money on "curb appeal" items which attract potential tenants rather than on security-related needs. These security and safety tips may help you in selecting your apartment home—then in being safe while you are in it.

- Before you begin to look for an apartment, try and find out as much as possible about the area of town you are considering. Places which may have useful information include police departments, chambers of commerce, apartment locator services, and local newspapers.

- When you are out looking for an apartment, pay particular attention to the surroundings. Beware of low-income housing projects, convenience stores, liquor stores, nightclubs, and other businesses that could attract would-be criminals.

- When you find an appealing apartment community, drive through the complex before going to the leasing office. Look at how well the grounds are maintained and the placement of lights. If the grounds appear to be unkempt and there are other tell-tale indicators of problems, such as abandoned vehicles in the parking lot, this may be a clue of how well the complex is managed. When speaking with a leasing agent, ask the following questions:

Q: What type of security measures does the complex take for the protection of its residents?

Q: What type of crimes have occurred at the complex?

Q: Have there ever been any rapes or sexual assaults committed at the complex?

Q: Do you have a security guard or security service that patrols the premises? If yes, what hours and days of the week do they patrol?

Q: How timely are repairs to lights, locks, and other security-related equipment?

Be cautious of responses such as:

"It is as safe here as anywhere."

"We have had some crimes, but no more than anywhere else."

"We have off-duty police officers that live on the premises."

"We have courtesy officers that make patrols."

If you receive such responses to your questions, make sure the leasing agent explains in detail what each means.

■ Ask to see the model apartment and have the leasing agent point out any security and safety measures therein.

■ When you are shown the apartment that is being rented to you, make sure that it is equipped with the same security and safety features that the model had.

■ Pay particular attention to the type of locks that are on the doors. Entry-way doors should be solid wood or metal, both of which will better resist external force.

The door should be equipped with a dead-bolt lock, with a minimum one-inch throw-bolt. There should also be a peephole and a security chain lock or U-bolt lock.

If the apartment has sliding-glass doors, they should be secured with a "Charlie Bar" device—a metal bar that sits in the door horizontally and secures the sliding portion of the door to the stationary wall—which is mounted in the center, or a wooden dowel which lays in the bottom track of the door. It is also recommended that the door be secured with a pin-type of lock that slides through the moving door and the stationary door. You should also request that the maintenance person install two or three screws in the top track of the sliding glass door to prevent its being lifted from its track.

If the apartment has French-style doors, they should have a double key-cylinder dead-bolt lock and a secondary lock such as a chain or U-bolt lock.

■ Look at the locks provided on windows. Like doors, windows should be equipped with secondary locking devices. These come in many different forms, from key locks and thumb screws to wooden pins or metal pins inserted through drilled holes to prevent their being forced open.

Once you move in, you many want to consider putting a small amount of Super Glue around the edges of the glass pane. This will add additional strength to the glass a burglar may be attempting to break.

■ If you are a single female or a male living with a female roommate, you should consider asking for a second- or third-story apartment. Rapists often target women living in downstairs apartments.

■ Ask the leasing agent what police agency serves the complex and how often they patrol the premises.

■ You may want to call the police agency servicing the complex and ask to speak with someone who can give you a feel for what type of complex it is.

■ Before making the decision to move into the complex, drive back at night and observe the lighting. Make sure that the parking lots, stairways, hallways, breezeways and areas at the rear of the apartment buildings are well lit.

■ On your return visit, you may want to stop and talk with a resident and asked what his or her experience has been at the complex.

- Look to see if the complex is fenced around the perimeter or if it has access-control gates. However, don't get a false sense of security if the complex has access-control gates. They offer very little security if not manned twenty-four hours a day and are often broken or in need of other repairs which render them worthless.

- If there is shrubbery planted near doors or windows, you should ask that it be trimmed or removed before you move in. Shrubbery often provides excellent hiding places for would-be criminals.

- If you like the complex, but it doesn't have the type of locking devices recommended above, read the lease to see if it prohibits you from installing them. If it does then you might want to consider another complex.

- Once you move in, consider installing a single-cylinder dead bolt with a one- to two-inch throw bolt on your bedroom door. This allows you additional security inside your apartment and provides a "safe room" in which to take refuge in the event of a break-in while you are at home. You should have a flashlight, telephone, and emergency phone numbers in this room as well.

- After moving in, mark valuable items that burglars are likely to steal. Record the serial numbers of your television and stereo equipment and engrave your social security number or driver's license number on the bottom. This will help the police to identify your property if stolen.

- You should keep expensive items such as jewelry in a bank safe-deposit box, not in your apartment.

- Request that the leasing office notify you before allowing maintenance men or service people into your apartment. Then request that they leave you written notification attesting to who entered your apartment and what type of work was performed.

- When leaving or returning to your apartment, always walk

briskly and with confidence. Keep your keys in your hand and remember they can make an excellent weapon in the event you are attacked.

- If you know you are going to be returning after dark, always make sure that you leave all your exterior lights and at least one interior light on. You should also consider leaving a radio or television set playing as well. Automatic timers can be used to vary turning lights, radios, or televisions on and off.

- Remember that most apartment front-door and patio-door lights operate by switches inside your apartment. Leave these lights on during the night.

- If you feel it is dark behind your apartment, request in writing that the complex add additional lights.

- Many apartments today are equipped with burglar alarms. Remember most are not operable unless you sign up with the company providing the system and pay a monthly fee for it to be monitored. If you elect to take the service, you should test your system at least once a month to insure that it is working properly. The company providing the alarm will provide you with the procedures for testing your alarm.

- Never allow entry into your apartment by an unexpected delivery person, salesman, or repairman. Always ask for positive identification, and if you still have suspicions, call the person's office for verification.

- Never allow someone to come into your apartment to use the telephone. Tell the person through the door that you will be happy to dial the number and relay a message. Never leave an extra key "hidden" outside your home. Smart criminals normally look in "hiding places" first before trying to break in.

- Never leave notes outside your door announcing your absence.

- If your name is required at the mailbox, always use your first initial instead of your name.

- Never leave your house keys with your car keys if you are

parking at a parking lot.

- If your complex has a "Neighborhood Watch" or "Crime Watch" program, participate and attend the meetings. It's good advice and gives you an opportunity to meet some of the other tenants at the complex.

- Try to familiarize yourself with what your immediate neighbors look like.

- Never hesitate to report to the leasing office or call the police about anything that appears to be suspicious. Something that looks slightly out of place may mean criminal activity.

- If you should become a victim of a crime, report it immediately to the police and then to the apartment management.

- The last thing you should do at night is check and make sure that all of your doors and windows are shut and locked and that your outside lights are on and operating.

- Never leave doors and windows open—even if you are at home. Screen doors or screens on your windows provide *no* protection against would-be criminals.

- If you should have your keys stolen or they are lost, immediately have your apartment locks changed before spending another night in your apartment.

- If you are a single female, and have a telephone answering machine, consider having a male friend record the outgoing message for you.

- If you are a single female, avoid publishing your first name in the telephone directory.

- If you notice any outside building lights or street lights that are not working, report them to the leasing office immediately. If they are not repaired within twenty-four hours, call and report them again.

- Never include your address in a newspaper advertisement.

- If the apartment complex publishes a newsletter, ask them

not to use your full name or list Mr. and Mrs. if they list new residents.

■ Check into taking out a renters' insurance policy to cover the loss of your property from theft. These policies are normally inexpensive and will provide you with added protection.

■ If you should receive suspicious calls, hang up, but take them seriously. If they continue, report them to the police and the telephone company.

■ If you walk or jog around your complex for exercise, be aware of your surroundings and never wear headphones; they block one of your most important self-defense senses, your hearing. If you walk or jog at night or in the early morning hours, stay in well-lit areas. Have a friend join you if possible.

■ Keep a record of any representations made by the apartment complex about security or safety issues or any requests that you make of the complex. Record the dates and the name of the person with whom you dealt. These could prove to be very helpful in finding the apartment owner liable in the event you should become a crime victim there.

These security and safety recommendations will help you select a new apartment home. If you practice them, they can decrease the likelihood of you becoming a victim of a crime. However, there are determined criminals who will find a way to commit crimes in the face of the most sophisticated security systems. Therefore, it is imperative that you always stay alert and practice reasonable security measures to protect yourself from the potential threat of a criminal attack.

■ ■ ■

Security and Safety Tips for Shoppers

EVERY DAY, MILLIONS OF MEN, WOMEN, AND CHILDREN VEN-
ture from their homes or from work to shop in area shopping malls, strip
shopping centers, or the corner convenience store. However, in today's
climate of random violence, the seemingly innocent act of shopping does
not guarantee safety from crimes such as car-jacking, robberies, and
assaults. Shoppers can be easy targets for criminals. By following these security and safety tips while shopping or walking or otherwise traveling to and
from home or work, your chances of becoming a victim of a crime will
decrease dramatically.

IF YOU ARE DRIVING

- Make sure that you keep your car in good repair.

- Always make sure that you have an adequate supply of gas
in your car.

- Plan your travel route ahead of time and don't stray into areas
of town with which you are not familiar.

- Remember: a car phone is an excellent security device.

- Always keep your car doors locked and windows rolled up,
especially in inner cities. Invite a family member or friend to

go shopping or run errands with you, if possible. If you are in your car and feel that you are being followed, drive to the nearest police station or fire station. If there are none nearby, you may want to consider driving into the entrance of a hospital emergency room.

- Walk to and from your car with your key in your hand. Remember, keys can make an excellent weapon against a sudden attack.

- During daylight hours, always try and park as close to the mall or store entrance as possible.

- At night, park in well-lit areas.

- Avoid poorly lit parking lots or parking decks. If you have to park in a parking deck, try and park on the lower decks and avoid using the elevators. Elevators in parking garages offer concealment for would-be assailants. Also, be watchful for anyone hiding between or behind parked cars.

- Always lock your car before walking into the mall or store.

- Many shopping malls have valet parking attendants; use them if at all possible.

- Always look around before getting out of your car. If you should see anything at all that makes you feel uncomfortable, don't get out. Always trust your instincts.

- If you think someone is following you to or from your car, turn around and look. A surprise hostile look or aggressive words might change a would-be assailant's mind.

- If someone should grab you, consider acting as if you are fainting, or scream "Fire!" which has proven to be more of an attention-getter than yelling "Help!"

- Try to avoid leaving packages or other valuables in plain sight in your car.

- Always look into your car before opening the door, to make sure that no one is hiding in your car to attack you.

IF YOU ARE WALKING

- Remember: the best choice is not to walk alone.

- Always stay on well-lit and well-populated streets.

- Don't stray into strange areas.

- Use well-traveled routes.

- Walk briskly and with confidence. Stay away from bushes, buildings, and entrances to alleyways.

- Be alert and aware of your surroundings. If you feel someone is following you, turn and look at them. Cross the street or change your pace, then look again. Remember, a hostile look or aggressive words may well change the mind of a would-be assailant.

- Never walk alone if you are upset, have been drinking, or are taking medications.

- Avoid using headphones. They make you more vulnerable to a surprise attack.

- If a car follows you or stops, change direction, and head for safety toward other people, stores, a house, or a church.

- Always carry enough change to use a pay phone in the event you need to call someone to pick you up. Remember, you don't need a quarter to call the operator or dial "911."

- Never hitchhike or accept a ride from a stranger, no matter how innocent the person or persons look who are offering the ride.

- If a driver of a car should pull over to the curb to ask you for directions, never walk over to the car. Stay in the center of the sidewalk and give the directions from there.

IF YOU ARE ATTACKED

- Remember: your best weapon is *common sense*.

- Trust your instincts.

- Try to control your emotions and remain calm.

- Can you fight back? If the person is armed with a weapon, don't ever think about resisting. Generally, if robbery is the motive, the robber will not harm you if you cooperate with his demands. Do exactly what he tells you, and don't resist or hesitate to give up any of your personal belongings he may ask for. Property can be replaced—your life cannot. If the attacker is unarmed and you feel confident that you can fight back and escape, then trust your instincts. Remember, areas such as the eyes, throat, temples, kneecaps, and groin are good targets. If the assailant has approached you from the back, hit him in the stomach with your elbow or stomp on his foot. Biting, scratching, and kicking are other defensive tactics.

- Scream as loud as possible. Remember, "Fire!" is more effective than "Help!"

- You may want to discourage your attacker by displaying anger, acting crazy, faking fainting, or acting as if you are going to throw up.

- Try and always think rationally and evaluate your resources and options. But always do what you feel is going to keep you alive.

GENERAL TIPS

- Never carry large sums of cash. If you do carry cash, avoid flashing it when paying for purchases.

- Avoid wearing flashy jewelry when you are out shopping.

- If you are a female and carrying a purse, always carry it securely against your body or clutch it firmly in your hands.

- You may want to consider carrying a personal protection alarm. These may deter or scare off would-be attackers, while alerting others that you are in need of help.

- A police whistle attached to your key chain may prove to be useful in summoning help, in the event you are attacked.

- If you need to use an automatic teller machine (ATM), you may want to consider using one that is located inside a mall or grocery store. A would-be criminal is less likely to attack you inside of a store than outside, where they can easily escape on foot or in a waiting car.

- If you decide to carry a weapon of any type, be familiar with its use, and be *mentally* prepared to use it. If you are not 100 percent mentally prepared to use a weapon, then it is best that you don't carry one. More likely than not, it can be taken away from you and used against you. It could also provoke a violent attack.

AFTER AN ATTACK

- Go to a safe place and call the police. Then call a friend or family member and let the person know what has happened and where you are.

- Try and remember as much as possible about the attacker—physical description, approximate age, dress, mode of escape, and anything he or she said to you during the attack.

- Do not disturb anything in the area where the attack occurred. It is important to preserve as much physical evidence as possible for court use if your attacker is identified.

- Reach out to others for help in dealing with the aftermath of an attack. Don't hesitate to seek professional help.

As with any security and safety tips, these precise rules may not prevent you from becoming a victim of a crime, but they may prevent or reduce the likelihood of your being injured during an attack.

■ ■ ■

CHAPTER SIXTEEN

What to Do if You Should Become a Victim of Rape

RAPE CONTINUES TO BE ONE OF THE FASTEST-GROWING VIO-
lent crimes in today's society. Women living alone in apartments, staying
in hotels/motels, out shopping, or traveling to and from work may be a
rapist's easiest targets. In order to better understand this heinous crime, it
may help to know a little more about a typical rapist and why and how
he chooses his victims.

Rapists are generally grouped into two basic categories: serial and
opportunistic.

Serial rapists by and large have above-average intelligence and stable
employment, are well groomed and take pride in their personal appearance. They exhibit a wide range of emotions from "caring and humorous"
to "cold and aloof." Most serial rapists tend to meet and interact with people easily in social settings; they will eventually attempt to dominate personal relationships by using manipulation and cunning. The vast majority of serial rapists were abused as children—a fact that may be one of the
major contributing factors in their becoming the violent people they
are. Their attacks are not sexually motivated.

Opportunistic rapists, on the other hand, may be the only class of sexual offenders whose primary motive is raping women for sexual gratification. The opportunistic rapist normally targets his victims during the commission of another crime, such as the burglary of an apartment or a
hotel/motel room. Often, while committing the crime, he discovers the

victim inside the dwelling or the victim walks in while the criminal is there. The criminal then finds the victim to be sexually attractive and proceeds to rape her impulsively.

Victims of serial and opportunistic rapists are generally strangers to them, and this fact accounts for why rapists are so easily able to evade being identified and arrested. Also, it is noteworthy that most rape victims are singled out more for their vulnerability than any other particular or personal characteristic. It is this fact that justifies a person's taking personal security and safety measures and practicing them both at home and away.

If you are attacked, the optimum time to defend yourself is normally within the first ten to twenty seconds. If you are not emotionally capable of inflicting harm on the rapist, then you should avoid resisting his attack by fighting. If you choose to fight back, there may be many items at your disposal that will make effective weapons in warding off your attacker. At home, things such as hair spray, bleach, fingernail polish remover, combs, a hot curling iron, hot water, and various kitchen tools may prove to be excellent weapons. Remember, trust your instincts. Areas such as the eyes, throat, temples, kneecaps, and groin are the best targets. If the assailant has approached you from the rear, hit him with your elbow to the stomach or stomp on his foot. Biting, scratching, and kicking are other defensive tactics.

If the rapist is armed with a weapon of any type, then resisting may only serve to bring harm to yourself. However, a rapist may be reluctant to have sex with someone who has fainted, confesses to having a venereal disease or AIDS, says she is menstruating, or has to relieve herself or vomit.

IF YOU ARE RAPED

If you are not able to get away and fall victim to a rape, remember that he is the criminal—not you. After the rapist has left, you should take the following steps:

- If you are in your apartment or home, immediately lock your doors and windows, then dial "911." If the rapist has disconnected your telephone, crack open a window and scream "Fire!" If you cannot summon help that way, you should arm yourself with a glass of bleach or hot water to throw in the eyes of your assailant if he should still be lurking in the area. Run to the nearest neighbor for help. This is why it is important to know your neighbors and know if they are home or not.

- If you are outside your home when the rape occurs, go to the nearest open business or pay phone and call the police.

- During the attack, try and get a good look at your attacker and remember as much as possible about him as you can. Things such as his speech, dress, etc., may provide useful information to the police in trying to identify him later.

- Don't use the bathroom, shower, bathe, douche, or comb your hair after the rape. Such activities may destroy valuable evidence which can help to identify your assailant. Preserve the clothing you were wearing during the attack.

- Don't clean up anything or disturb the scene of the attack.

- Don't touch anything that the assailant may have touched.

- If possible, immediately write down or tape record all the details of the attack. Don't leave anything out—no matter how insignificant it may seem to you.

- After the police arrive, it is likely they will transport you to a hospital for an examination. If they don't, demand that you be taken and that a "rape test," something with which they should be familiar, be performed.

- Before leaving for the hospital, call a family member or close friend and ask him or her to meet you at the hospital. This support is very important and greatly needed.

- At the hospital, make sure that you get medical treatment for any injuries and are tested for venereal diseases and pregnancy.

- Demand that they test you for AIDS and ask how often you should be tested in the future.

- If you live in an apartment, make sure that either the police or you notify the apartment management as soon as possible with the details of the attack so they can warn others in the complex.

- Share your feelings with your family, close friends, and co-workers.

AFTER THE ATTACK: REACHING OUT FOR HELP

Being a victim of a crime such as rape takes a tremendous psychological toll, and many rape victims feel rage, anger, guilt, and helplessness. Some rape victims blame themselves for what happened to them. Only recently have researchers found that many rape victims suffer as victims of war, natural disasters, and catastrophic illness do. In addition, the fear and emotional distress of the rape victim often extends to the victim's family and friends. These traumatic effects on victims of rape can last for months, years, or a lifetime. That's why it is important that you don't try and deal with the aftermath of a rape by yourself.

There are many avenues available to you, but you must first realize that you need the help and support these groups have to offer. The first level of support and understanding normally comes from family and friends, but they may not be professionally trained to give you the long-term counseling and treatment you need. Most major hospitals or communities have Rape Crisis Centers staffed with professional counselors trained to deal specifically with the trauma associated with being raped. If the counselors at the rape crisis center feel they are not providing the type of help you need, they will know other professionals in the community they can refer you to.

Some rape victims have found that getting involved with volunteer work in the local rape crisis centers or crime-victims advocacy groups is a way to help deal with their own healing process.

Most people don't want to think that they can become a victim of a crime such as rape. If we hear about someone being raped in the news, it easy to say to ourselves, "It's not going to happen to me." But the reality, as demonstrated in the chapters of this book, is that crime can occur any place and any time, and all of us can become its victims.

Afterword

The acts of violence depicted in this book continue to occur in our society on a daily basis. In recent months, the nation has been stunned by the shooting rampage of Colin Ferguson, a Jamaican immigrant who opened fire with a semi-automatic handgun on a crowded New York commuter train, killing and injuring dozens of people as the train pulled into a suburban station during the afternoon rush hour. In a small California town, 12-year-old Polly Klaas was kidnapped from her home during a slumber party and brutally murdered by a paroled convict. In St. Louis, a frightened community mourns the death of two young girls abducted and murdered as they returned from school. Police fear that a child serial killer is stalking their streets. In Atlanta, a college freshman home for the holidays (and son of an Atlanta police detective) was gunned down in the driveway of a friend's home, a victim of a car-jacking.

When such acts occur, we are saddened and paralyzed by their senseless nature, and trying to understand them only boggles the mind. These crimes give politicians, from the president of the United States to local city council members, plenty to talk about—from gun control to more police, from more judges to more prisons, and above all, harsher sentences. However, these reactions of politicians are only one answer to the very complex issue of violence in our country. We, the people of this country, must take off the blinders and realize that we, too, could become the topic of the evening news and that these horrible acts of crime can reach out and claim another victim at any place and any time.

As this book demonstrates, we must take all the necessary precautions to protect ourselves and our loved ones. We do not have to be willing victims. But most of all, we need to examine the moral issues surrounding us, such as the glorified violence our children are subjected to in the movies, television and video games, and the fact that kids carry guns and other weapons to school because it is the "in-thing" to do. We need to teach our children that being bad is wrong, drugs are not "cool," and weapons of death should not be used to take another human being's life.

There are answers to these problems, but they start at home and with each of us.

Nietzsche's Dance

Nietzsche's Dance

*Resentment, Reciprocity and Resistance
in Social Life*

GEORG STAUTH and BRYAN S. TURNER

Basil Blackwell

British Library Cataloguing in Publication Data

Stauth, Georg
Nietzsche's dance: resentment, reciprocity and resistance in social life.
1. Nietzsche, Friedrich
I. Title   II. Turner, Bryan S.
193   B3317

ISBN 0–631–15407–8

Library of Congress Cataloging in Publication Data

Typeset in 10.5 on 12 pt Ehrhardt
by Columns of Reading
Printed in Great Britain

Contents

Acknowledgement

This book was partly conceived and partly written on the Murray River in 1985. We would like to thank Liba Liba for providing the houseboat and extend our grateful thanks to the crew members, both willing and unwilling: Joy Parham and Tony Parham, Adrian Vickery and Bozina Vickery, Karen Lane and Mona Abaza, Lena Sudano and Renato Novelli. We believe it entirely appropriate that a book on Friedrich Nietzsche should have been pursued on the banks of the Murray in South Australia since this book is about dancing and eating as modes of the everyday life which are often submerged within scientific sociology. While Nietzsche searched for health on the tops of mountains, we sought a new way in sociology on the banks of a river.

Various aspects of this book have been presented at seminars and conferences at Flinders University, La Trobe University and at the Conference on French Thought organized by the journal *Theory, Culture and Society*. We are grateful to Mike Featherstone and Roland Robertson for comments on an early draft of chapter 6. A version of chapter 3 was first published in the *Zeitschrift für Soziologie*, volume 15(2), 1986. We are particularly grateful to Sue Manser who typed the entire manuscript.

Abbreviations

and works by principal authors cited or referred to in the text

Works of T. W. Adorno

AE   *Against Epistemology: A Meta-Critique*, Oxford, Oxford University Press, 1982.

AT   *Aesthetic Theory*, London, Routledge and Kegan Paul, 1985.

DE   *Dialectic of Enlightenment* (with Max Horkheimer), New York, Herder and Herder, 1972.

INH   'The idea of natural history', *Telos*, 60, 1984, pp. 111–24.

JA   *The Jargon of Authenticity*, London, Routledge and Kegan Paul, 1973.

MM   *Minima Moralia: Reflections from Damaged Life*, London, New Left Books, 1974.

ND   *Negative Dialects*, London, Routledge and Kegan Paul, 1973.

P   *Prisms: Cultural Criticism and Society*, Cambridge, Mass., The MIT Press, 1981.

Works of M. Foucault

AK   *The Archaeology of Knowledge*, (1966), London Tavistock, 1974.

BC   *The Birth of the Clinic*, (1963), London, Tavistock, 1973.

DP   *Discipline and Punish, the birth of the prison*, (1975), London, Allen Lane, Penguin, 1977.

HB   *Herculine Barbin, being the recently discovered memoirs of a nineteenth-century French hermaphrodite*, (1978), Brighton, Harvester Press, 1980.

HS   *The History of Sexuality, vol. 1, an introduction*, (1976), Harmondsworth, Penguin, 1981.

IP   *I, Pierre Riviere, having slaughtered my mother, my sister and my brother. A case of parricide in the nineteenth century*, (1973), London, Tavistock, 1978.

LCM *Language, Counter-Memory, Practice*, Oxford, Basil Blackwell, 1977.

MC   *Madness and Civilization*, (1961), London, Tavistock, 1971.

NAP *This is not a Pipe*, (1982), Berkeley, University of California Press, 1983.

OT   *The Order of Things, an archaeology of the human sciences*, (1966), London, Tavistock, 1974.

PK   *Power/Knowledge, selected interviews and other writings 1972-1977*, edited by Colin Gordon, Brighton, Harvester Press, 1980.
     'The subject and power', (1982). In H. L. Dreyfus and P. Rabinow, *Michel Foucault, beyond structuralism and hermeneutics*, Brighton, Harvester Press, pp. 208-26.

Works of S. Freud

The Standard Edition of the Complete Works of Sigmund Freud, trans. and ed. James Strachey, London, Hogarth Press, 1953-66, 24 vols.
Totem and Taboo, (1913), vol. 13, 1953, pp. 1-161.
The Future of an Illusion, (1927), vol. 21, 1961, pp. 1-56.
Civilization and its Discontents, (1930), vol. 21, pp. 57-145.
Moses and Monotheism, (1939), vol. 23.
Leonardo da Vinci, a memory of his childhood, London, Routledge and Kegan Paul, 1957.

Works of J. Habermas

KHI *Knowledge and Human Interests*, (1968), trans. J. Shapiro, London, Heinemann, 1971.
     The Theory of Communicative Action, (1984), trans. T. McCarthy, Boston, Beacon Press, vol. 1.
     Der philosophische Diskurs der Moderne, (1985), Frankfurt, Zwölf Vorlesungen.

Works of F. Nietzsche

The Complete Works of Friedrich Nietzsche, ed. Oscar Levy, New York, Macmillan, 1909-11, 18 vols.

Abbreviations

AC   *The Anti-Christ*, (1888), trans. W. Kaufmann, *The Portable Nietzsche*, (New York, Viking, 1954); trans. with R. J. Hollingdale, with *Twilight*, Harmondsworth, Penguin, 1968.
BGE   *Beyond Good and Evil*, (1886), trans. R. J. Hollingdale, Harmondsworth, Penguin, 1973).
BT   *The Birth of Tragedy*, (1982), trans. W. Kaufmann, with *The Case of Wagner*, New York, Vintage, 1966.
CW   *The Case of Wagner*, (1888), trans. W. Kaufmann, with *The Birth of Tragedy*, New York, Vintage, 1966.
EH   *Ecce Homo*, (1888), trans. W. Kaufmann, with *Genealogy*, (New York, Vintage, 1968); trans. R. J. Hollingdale, Harmondsworth, Penguin, 1979.
GM   *On the Genealogy of Morals*, (1887), trans. W. Kaufmann and R. J. Hollingdale, New York, Vintage, 1968.
HAH   *Human, All Too Human*, (1878), trans. H. Zimmern and P. V. Cohn, *Complete Works*, vol. VI.
NCW   *Nietzsche contra Wagner*, (1888), trans. W. Kaufmann, *The Portable Nietzsche*, New York, Viking, 1954.

TI   *Twilight of the Idols*, (1888), trans. W. Kaufmann, *The Portable Nietzsche*, (New York, Viking, 1954); trans. R. J. Hollingdale, *The Anti-Christ*, Harmondsworth, Penguin, 1968.
TOS   *Thoughts Out of Season*, (1873-6), also referred to as *Untimely Meditations, four essays on the advantage and disadvantage of history for life*, trans. P. Preuss, Indianapolis, Hackett, 1980.
WP   *The Will to Power* (1883-8), trans, W. Kaufmann and R. J. Hollingdale, New York, Vintage, 1968.
Z   *Thus Spoke Zarathustra*, (1883-5), trans. R. J. Hollingdale, Harmondsworth, Penguin, 1973.

Works of M. Weber

ES   *Economy and Society*, trans. G. Roth and C. Wittich, Berkeley, University of California Press, 1978, 2 vols.
FW   *From Weber, essays in sociology*, ed. and trans. H. H. Gerth and C. Wright Mills, London, Routledge and Kegan Paul, 1961.
GEH   *General Economic History*, New Brunswick, Collier, 1981, p. ix.
PE   *The Protestant Ethic and the Spirit of Capitalism*, trans. Talcott Parsons, London, Unwin University Books. 1930.
SR   *The Sociology of Religion*, trans. Ephraim Fischoff, London, Methuen, 1966.

Introduction: Nietzsche's Dance

Nostalgia

There is a profound crisis within contemporary social philosophy which merely reflects the deeper problems of modern culture. This crisis is in part a crisis of reason itself. It is commonplace to talk about the end of the rationalist project and the collapse of modernity. This transformation of European consciousness is clearly identified with the philosophy and outlook of Nietzsche. In the nineteenth century, Nietzsche had proclaimed that God was dead and that the value system of traditional Christianity had been dissolved. In the gap left by God, sociology and other new forms of thought constituted an alternative to absolutism. According to Weber, we live in a world of increasing rationalization but this rationalization relates to technique and the means to achieving social goals. However, the values which are required by rationalism itself are opaque.

In the contemporary world, the project of modernity has become the crisis of post-modernity, because the confidence in a world which was predictable, orderly and rational has given way to the celebration of disorder and the non-rational. Once more, Nietzsche's name is evoked in order to justify the end of all projects. It is Nietzsche, the anti-rationalist and the priest of discontinuity, who presides over the post-structuralist world. This development is particularly important in the French post-structuralist movement led by Deleuze, Lyotard, Guattari and above all by Foucault.

The issue of post-modernism has not, as yet, clearly found a place in American sociology. The problem of rationalism is nevertheless widespread within contemporary American thought. It is evident, for example, that the whole problem of Nietzsche, nihilism and rationality is about to sweep across the American intellectual system with the appearance of *Beyond Nihilsm* (Schutte, 1984) and *Prophets of Extremity* (Megill, 1985). In one of the most influential studies of the modern period, Marshall Berman (1982, p. 15) observed that 'to be modern is to find ourselves in an environment that promises us adventure, power, joy, growth, transformation of our souls and the world – and, at the same time, that threatens to destroy everything we have, everything we know, everything we are.' In the words of Karl Marx we live in a world where 'all that is solid melts into air.' Of course, this crisis of knowledge and rationalism was quite familiar to writers like Tönnies, Weber and Simmel, but in the contemporary environment we have the added problems of ecological disaster, economic collapse and nuclear destruction. The scale of our dilemma is increasingly complex and increasingly out of control. In a period of crisis and confusion, it is perhaps not unexpected that Nietzsche should return to social and philosophical dominance in the contemporary intellectual movement.

If we live in a world of modernistic crisis, then we might expect, and we do perceive, a certain nostalgic movement in the contemporary view of society, nature and the individual. The loss of community, moral certainty and genuine experience of culture has led social philosophers to search for more secure foundations for identity and personal continuity in traditional cultures and institutions. The problem of nostalgia has a long history in western thought and medical science. Nostalgia is the pain for home which, as a medical condition, was well known in medieval science, but it was the Swiss physician Johannes Hofer who, in the seventeenth century, applied the term to Swiss mercenaries fighting far from their homeland. Their symptoms included despondency, melancholy, anorexia and often suicide attempts (Davis, 1974). A disease was created as a scientific label for the traditional English notion of homesickness, the German feeling of *Heimweh* and the French *maladie du pays*. In our time the word has drifted away from its pathological bases to find a location in a cultural reaction to the loss of social stability and comfort in the contemporary urban environment of endless social change and disruption (Davis, 1974). Of course, the death of God is precisely part of this homelessness.

Nietzsche is characteristically connected with the modern crisis because, it is argued, he identified the problem of uncertainty in a theory of language. In this perspective, our certainty about the world evaporates in the knowledge that all thought is merely metaphorical, including our thinking about thought. Since our confidence in the world disappears down an infinite regress of metaphors, we are utterly alone both in culture and in consciousness. While there is much in

Nietzsche's commentary on the modern world to justify such a position, it is a misleading analysis of Nietzsche's philosophy, which was fundamentally committed to the process of revaluation of values. It is not enough, therefore, merely to wallow in nihilism; indeed, Nietzsche was one of the most profound critics of such loss of direction. Nietzsche's project was to develop a new morality, but a new morality anchored in the prominence of our physical embodiment in the world. In this study, therefore, we emphasize first the importance of revaluation and Utopian thought against nihilism. Secondly, we argue that for Nietzsche the body and human embodiment were crucial to his whole philosophical and artistic response to the problem of nihilism and the collapse of traditional morality. Thirdly, it is argued via Nietzsche that the everyday world is the *habitus* for this embodied experience which provides the foundation for a critique of abstract rationalism detached from life. This project provides the basis for a Nietzschean criticism of institutional power over the everyday life, rational knowledge over the body and the artificial world of the state over the reality of everyday interaction and reciprocity. This study is, in short, an attempt to bring sociology back to its origins, namely an exploration of fellowship (*socius*) through the analysis of reciprocity against the revenge of institutions and rationalism.

The Reciprocity of Nietzsche

Conventional textbooks in sociology normally identify Marx, Durkheim and Weber as founding fathers of the discipline. Where there is a search for more distant foundations, some historians of sociology would locate the origins of sociological inquiry with St. Simon and Comte. These origins of sociology are, of course, the objects of considerable dispute; the dispute being typically organised around the Marx/Weber divergence. Occasionally, there are attempts to expand this list of founders and, in recent years, Simmel has been identified as a neglected figure in the development of social theory (Frisby, 1981; 1984). This study is based upon the argument that Nietzsche is the absent giant of contemporary social thought and that Nietzsche's contribution to contemporary social analysis has been systematically negated and suppressed. In particular, the discourse on rationalism has intentionally suppressed the major part played by Nietzsche's cultural criticism in our understanding of the modern world.

There is, however, a minor commentary on the relationship between Nietzsche and Weber (Fleischmann, 1964; Kent, 1983). Nietzsche's

3

influence on Weber is typically seen to be dominant in the area of political sociology where Nietzsche's conception of conflict and opposition was influential in the development of Weber's view of power politics (Turner, 1982). There is a view that Nietzsche's views on the superman provided part of the background for Weber's concept of charisma and the importance of Nietzsche on Weber's analysis of leadership has also been the subject of some recent discussion (Eden, 1984). It could also be suggested that Nietzsche's concept of resentment was influential in Weber's sociology and specifically in his sociology of religion where the concept played a part in the elaboration of the notion of pariah people in connection with the social location of Judaism (Sigrist, 1971; Turner, 1983; Zeitlin, 1984). These comment-aries do not, however, constitute a systematic evaluation of Nietzsche's impact on Weber. We argue that Weber implicitly disguised the Nietzschean themes which in fact characterized his total sociological perspective. Nietzsche's views on the death of God, perspectivism and relativity fundamentally conditioned Weber's epistemology and philos-ophy of social science. The whole theme of rationalization was derivative and parasitic upon Nietzsche's own treatment of the relationship between knowledge, institutions and power. The theme of resentment was constitutive of Weber's sociology of religion, but within a broader canvas this theme determined Weber's attitude towards morality and modernity.

Nietzsche's influence on Weber was also mediated through the work of Simmel who was a serious student of Nietzsche's legacy. For example, Simmel published a book on Schopenhauer and Nietzsche in 1907 and defended Nietzsche against Tönnies's attack in *The Nietzsche Cult* in 1897. Nietzsche also influenced Simmel's approach to the problem of abstraction and rationalization in his philosophy of money; this treatment of intellectualism and exchange was clearly in line with Weber's development of the themes of abstraction in law, religion and economic relations. More generally, Nietzsche's attempt to rethink the problem of the individual was also influential in Simmel's approach and analysis of the individual and society. Simmel sought to avoid any reification of society through the development of the notion of sociation. Nietzsche was part of the background to Simmel's attempt to formulate a theory of modernism, but this influence has been inadequately discussed and appreciated in the literature on Simmel. There is no question, therefore, that both Weber and Simmel attempted to develop the modern discipline of sociology under the philosophical influence of Nietzsche but the extent and character of that influence has yet to be fully explored and documented.

4

In the German context, Tönnies, Weber and Simmel should be interpreted as will-to-life philosophers, responding to social changes which they regarded as negative and artificial. Their will-to-life perspective was shaped primarily by Schopenhauer and Nietzsche. In particular, we can trace Nietzsche's will-to-power through the whole movement of German social science as a reaction to the social destruction brought about by State capitalism and as an intellectual response to the system-building of Hegel. This reaction is especially prominent in Tönnies's distinction between *Gemeinschaft* and *Gesellschaft* as two forms of will (Atoji, 1984).

Although Freud is rarely regarded as a primary founder of social science, it is clear that Freudian psycho-analytic theory has played a significant part in the development of, for example Parsons' sociology and treatment of personality, as well as influencing the work of the Frankfurt School who saw, in Freud, a useful point of departure for the development of a critical theory of psychology and personality. Freud was important for Parsons in the development of the theory of the social system in 1951 but this impact became increasingly significant as Parsons went on to develop the theory of action in relation to the family, socialization and interaction. In addition Freud was important in the development of Adorno's view of enlightenment, Marcuse's theory of sexuality and the development in critical theory of the notion of the 'authoritarian personality'. In *Eros and Civilisation*, Marcuse identified Nietzsche as a significant turning point in the history of western philosophy, since it was Nietzsche who exposed the pretentions of the rationalization of the world through reason. In Marcuse's interpretation of Nietzsche, the false moralities of the world have the function of justifying and compensating the underprivileged while protecting their overlords from any recognition of genuine existence. These false philosophies brought about the eventual degeneration of life instincts, that is, the decline of man as such (Marcuse, 1969). In Marcuse, therefore, the work of Freud and Nietzsche was brought together to provide a critique of the one-dimensionality of the modern world. Freud's psychoanalytical method was also adopted by Habermas in the notion of free exchange and the emergence of true forms of knowledge. In Habermas' critical theory, Freudian analysis was identified as a model of valid enquiry into the condition of human beings through the free exchange of information. At a more profound level, Freud provided part of the essential framework of Rief's critique of modern morality (Fromm, 1980). More recently, Freud has been appropriated by a diversity of writers including Althusser and Lacan who have attempted to rediscover and relocate the radical features of Freudian analysis (Kurzweil, 1980), but this rediscovery did not lead directly to a re-evaluation of Nietzsche.

Freud's influence, both in terms of theory and practice, is obviously extensive and fundamental to various perspectives on modern society and sexuality, but Freud's dependence on Nietzsche has been inadequately recognised and analysed in contemporary social theory. This neglect of the Nietzschean background to Freud may be, itself, an effect of Freud's denial of Nietzsche. Freud persistently contrasted the importance of his own scientific and 'laborious' investigations with Nietzsche's flashes of insight which did not amount to a significant development of psycho-analysis (Anderson, 1980). Freud's labour was very different from Nietzsche's dance. On other occasions, Freud in, for example, *History of the Psycho-Analytic Movement*, argued that he had denied himself the pleasure of reading the works of Nietzsche since he did not want to hamper his own intellectual development. In his autobiographical study of 1925, Freud went on to recognize, indirectly, that what he called the 'premonitions and insights' of Nietzsche often paralleled his own achievements in psycho-analysis. Freud, therefore, opposed his science, work and objectivity against Nietzsche's art, play and subjectivity. Freud also undermined the stature of Nietzsche indirectly by various unwarranted commentaries on Nietzsche's alleged homosexuality when Freud suggested that the enigma of Nietzsche was bound up with his passive and deviant sexuality. Specifically, Freud alleged that Nietzsche had contracted syphilis in a male brothel in Italy.

In reality, it is clear that Freud was aware, in the most systematic manner, of Nietzsche's philosophy. For example, Freud was a member at the University of Vienna between 1873 and 1877 of the Society for German Students where he specifically studied the works of Schopenhauer, Wagner and Nietzsche. Joseph Paneth, who was a close friend of Freud, had also studied Nietzsche's philosophy in Brentano's lectures in 1874. Freud also admitted to Fliess in February, 1900, that he had purchased the works of Nietzsche and finally we should note that Freud became a close friend of Lou Andreas-Salomé who came to Vienna to study with Freud in 1912. Salomé had met Nietzsche in May, 1882, and shortly afterwards Nietzsche had proposed that they should be married.

These biographical details are interesting but not necessarily crucial. What we should note is that the basic assumptions of Freud's psycho-analytical theory had been clearly worked out by Nietzsche long before Freud formalized his clinical experience into a theory of the psyche, society and civilization. Nietzsche's views on the tension, conflicts and resolutions between Apollo and Dionysus anticipated and provided a basis for Freud's view of the conflict between sexuality and civilization. Nietzsche's notion in the analysis of resentment that the weak disguise their real feelings of anger and resentment behind the veneer of false morality laid some of the foundations for Freud's view on transference and sublimation. Because the weak cannot express their violence in public, they generate neuroses and illness as a substitute for genuine expression. More importantly, Nietzsche developed the notion of the bad conscience (that is, guilt) and treated that conscience as the source of illness, where men could not resolve the conflict between their instinctual life and social demands. Nietzsche went on to argue that instincts that do not discharge themselves outwardly must turn inward through a process of internalization to generate neurosis and disease. The denial of enjoyment became the basis of guilt and what we call 'civilization.' Nietzsche's contribution to the historical analysis of guilt in the generation of civilization has not been fully appreciated in the recent literature on the culture of guilt (Carroll, 1985). There was also a substantial overlap between Nietzsche's treatment of religion as the denial of instinct and Freud's own view of the relationship between civilized restraint, religion and illness. In short, Nietzsche's analysis of human personality and society provided the general framework for Freudian psycho-analysis.

Nietzsche's views on knowledge, power and society were influential in the development of the Frankfurt School and of critical theory, although Nietzsche's relationship to this group of writers is complex. Much of the Frankfurt School's understanding of Nietzsche was filtered through the debates amongst neo-Kantianism (as in Rickert) and the phenomenological schools of thought (specifically with the work of Scheler). The intellectual offspring of these schools (such as Klages, Lessing and Lukács), in their reading of Nietzsche, had a strong influence on the work of Adorno. Although Nietzsche's critique of modernity in relationship to the Frankfurt school has been acknowledged, the treatment of this relationship has been somewhat superficial. We should also note that Nietzsche was extensively quoted in the *Dialectic of Enlightenment* which was one of the fundamental texts of the critical school by Horkheimer and Adorno. Although Adorno was obviously and overtly influenced by Nietzsche, we argue that the appropriation of Nietzsche by the critical theorists in fact denied and distorted the real importance of Nietzsche for an analysis of modern society. That is, the critical theorists were unable to come to terms with Nietzsche's powerful critique of rational thought from the standpoint of physiology and genealogy or, more accurately, from the standpoint of social embodiment in the everyday world.

7

Nevertheless, Adorno came closest to the type of critique with which we want to explore in moral social life, especially through his aesthetic outlook. If we do not refer constantly to the writings of Adorno in detail, it is because we are more concerned with general sociological questions than with an exegetical interpretation of Adorno. Although Adorno's notion of aesthetics remains somewhat structuralist and separated from the creativity of sociality, we attempt to explore this creativity in terms of its material and practical basis. Social attitudes, as we wish to explore them here, are attitudes of modernity. Within the modernist perspective on Nietzsche, social attitudes are attitudes of taste, of stylish movements, and of art. Adorno's aesthetic redemption remains in the last instance – against Nietzsche's critique – a quest for high culture; this aesthetic was, therefore, never grounded in the senses and practice of social life.

We have suggested that Nietzsche has been profoundly important in the development of the thought of Weber, Freud and Adorno. Furthermore, it has been claimed that this influence was either disguised or subordinated by writers who, amongst other things, sought to emphasize their own originality and independence from Nietzsche. In the post-war period, however, there has been a revival of Nietzsche and this revival has been associated with existentialism through the writing of Sartre and under the influence of phenomenology especially through the philosophical analysis of Heidegger. Over a longer period, philosophical interest in Nietzsche has been kept alive by the careful and sympathetic exegesis of Kaufmann (1974). Within the English speaking context, the interpretation of Nietzsche has also been usefully guided by Hollingdale (1973) and Stern (1979).

However, the impact of Nietzsche on contemporary sociology has been closely and significantly associated both with the development and with the reaction against so-called French structuralism. In addition to Michel Foucault, Nietzsche's philosophy has been important in the intellectual development of Maurice Blanchot, Jacques Derrida, Pierre Klossowski, Philippe Lacoue-Labarthe, Jean-Luc Nancy and Bernard Pautrat. Various aspects of Nietzsche's thought have been important in the development of contemporary French social philosophy. The first is Nietzsche's analysis of language and thought as metaphor. The centrality which Nietzsche gave to language in the appropriation of reality and his analysis of grammar have contributed to the development of a distinctively French understanding of language and discourse. Another aspect of this is the apparent relativism of Nietzsche's emphasis on perspective in respect to analysis of reality. The second is Nietzsche's profound critique of the pretentions of rationalism in

8

exposing the metaphoricality of reasoning itself. Nietzsche's analysis of metaphor provided the basis for a rejection of Cartesian rationalism which had been the foundation of traditional positivism in French social thought. Within these two features of Nietzsche's thought, French social theorists were able to develop a significant and rigorous criticism of the determinism which was present in the thought of Marx and also of Marxist structuralism. Against determinism and positivism, French social theory has looked towards the body and desire as a critique of the instrumental-rational basis of industrial societies. With the collapse of Marxist thought in France as a major element of social theory, Nietzsche has increasingly emerged as a profound critic of the rationalist assumptions which lie behind both capitalism and state socialism. We can see these influences specifically in the work of Foucault, Derrida and Deleuze, although the impact of Nietzsche has been extensive across a far wider range of French thinkers (Allison, 1977).

Foucault's contribution to contemporary sociology has been significant and profound. He has also been important in the development of alternative historical and epistemological views on science, philosophy and art. The revival of sociological interest in Nietzsche is thus somewhat indirect, being in part the consequence of the impact on contemporary social theory of French philosophy. Foucault, for example, adopted several features of Nietzsche's perspective and philosophy, although he has often been somewhat guarded in his references to Nietzsche. Foucault's development of the notions of genealogy and archaeology was the direct outcome of his engagement with Nietzsche's treatment of history and philosophy (Rorty, 1986). Foucault adopted the principle that 'history' is incoherent, contingent and lacks teleological development. Therefore, historians who try to make history familiar simply construct an artificial mythology by imposing a reasonable order on that which is unreasonable and unfamiliar (Turner, 1985c). Foucault showed the force of these arguments in his analysis of madness where he identified the problem of writing about unreason from the standpoint of reason. However, in this study, we are primarily concerned with Foucault's analysis of the body and with his use of Nietzsche in the development of the analysis of discipline, sexuality, social control and bio-politics.

The core of Foucault's social theory is specifically Nietzschean, being an analysis of the inter-relationships between knowledge and power, where both knowledge and power are focused upon the body, conceived as population and as individual. Indeed, in Foucault's analysis of discipline, the body is specifically the effect of modern forms of power and knowledge. The human body is the outcome of a complex history of medical power and knowledge, an effect of medical discourse and institutions. As we will see, one problem with Foucault's analysis is that the body is simply the passive recipient of social processes and the product of knowledge/power, whereas we need a theory of bodily resistance and the resilience of embodiment to social regulation and control (Lash, 1984). We need a theory of active embodiment. In this study, we give a special emphasis to the relationships between the dense world of reciprocity and social experience through the lived body, since we wish to reject the remaining structuralism within Foucault's approach to the body which gives a priority to the rigid determination of experience by powerful discourses.

Nietzsche's philosophy of the body, knowledge and power has also significantly influenced writers such as Derrida. Derrida's reading of Nietzsche can be seen as part of a wider project which is concerned with the de-construction of the presumptions of rationalism and with the assumptions of literary criticism. Derrida's attack upon hermeneutic interpretation was clearly illustrated by his commentary on a fragment from Nietzsche in his book *Spurs, Nietzsche's styles* (1979). The point of Derrida's playful interpretation was to call into question all normal conventions of relevance and contextualism.

We should also note the importance of Nietzsche in the work of Deleuze and Guattari in their study of anti-Oedipus (1977) where they outlined an important theory of desire. Deleuze, following Merleau-Ponty, attempted to develop the idea of a body without organs since he wished to emphasize the importance of phenomenology of the body as against material interpretations of biological reality. Our bodies and our experience of them are focused around the question of desire, and it is through this notion that Deleuze is able to develop certain ideas about resistance and opposition to institutionalized control. Against Foucault's implicit view of the passive body, Deleuze (1983) emphasized the importance of the forces of desire.

Whereas Marxist theory has typically concentrated on the problem of needs which can either be satisfied or denied by the social processes of capitalist production, French social theory has increasingly placed an emphasis on desire and pleasure as critical principles in a world of institutionalized conformity and instrumental rationality. The conservative phenomenology of Heidegger, and the critical thinking of Foucault and Derrida can be seen as the working out of a project which has its origins in Nietzsche's response to modernity in terms of a rejection of the narrow presumptions of instrumental-rational thought in the service of state power. Nietzsche identified a crisis in the world which he described in various ways but primarily under the label of nihilism; this crisis provided the starting point for contemporary French social theory (Megill, 1985); this crisis in thought and society is fundamental to an understanding of the uniqueness of modern dilemmas.

The revival of Nietzsche's social philosophy and the mounting interest in the problems which he addressed may be both part of a new direction in social thought, namely towards a genuine social interpretation of the body as opposed to the positivistic interpretations of socio-biology, and part of a new direction in the organization of contemporary society with respect to the problem of bio-politics. It is also an effect of the wider social condition of post-modernism. The Nietzsche revival has been particularly important in the growing attention to the sociology of the body: *Political Anatomy of the Body* (Armstrong, 1983), *The Civilized Body* (Freund, 1982), *Bodies of Knowledge* (Hudson, 1982), *The Body's Recollection of Being* (Levin, 1985), *Five Bodies* (O'Neill, 1985), *The Body and Society* (Turner, 1984) and *The Tremulous Private Body* (Barker, 1984). This renewal of interest in the body is, in part, a reflection of a certain theoretical dissatisfaction with the positivistic analysis of the body in medicine and socio-biology, but it also reflects a growing debate about the nature of the agent in the traditional problem of agency. The origins of this interest are complex and varied, but within the French context the work of Sartre has been of particular importance; however, Sartre's own work reflected the impact of the philosophy of Heidegger (Warnock, 1965). It is evident that an analysis of biology and social embodiment has also become important as a consequence of the feminist critique of the notion of nature, human nature and biological destiny. This feminist critique has given a new direction to certain issues in philosophical anthropology, namely the relationship between anatomy, culture and social roles. This debate, in turn, is critically related to the issue of what is a person, that is, whether being a person involves continuous social experiences of embodiment or not.

Within a wider sociological framework, we must assume that the problem of the body is an effect of changes in the character of consumption and production in modern societies where the new ethic of hedonistic consumption is focused on the pleasures of the surface of the body. In addition, the changing demographic structure of society has brought into political focus the critical problems of ageing, the stigmatization of age and the dependence of the aged upon the state. Pain, ageing and death have been major issues in traditional theology; they also raise important issues with respect to certain philosophical problems of personality and personhood. They have, however, gained a

11

new significance in modern secular society. Furthermore, changing norms with respect to sexuality have drawn attention to the 'issues' of homosexuality, the family, the rights of children and problems relating to abortion and euthanasia. Scientific developments in medicine have changed the parameters of the analysis of what life is, what health is and what death is. New technical possibilities in medicine of reproducing life artificially have reorganized the political, social and philosophical relationships between the body, mind and society. These processes can be seen as dimensions to the crisis of modernity and post-modernity because they make problematic, as Heidegger clearly recognized, the very nature of being. Our anxieties about the end of the self have been linked necessarily with the end of the body.

The point of this study, however, is not simply to offer an analysis of Nietzsche's influence on Weberian sociology or to trace out in detail his presence in the work of Freud, or finally to show how Nietzsche provided the background for critical theory. This study does not seek necessarily to reflect directly on the revival of Nietzsche in French social thought, or more recently in German social philosophy. We do not attempt in any detail to provide an analysis of the causes behind the Nietzsche revival in social theory. These textual exercises are not necessarily the most effective method for developing social theory. Social theory often turns out to be simply a re-interpretation of existing lines of argument and assumes, therefore, a repetitive and parasitic character.

The aim of this study is to retrieve the influence of Nietzsche by attempting to provide the outlines of a theory of society which would be consistent with some original perspectives laid down by Nietzsche on the relationship between language and body, society and self, thinking and being. If this study diverges from certain perspectives of Nietzsche, then this is to be expected, since our aim is to promote new developments in social theory rather than simply to adhere slavishly to certain well-known themes in Nietzschean philosophy. By developing a position which responds to and reflects on Nietzsche, we hope to advance the analysis of modernity. It is the case, however, that in our view much contemporary writing about Nietzsche intellectualizes the spontaneity and robustness of his approach. One illustration of this approach would be Richard Schacht's *Nietzsche* (1983) which presents a sophisticated philosophical exegesis of Nietzsche's thought. However, the consequence is to domesticate Nietzsche, in a way which neutralizes the challenge of Nietzsche's dance. We must pay attention constantly to the irony of Nietzsche's argument.

By emphasizing the importance of medical metaphors, social

12

embodiment and the everyday world in the thought of Nietzsche, we hope to correct this emphasis on cognitive norms which appears to be particularly influential in the work of Habermas. Given Nietzsche's scepticism with respect to the validity and value of merely rational thought and cognitive perspectives which deny the sensuous reality of human practice and human engagement in the everyday world, it is curious that much of the so-called Nietzschean revival should focus so persistently on problems in the relativity of knowledge, perspectivism and rational discourse. We also wish to depart, ultimately, from the aesthetic analysis, since, in our view, this aestheticism fails to grasp the sensuous emphasis in Nietzsche's work (Megill, 1985). Eating as well as painting are sensuously practical activities which are life-enhancing.

A Table of Contents

In chapter 1 we explore the metaphors of nostalgia in sociological theory from the classical reflection on the loss of community to contemporary commentaries on the loss of virtue in moral systems, especially in the work of Alasdair MacIntyre. This inquiry provides a critical evaluation of the role of concepts like community and the sacred in the sociological imagination.

In chapter 2 we start with the facts of human embodiment which, we argue, create certain dependencies on society, especially where there is a high division of labour. That is, given human embodiment, we are unable to satisfy either our needs or our desires without some encounter with other social actors within existing social relations. While embodiment creates dependency, it is also the site of resistance. We enjoy a certain sovereignty and immediacy over our phenomenal embodiment, and there is consequently a contradictory or dialectical relationship between our dependency and our resistance. The second level which we discuss is the inter-subjective everyday world of reciprocity which is characterized by an endless series of exchanges, both symbolic and material. That is, the life-world is the site of endless concrete exchanges of material and symbolic objects which constitute the web of society itself.

Sociology is literally the study or knowledge of friendship and consequently the study of exchange within the life-world is fundamental to the whole sociological project. This reciprocal reality leads us into a consideration of the fundamental importance of fellowship, sympathy and empathy as basic social attitudes. We treat the larger institutional reality of society as parasitic upon this dense world of exchange. There is, however, also something ambiguous about this world of reciprocity in the fact that it can be denied, betrayed, redirected and imaginatively reconstructed. Within this ambiguity, reciprocal relations are the hidden locus of bondage of the socializing self. This world of reciprocity figures in discourse as both myth and nature. Against the mystifying of reciprocity in the discourse of modernization, we wish to show the primary feature of everyday reciprocity against organized modernity. The world of industrial modernity is simply a replica and a dependent growth upon basic forms of human reciprocity. Although the view of the merely cognitive modernizing self might wish to suppress this fact of modernity's dependence upon social reciprocity, its bondage to reciprocity becomes clear only through unmasking the ideological preference of macro-institutions. However, merging within it, modernity also entails forces of rational-cultural formation, namely the creation of cultural pretensions and intensities. With the exception of Scheler's re-interpretation, resentment has been completely suppressed as a sociological category of social attitudes for the analysis of modernity; it became clear that Nietzsche's sensuous-practical solution (of 'intentional non-intentionality' towards the 'nearest things', persons and the everyday world) remains largely unrecognised and misleadingly interpreted as an artistic meta-physics within the discourse of modernity. In short, we reject the aestheticization of Nietzsche's practical ethics of reciprocity.

The final level of the social world is the reality of regulating institutions which attempt to organize the inter-subjective world and the world of social embodiment. We treat these institutions as social bodies which, through an intellectual stratum (the professional men of learning and taste), seek legitimation over the world of communal reciprocity and individual embodiment. This 'higher' social world can be conceptualized as a form of institutionalized resentment which requires intellectuals, professional men and priests to smooth out its operation; they exist to render the world either acceptable or efficient. This culture of resentment stands in opposition to the human world of sensualism, practice and feeling.

In chapter 3 we are specifically concerned with the sociology of Max Weber which we analyse through a study of cultural control in the form of religion. This provides the opportunity for a detailed consideration of religion as resentment and we look at various social forms whereby religion is constituted. In this chapter we consider the contradictory relationship between bureaucracy and charisma, and we analyse the various dimensions of rationalization and nihilism. In certain respects, religion can be conceived as a particularly primitive institution in the

14

sense of elementary forms of regulation and cultural control over feeling and sexuality. Nietzsche described Christianity as 'a piece of antiquity intruding out of distant ages' (*HAH*, section 113). In historical terms, religion has played a crucial role in the regularization of sexuality, and particularly in the constitution of female desire in the interests of power and property. The word 'religion' itself is derived from 'religio' which signifies both rule and regulation, which have the effect of binding persons to the social body. Although religion may express certain primeval and primary emotions, religion becomes intellectualized through the work of theologians who redirect religion away from the binding of the everyday world through reciprocity to a new level of institutional cultural control.

In chapter 4 we extend our critique of Weber through a consideration of Freud's 'laborious' science of human psychology. It is argued that Freud's social theory, psychology and therapy had simultaneously radical and conservative implications, especially as an analysis of the non-rational. Freud's reception in social science is considered with respect to this ambiguity. In order to follow this implication of his work in detail, we compare and contrast Nietzsche and Freud on the social functions of religion. We argue in favour of the radical and playful character of the Nietzschean critique of religious culture and conclude with an outline of Nietzschean psycho-analysis as a theory of language.

In chapter 5 we turn to ideology as a form of institutionalized regulation and, by an examination of the critical theorists, we explore the origins and character of the administered society. With special reference to the work of Adorno, we look at the opposition between critical reason and the administered world of capitalism. Contemporary society has been described from a variety of positions as a world dominated by bureaucracy, by discipline and by administration. These bureaucratic forms of capitalism represent a new epoch of regulation which has profound implications for individual autonomy and social reciprocity. This chapter allows us to develop further the concepts of revenge and reversibility as sociological perspectives.

In chapter 6 we take up the question of embodiment through the study of the work of Foucault and his followers. We show how Foucault develops certain aspects of Nietzsche's philosophy, but also how he departs from Nietzsche's emphasis on the sensuality of the 'little things' of the everyday world. We attempt to develop the idea that knowledge and power are focused on the body by looking at various forms of regularity and rationalization which impinge upon our sensuous embodiment in social relations. Although we concentrate on the

15

questions of language, perspectivism, repetition and regularity, we wish to emphasize the importance of sensuous-practical experience within Nietzschean sociology. This chapter also considers the parallel relationships between Weber's metaphor of the 'iron cage', Adorno's concept of the administered society and Foucault's emphasis on panopticism. While the body can be regarded as the target of modern forms of rationalization and regulation, we also attempt to elaborate the idea of resistance to incorporation within an administered world. Finally, we consider the problem that Nietzsche's view of the nature of the individual and society might be entirely incompatible with the sociological project which, since the time of Durkheim, has emphasized the social determination of the individual. Within the post-modernist perspective, there is much greater emphasis on subjectivity (in which an ethic of taste replaces an ethic of good actions), and we have to confront the problem that Nietzsche's 'sociology' might be entirely incompatible with all previous forms of sociological theorizing. This possible contradiction leads us finally into a brief reconsideration of the work of Simmel who may be regarded as the first sociologist of post-modernity.

In chapter 7 we review the theoretical framework which has been elaborated in the central chapters of this study and attempt to formalize some of these conclusions by systematically considering the relationships between resentment, revenge, reciprocity and resistance. We also attempt to demonstrate how this perspective becomes an important feature of the critique of modernity. The question behind this entire discourse is whether it is possible or desirable to discover universal foundations for a morally good life in a global system dominated by rational discourse and practice. This final chapter also provides the basis for examining the globalization of modernity and its paradoxical relationship to traditional forms of reciprocity and exchange. We will now anticipate some aspects of this conclusion.

An Overview

The modern reception of Nietzsche in social theory has often emphasized his treatment of the problem of knowledge in a world where absolute values have collapsed. In this respect, Nietzsche entered modern sociology via Weber's commentary on the so-called polytheism of values in contemporary society. Our approach to Nietzsche starts at the other end of the problem, as it were, namely with the issue of the body, the everyday world, inter-subjectivity and the issue of 'health' in

16

social and individual existence. One theme of this study is the role of physiology in Nietzsche's outlook, his emphasis on the centrality of everyday experience, his critique of the intellectualization of mundane reality, and his celebration of 'polytheism' in morality and culture as a condition for individuality. For Nietzsche, the collapse of a conventional God-centred morality created new possibilities for individual authenticity.

One aspect of Nietzsche's concern with embodiment was the search for personal health and social well-being. Nietzsche's own life was dominated by the search for personal stability and health, and he was forced to relinquish his professorial chair in 1879 partly as a consequence of illness. The quest for health was the central motif not only of his life but of his philosophy. Nietzsche, of course, saw Germany itself as a sick society and interpreted his own role as a cultural psychologist whose task was to understand the social virus of his period. His writing constantly employed the metaphors of illness and health in the analysis of society and the individual (Pasley, 1978). By contrast with modern society, Nietzsche frequently referred to Greek society and people as fundamentally healthy, in their quest for personal autonomy within the competitive arena of sport and politics. Another dimension to his interest in bodily metaphors was his use of a parallel between the mind as an organ which consumes ideas and the digestive system as an organ which processes food for energy. In a way which paralleled Marx's view of alienation, Nietzsche often referred to religion as a narcotic which was a palliative for those who were already sick, but fundamentally damaging when administered to a healthy society. Nietzsche also saw sickness as a potentially positive challenge which stimulated the body into action, just as dangerous ideas forced the mind to confront in a progressive way a new domain of experience. One should also explore Nietzsche's view of himself as a physiologist of morals whose function it was to identify and transform the disorders of society. Those commentators who focus almost exclusively on Nietzsche's aesthetic perspectivism should reflect more systematically upon the presence of the body and its maladies in his philosophical outlook on the individual and society.

Nietzsche's treatment of the relationship between body and mind, self and society, nature and culture has been neglected and provides an important input into the development of a sociology of embodiment, since Nietzsche, unlike Foucault, presents a view of the body which is active, reactive and resistant rather than supine and incorporated. We wish to retain th'ُ view of Foucault, although we recognize that in the later volumes ﻭ‎ the *History of Sexuality* Foucault provided a basis for the notion of active resistance through an inquiry into the technologies

17

of the self. Nietzsche's view, as we have already suggested, represents a significant opposition to structuralist analysis of the body as an effect of discourse. Contemporary social theory typically treats embodiment as the socio-biological grounds for enslavement within consumerism and hedonism, but the body's presence in society is always dialectical and contradictory as Nietzsche expressed well in his own complex writing on the relationship between physiological and cultural processes.

Nietzsche has typically been associated with reactionary tendencies in politics and conservative processes in social theory. Of course, much of Nietzsche's writing overtly lends itself to this interpretation, but there has also been significant misinterpretation of Nietzsche's purpose. Nietzsche was a major critic of nationalism in the German state and the assumptions of bourgeois German dominance. In fact, Nietzsche's views on the state and politics do not necessarily lend themselves to fascism and they do not support a Darwinistic view of human survival; indeed, Nietzsche was a major critic of Darwinism in his time (Turner, 1982a). Nietzsche's moral position called for the end of hypocrisy and his ideas were not cynical or nihilistic, since he called for the revaluation of values (Stern, 1978). Recent interpretations of Nietzsche have noted the great distance between Nietzsche's philosophy and fascism. It is also evident that Nietzsche's philosophy cannot be easily interpreted as a form of anti-feminism (Thomas, 1983).

By placing an emphasis on Nietzsche's interest in sensual reality and embodiment, we draw attention to a theoretical convergence between the work of Marx and Feuerbach. Within Marxism, there is a tradition which gives centrality to praxis and our sensual engagement with nature. This humanistic tradition does converge, in many respects, with Nietzsche's own emphasis on the primacy of experience of reality in the everyday world over the abstract theorization of that experience in the language of high culture. Nietzsche humorously compared the superficiality of language with the reality of the digestive system. In this regard, Nietzsche is fundamentally a materialistic thinker insofar as he gave emphasis to material embodiment and experience in the life-world, seeing culture and institutions as merely reflections upon that primary act. Our being-in-the-world is essentially a being-in-embodiment.

In this study, the nature of the individual becomes a recurrent issue in our commentary on Nietzsche's thought and its implications for the analysis of the social world. We wish to avoid the conclusion that we are simply rewriting a form of liberalism or anarchism, where the autonomous individual is posed against the state. In other words, we emphasize the distance between our analysis of the problem of the

18

individual and earlier thinkers like J. S. Mill, Spencer and other nineteenth-century individualistic thinkers. Nietzsche's concept of the individual was part of a broader critique of the idea of rationalization and the cognitive construction of entities divorced from praxis. By contrast, Nietzsche saw the individual as a sort of negation of the importance of life processes. For Nietzsche, and for our own position, the individual is seen to be a construct of western society and, therefore, to defend the individual against social processes is merely to reproduce a rather limited view of the society-individual complex and to express a petty-bourgeois anxiety concerning the role of bureaucracy in industrial social systems. Our intention is to locate this discussion within the more general argument about agency and structure. In our perspective, sociology has inadequately conceptualized the notion of the agent, but in taking note of this limitation we do not wish to suggest that our argument is one in favour of the autonomous, separate and private individual. We do not wish to replace the absolutism of 'society' with the absolutism of 'sovereign individuals'. We develop the argument that the individual, like other ideal typical cognitive constructs, is simply a negation of the more fundamental issues which Nietzsche sought to present, namely the importance of the will-to-power, that is the will-to-life.

Rather than developing categories around the individual and individuality, which we regard as limited, life-denying concepts, we attempt to develop a sociology which is grounded in social categories which relate primarily to the fact of embodiment and the life experience of this embodiment. A sociology following Nietzsche's philosophy should deal with sensual, practical, this-worldly experiences, attitudes and dispositions. We want to avoid theory which brings about an isolation and separation of these experiences into something abstract called the 'individual'. Indeed, the whole implication of Nietzsche's argument is that abstraction is rationalization, rationalization is reification, and reification is political control. Sociology, in embracing the idea of the individual versus structure, is merely representing and reproducing these limited state concepts.

Our argument is, following Nietzsche, that the 'individual' is an artificial and a superficial construct which we wish to contrast with the genuine experiences of social reciprocity and sensual embodiment. Our constant emphasis is on the genuineness of mundane, everyday experiences rather than on the artificiality of liberal-bourgeois 'individual' experience. Our object is similar in intention to Agnes Heller's *Everyday Life* (1984), namely to provide an understanding of the world of artefacts, customary habit and language through a study of the everyday reality as the locus of human reciprocity. Here again, the notion of modernity is complex and ambiguous. Modern, modernity and modernization can be seen to be cultures or social processes which elaborate and emphasize artificiality and superficiality over the genuine experience of everyday reciprocities.

In attempting to provide the framework for a theory of social relations, we attempt to avoid a contradiction between arguing the case for the individual and arguing for some notion of the self. There are various ways by which we could distinguish these two notions. Essentially, we attempt to avoid the notion of a bourgeois individual as a thinking and owning self (a 'sovereign individual'), and to emphasize, by contrast, the idea of sensuous, practical activity. Nietzsche was overtly critical of the notion of possessive individualism; he wanted to help the development of personal autonomy, not personal property. Our notion of the self has to be located within our discussion of empowerment, embodiment and enselfment, that is with a notion of social embodiment and the social self. In the study of the will-to-power Nietzsche was hostile to the notion of Descartes's philosophy, especially to the idea that 'I think therefore I am.' By contrast, Nietzsche wanted to stress the will-to-power, that is the will-to-life as the essential force behind human action and social relations. We attempt to distinguish our notion of practicality from the narrow notion of labour, especially where this notion is associated with economic practice. We want to distinguish our position from that of an economic and bourgeois sense of the appropriation of nature through the owning and possessing self; we are clearly not presenting a normative theory of possessive individualism (Macpherson, 1962). Like Adorno, we see the ethic of world-mastery as a negative force of enslavement. We want to develop a Nietzschean sociology which would stand against both Descartes' cognitive self and Marx's labouring agent. Our perspective is thus to be distinguished from that of working-class, labour politics in which labour assumes heroic character when associated with the proletariat. We do not present a socialist position with respect to labour, since our concept of 'practice' goes back again to some notion of embodment, not to political and economic actions. It is ironic that modern Marxism in fact has no real theory of materiality.

Practice is essentially embodied, but here again we are not just arguing for a theoretical return to the young Marx. We want to develop a conception of practicality which grows out of Nietzsche's own perspective. His idea of practicality and life achievement breaks the dichotomy between mind and body, theory and practice, culture and nature, self and society. We do not have to chose between theoretical practice and other forms of practice, since the idea of embodiment draws these two inextricably together. Dichotomies are, of course, grounded in certain institutions which formalize and reify these distinctions. The final aim of our reflections on Nietzsche would be to develop a notion of practice which transforms and transposes these dichotomies through the notion of embodied practices. To accept an institutionalized separation of thought and practice, or to accept blindly institutions of control and regulation means that one becomes totalized within that framework. However, to depart from, or to avoid, or in some way to escape institutions is merely to adopt the mirror image set of problems, whereby one cannot live an authentic position, since one's opposition is itself determined by the institutions one seeks to reject. The idea of practicality as self-affirming and affirmative activity would provide a middle course which would avoid both the pragmatism of the institution and the romanticism of anti-institution. Nietzsche, of course, had argued that God was dead, but the implication of that argument was that one should not place a substitute in God's empty space. Sociological theory has often found a convenient substitute for God in such comfortable concepts as 'community', social determining 'institutions', 'autonomous man', 'labour' or some such absolute concept. This is to reify constructs. The final purpose of our theory is not to fill the gap left by God with some new construction, but to emphasize the trial-and-error nature of practicality and to assert the primacy of what Nietzsche called 'the little things' in order to develop a sociological theory which would be grounded in the reciprocity and practicality of the affirming, socializing individual.

Furthermore, we can argue that standardization of behaviour has been achieved through regularization, the uniform construction of taste and evaluation, individuation, and the imposition of rules. This imposition takes place within the political framework of the nation-state and, as a consequence, there is, as it were, a globalization of routine regularization and rule-bound behaviour. This iron cage of contemporary administration is incompatible with the idea of high morality, life-affirming behaviour of a genuine aesthetic of happiness, and self-actualization. There is a certain necessity about administration, but this is masked by the presence of an ideology of the state which renders these forms of institution opaque to inspection and criticism.

Nietzsche argued that, given our embodiment, there is no such thing as a general standard of health, but only unique forms of health. By extending this notion, we can criticize any attempt at a standardization of well-being or health through state legislation and regularization of individual life-style and *habitus*. Our notion of embodiment, once again, provides a useful point of departure for the critique of rules, regulation and state control. The notion of embodiment and our treatment of practicality points to a certain uniqueness in the self-affirming individual as particular and peculiar.

Following Nietzsche's notion of *Die Fröhliche Wissenschaft*, joyful sociology is a critique of standard sociology, that is a sociology which attempts to render new forms of regularity and uniformity legitimate without reflection through such concepts as 'role' or 'institution' or 'social system'. Even those sociologists who argue the case for the notion of life-world render our 'peculiarity' into some new form of regularity by arguing that there are certain uniform and standard processes within reciprocity within the life-world. We attempt to provide certain openings for not only a critique of the state, but a critique of sociology which, however unwittingly, is still a servant of the regulating state as it renders the particularity of our social relations into understandable generalizations which are abstract and, therefore, standardized. The standard then becomes a direct target of state-action. The notion of the ideal type is a classic illustration of the regularization of life through a sociology which itself embodies the process of rationalization and the subordination of life-worlds to technology and instrumental rationality. In the absence of God, the life-world philosophies only re-analyse the institutions of the regular administered society in an old language. The institution remains intact, but is transposed to a different area and is legitimated in new forms.

In this study we are concerned to introduce Nietzsche's own conception of health and illness in relation to his social theory and his perspective on the problems of modern societies with special reference to science and the state. The quest for health in Nietzsche's work was not simply a medical activity, but represented a more general, complete approach and attitude towards the good life and a *habitus* which would be congenial and compatible with the needs of the social individual. Here again, Nietzsche's emphasis on self-health and self-actualization is important in developing a critique of consumerism which we see often as a rather shallow, standardizing approach to need and its satisfaction. The programme which follows from Nietzsche would not be a general programme for society, but again would involve an emphasis on the importance of the social individual of finding good food, congenial ideas, satisfying music and supportive social relations in order to develop themselves over a life span.

In this study we do not wish to enter into a discussion about Nietzsche's method; we take the position that his method is, in fact, very close to that of Marx. Nietzsche employs the technique of a dialectical critique of values and institutions and, by tracing out their history through genealogy, shows the original purpose and function for which these values were established and how, over time, they are decomposed, destroyed and fragmented. We note that Foucault has made much of Nietzsche's method, but in this study we take the opportunity of criticizing Foucault on a variety of grounds. Nietzsche's perspectivism in the hands of Foucault becomes a relativistic standpoint which does not, in any direct way, lend itself to a critique of existing social relations. We would agree with Gillian Rose (1984, p. 183) that Nietzsche unlike Foucault did not attempt to separate politics from knowledge; his aim was not retreatism but to secure personal independence without *ressentiment* and to develop a new politics. To some extent, Foucault's position rules out utopia as a critique of the status quo. However, we argue that utopia may have a positive function in social life. It is not the possibility of utopia as such but the idea of utopia which plays a critical role in social relations. By way of analogy, we would argue that the formation of astrologies has a somewhat negative function, because astrology sees social relations and human beings as determined by forces over which they have no control at all. Nietzsche proclaimed that God was dead but the modern astrologies of social analysis simply seek to substitute a new form of determinism for the old discourse of God. By using the notion of astrology, we can criticize Weber's fatalism in social relations, Freud's notion that we are determined by the forces of the unconscious and Marx's more vulgar notions concerning the determination of need through the economy. Against these determinisms, we seek to find methods for developing a joyful sociology of utopian critique and the pleasures of embodiment. This is the meaning of Nietzsche's dance.

We might contrast this notion of astrological determinism with the idea of astronomy which would be the creation of utopias in a distant place in order to mount a critique of current social relations. Astronomy would provide open-ended, future-orientated critique of modernity by suggesting alternative universes which would be escapes from and alternatives to this world. We would emphasize, of course, that utopias are utopias and that it is merely the idea of alternatives which generates social and political action to change the world we inhabit.

By comparing and contrasting the astronomy and astrology of modern societies, we seek to avoid the idea that we are simply cynical or nihilistic critics of modern conditions. We have a positive critique to mount because we are arguing the case for the importance of the centrality of social embodiment, reciprocity, inter-subjectivity and self-actualization against the processes of uniformity, standardization and regularization. We define the state as generally an institution which seeks the destruction of the life-world. In addition, we have already argued that we are committed to the idea of utopian conceptions of community and self-actualization through social embodiment and practice, not in the sense that we would expect these Utopias to be realized, but simply as providing an alternative picture or perspective on existing social relations.

This approach then leads us back to a critique of false consumerism, the State and existing productive relations, all of which form a social unity, however unstable. The critique of consumerism, therefore, flows out of an argument in favour of astronomy over astrology, of practical action against uniform determinations, of uniqueness against administration. Of course, the point of developing this position is to provide a critique of Foucault who uses archaeology as a retrospective critique of values, a critique of Marx's metaphor of economic determination and Adorno's picture of the administered world as the iron cage of instrumental reason. The notion of astronomy is a forward projecting Utopian critique which avoids the deterministic metaphors and the fatalistic meta-physics of Weber, Adorno and Foucault. By calling traditional social theory an astrology of practice, we take a position that classical theorists were merely describing the iron cage with its deterministic social relations rather than providing an alternative picture of genuine social practices which would bring about a revaluation of values.

The Doctrine of the Little Things

Our aim in this study is not primarily to produce an interpretation of Nietzsche; it is not to write a book about a book. Our concern is to outline an approach to resentment, resistance and reciprocity for sociology which is broadly consistent with Nietzsche's playful, danceful critique of the modern state and its ideologies or idolatries. However, in order to examine that playfulness, we are logically bound to assume a perspective on Nietzsche. In this text, we argue that Nietzsche criticized formal rationality in its Socratic forms as antagonistic to life; rationalization under the regulation of state philosophers was part of modern nihilism which constituted a process of institutionalized revenge. In short, we do not fully support the view that Nietzsche's philosophy represented an aesthetic response to modernistic nihilism and decadence. In our schematic interpretation of Nietzsche's work, we argue that he sought primarily a revaluation of values at the level of reciprocal relations within everyday life; in particular, he attempted to re-assert sense, emotion, touch and feeling over reason and cognitive abstraction. Following some recent interpretations of Foucault (Jay, 1986), it can be noted that Nietzsche's philosophy, in questioning conventional forms of philosophical investigation, was not offering a privileged location for vision, for the authority of the gaze, or for any controlling optics. Instead, he argued that we should rediscover the senses in the naivety of the everyday world. In this study of Nietzsche's dancing lesson, we refer to this perspective on life as his 'doctrine of the little things'. Because we depend on a particular passage in *Ecce Homo* (*EH*, pp. 66–7) for developing a critique of state-formation, decadent moralities and the dominance of the 'theoretical man', it is important to quote this passage at some length at the beginning of our study. We take *Ecce Homo* to be Nietzsche's last testament and the definitive proclamation of the project of revaluation. Furthermore, this doctrine appears in the middle of an autobiographical reflection (on 'the little things' in his own life which are essential for what he regards as the great tasks of his life-work), where Nietzsche underlined the importance of every detail of his life. His praise of the little things ('nutriment, place, climate, recreation, the whole casuistry of selfishness') in opposition to abstract virtues ('God', 'soul', 'virtue', 'sin', 'the Beyond', 'truth', 'eternal life') was part of his final defence of *amor fati*; this was Nietzsche's formula, namely the Dionysian affirmation of life as it is and always will be (*WP*, Section 1041). This affirmation of the little things of life was a central part of his rejection of no-saying philosophies from Socrates through to Schopenhauer. Although interpretations of Nietzsche have in the past drawn attention to the importance of the *amor fati* formula (Kaufmann, 1974; Schacht, 1983; Schutte, 1984), in our view insufficient weight has been given to Nietzsche's commentary on little things as a feature of his joyful science. This formula was basic to his rejection of pessimism, asceticism, theoreticism and negation.

I want to learn more and more to see as beautiful what is necessary in things; then I shall be one of those who make things beautiful. *Amor fati*: let that be my love henceforth! (*GS*, section 276.)

This affirmation of life was a continuous theme in Nietzsche's response to modernity, providing a link between *The Gay Science* of 1882, *Zarathustra* (1883 to 1885) and *Ecce Homo* in 1888. The corner-stone of this doctrine of *amor fati* is here:

All questions of politics, the ordering of society, education have been falsified

25

down to their foundations because the most injurious men have been taken for great men – because contempt has been taught for the 'little' things, which is to say for the fundamental affairs of life . . .

Now, when I compare myself with the men who have hitherto been honoured as *pre-eminent* men the distinction is palpable. I do not count these supposed 'pre-eminent men' as belonging to mankind at all – to me they are the refuse of mankind, abortive offspring of sickness, and revengeful instincts: they are nothing but pernicious, fundamentally incurable monsters who take revenge on life . . . My formula for greatness in a human being is *amor fati*: that one wants nothing to be other than it is, not in the future, not in the past, not in all eternity. (*EH*, pp. 67-8.)

We take this formula to lay the foundations for a joyful sociology of revaluation.

1
The Moral Sociology of Nostalgia

Introduction: The Sociological Tradition

Various attempts have been made to establish the main contours of the history of sociology. One central theme of these attempts to reconstruct the history of sociology has been the question of tradition and community under the impact of utilitarian individualism with the expansion of economic exchange associated with modern capitalism. Sociology itself can be seen as a response to the decline of communal relations. An important contribution to this debate was made by Robert A. Nisbet (1953; 1967). Nisbet argued that the core of sociology was constituted by a number of 'unit-ideas'; these included the concepts of community, authority, status, the sacred and alienation. In *The Sociological Tradition*, he suggested that sociology had been constituted by three ideological and philosophical traditions (conservatism, liberalism and radicalism) which were responses to two major transformations of the European social structure, namely the French Revolution and the Industrial Revolution. The intriguing feature of Nisbet's argument was that the predominant metaphors and perspectives of sociology had been derived from conservatism, since the central themes of sociology were concerned with the problem of order and the corresponding loss of community. The sociological response to the problem of order was couched in terms of a conservative diagnosis of the importance of values, shared assumptions and a range of institutions which guaranteed some form of social stability. Nisbet's thesis was important in a public context, because sociology had often been associated with socialism. By associating sociology with conservatism, Nisbet had raised a range of important issues in the unfolding of sociology as a perspective on contemporary society. Nisbet's thesis was to some extent confirmed by the ensuing debate in European sociology in the 1970s concerning the relationship between radical Marxist perspectives and sociological approaches. Under the influence of writers like L. Althusser and N. Poulantzas, European sociologists began to argue that sociology should be radically distinguished from the scientific perspective of Marxism (Therborn, 1976; Shaw, 1985).

Although the Nisbet thesis was an important framework for sociology, it was criticized on a variety of grounds. Capitalist industrialization and political change took rather different forms and different sequences in European society. While Nisbet put a special emphasis on the consequences of the Industrial Revolution, the timing of industrial change was very different in France, Germany and Britain. Nisbet's argument was to some extent primarily focused on the French experience, but in the French case industrialization was slow and uncertain. There was a significant historical gap between the close of the French Revolution and the final development of French industrial society. By contrast, in the English case, the major political transforma-tions of feudalism were over by the end of the seventeenth century whereas the final stages of industrialization were completed in the 1850s. The social structure and characteristics of change in the German case were again quite distinctive and unusual. Germany achieved industrial development from above as the consequences of the intervention of the state in a society where the traditional land-owning class (the Junkers) had retained a monopoly over political power long after the emergence of an industrial bourgeoisie (Cipolla, 1973a and 1973b). Since there was no uniform experience of political and industrial change, it is not surprising that there was no uniform sociological tradition. There are important differences between French, German and British sociologies which are themselves consequences of separate and distinctive paths of industrialization and state-formation. Nisbet's thesis can also be criticized on a variety of less significant grounds, relating to the interpretation of specific sociologists. For example, it is somewhat doubtful that Nisbet's interpretation of Durkheim can be sustained, since Durkheim had a much closer relationship to radical ideologies than Nisbet's thesis would suggest.

Although it is possible to challenge the Nisbet thesis, it provides an important starting point for a consideration of the meta-theoretical and metaphorical background assumptions of the discipline. One of the most powerful metaphors of sociological analysis is that of nostalgia. A variety of different and distinctive sociological perspectives can be seen as simply variations upon a theme of nostalgia which has its focal point in the sense of a loss of community. This sense of loss relates in particular to the moral, religious and cultural world, although it

28

embraces a perspective on politics and urban life. While the various sociological traditions in separate nation-States have their own language, topics for research and orientations, it can be shown that these separate traditions are in part reflections upon a common metaphor, that is the metaphor of lost space and time.

Using the terminology of Foucault, sociology is dominated by a common episteme which provides the leading motif for the separate and jarring discourses of various sociological approaches. While the actual terminology of these sociologies is quite separate, the various terminologies are actually dominated by a uniform problem, which is the problem of nostalgic memory. The point of this argument is not simply to describe the nostalgic metaphors of sociology, but to provide a critique of nostalgia in order to set sociology on a different course. This nostalgic metaphor is a form of social theology in which most of the traditional themes and issues of Christian theology are transformed and transposed into a secular terminology, but the underlying meta-physics of nostalgic sociology are essentially sacred. This form of nostalgia is consequently incompatible with Nietzsche's death-of-God theme and with the project of moral revaluation.

The Nostalgic Paradigm

In order to understand the nostalgic discourse of sociology we should first consider the medical history of the concept of nostalgia. Nostalgia began its career as the moral problem of isolated monks who experienced various forms of melancholy described as 'tristitia' or 'acedia' (Jackson, 1981; McNeil, 1932). Nostalgia as a complaint of monks and intellectuals was associated with dryness and withdrawal from activity. The remedy for this complaint was increased prayer and commitment, that is a renewal of religious vows. In literature, the most prominent representative of the nostalgic disposition was Hamlet; there is evidence that Shakespeare based the character of Hamlet on a medical treatise by Timothy Bright who published *A Treatise of Melancholie* in 1586 (Wilson, 1935). Hamlet has subsequently been closely associated with the problem of modernity, since *Hamlet* explores many of the dominant themes of modern culture including the Oedipal complex and the crisis of sexuality. Hamlet's crisis was also linguistic, since for Hamlet a gap had grown up between language and things which is signified in his complaint 'words, words, words'. Hamlet's problem was also associated with role-playing; he is forced to assume a variety of parts and roles which also distance him from a sense of reality. This idea, that melancholy is associated with masks and disguise, came to full expression in Robert Burton's *The Anatomy of Melancholy* in 1621 (Skultans, 1979). In summary we can say that the melancholic sufferer from nostalgia no longer feels comfortable in the world because he experiences reality as an illusion which cannot be managed by either language or practice. The term in medical analysis was first used, as we have seen, by Johannes Hofer in the seventeenth century. Because modern men are not comfortable in their social roles, we can say that they are no longer at home in the world; this is the basis of the more contemporary meaning of nostalgia as literally a painful sense of homelessness.

While nostalgia is part of medical history, we can usefully transform the concept into the notion of a nostalgic paradigm dominating sociology. This paradigm has four major components. First, there is the view of history as decline and loss, being a departure from some golden age of 'homefulness'. Social teleology is seen to be in reverse whereby modern institutions are a winding down from a previous period of progress and development. At the individual level this history is one of despair and hopelessness, since the pessimistic element of nostalgia suggests that the future will be not only a continuity of decline but an intensification of it. In social theory this sense of despair was prominent in Weber's sociology of fate (Turner, 1981) because Weber said that the future would be a polar night of icy darkness; E. Troeltsch in 1896 proclaimed to a gathering of theologians at Eisenach 'gentlemen, everything is tottering' (Hughes, 1959).

The second component of the nostalgic paradigm is a sense of the loss of wholeness and moral certainty. History is seen to be a collapse of values which had once provided the unity of social relations and personal experience. This nostalgic theme contains a strong theory of secularization in which the overarching canopy of religious and sacral values has been undermined by some catastrophic social process, such as capitalist industrialization, the collapse of rural communities, the spread of scientific knowledge or the increasing differentiation and complexity of the social structure. It is difficult to commit oneself to a moral scheme of life or to a general philosophy of social reality, because we live in a world of competing and conflicting perspectives. As Nisbet argued, the principal exponent of this perspective in classical sociology was Durkheim who in *The Division of Labour in Society* presented the major division between mechanical and organic solidarity as a theoretical account of the transformation of social structures by differentiation. The moral coherence of mechanical solidarity had given way to a more complex and uncertain world of reciprocity where the collective consciousness had become generally thin and dispersed through social space. Although Durkheim in this particular study had been relatively confident about the prospects for social unity, this sociological certainty had declined by the time he published *The Elementary Forms of the Religious Life* in 1912 and by the advent of the First World War when Durkheim turned to the question of nationalist symbolism and social ritual as the basis of social unity. The loss of moral unity results in a world characterized by extreme relativism in ethics and a general sense of the problem of perspectivism in philosophy. Weber described this world as polytheistic because he viewed the modern world as one of perpetual conflict between philosophical frameworks which could not be resolved.

The third dimension of the nostalgic paradigm is the loss of individual autonomy and the collapse of genuine social relationships. Given the loss of moral unity, the individual is increasingly exposed to macro-social processes and institutions which slowly undermine the individual and strangle him in a world of bureaucratic state dominance. This theme of individual regulation and loss of autonomy has a number of intellectual roots. For example, there is a clear tradition from J-J. Rousseau which sees all social development as the negation of individual autonomy and moral coherence. It was Rousseau who compared the autonomous savage (whom he described as 'solitary, indolent and perpetually accompanied by danger') in a state of nature with urban individuals in civil society whom he saw as dominated by fashion, public opinion and malicious gossip. In Weberian sociology, this increasing subordination of the individual to social bureaucratic relations was conceptualized in the now famous metaphor of the iron cage. This tradition was inherited by the critical theorists who came to describe modern society as an administered world where the fragmented individual is subordinated to the perverse logic of instrumental rationality. There is an important relationship between Adorno's notion of 'the administered society' (Jay, 1984) and Foucault's notion of the carceral. Within sociology, it is normally argued that bourgeois capitalism produces individualism as an ideology while undermining the genuine individual as a consequence of the division of labour, the dominance of the discipline, the spread of bureaucracy and the regulation of persons by the State. Certainly there is in contemporary social thought a common emphasis on the notion that we live in a world which is increasingly regulated and dominated by an overarching bureaucratic structure which threatens privacy.

The final component of the nostalgic paradigm is the sense of a loss of simplicity, spontaneity and authenticity. The individual is not only

31

regulated in terms of administration, but also in terms of certain micro-moralities of behaviour which prohibit autonomous expression of feeling. Althouth we live in a world of macro-conflicts and violence, the everyday world is mediated and regulated by the micro-moralities of the *habitus* which deny and prohibit strong passionate emotions. The individual is seen to be regulated by certain forms of conduct which are manipulated by the world in which consumer culture is increasingly dominant. In the work of Norbert Elias, there is an account of how the process of civilization brings about a transformation of savage emotions by an etiquette of everyday behaviour. Although the world lacks an overarching moral coherence, there are certain everyday practices which deny expression of strong libidinous emotions. In *All Manners of Food*, S. Mennell (1985) has shown how primitive gluttony and abandonment gave way through the civilization of appetite to refined manners and personal restraint with the cultivation of the gastronomy of taste. The social order depends, not upon common collective practices and moral schemes, but upon certain fragmented and fractured assumptions about everyday behaviour which individualize experience without providing individual autonomy. In Freudian terms the development of civilization is brought at the cost of individual feeling and emotion because social relations require the regulation of the id and the control of libidinous powers. This theme is also found in critical theory especially in the work of Marcuse (1955) who saw contemporary capitalism as a social system based upon a surplus repression of instinctual behaviours.

In summary, the nostalgic metaphor suggests that we live in a world which lacks moral unity, in which individual autonomy is overwhelmed by administrative rules from a centralized state, and where direct expression of feeling is no longer possible, because need and desire have been rendered artificial and superficial by the spread of a consumer culture which exploits false needs. The modern world represents a fusion of Weberian bureaucracy and Foucaultian discipline in a system of personal controls (O'Neill, 1986). These four components provide the dominant metaphors and meta-physics of classical and contemporary sociology; this nostalgic episteme embraces a variety of sociological and political traditions which are overtly far removed from each other and which are conventionally regarded as quite distinct and distinctive.

The German Version of Nostalgia

Classical sociology in Europe was shaped by a sense of the erosion of religious values. This crisis was especially prominent in Germany and in German social theory. The philosophy of Hegel, Strauss and Feuerbach provided the general background for the growth of Marxism and the Marxist critique of religion. However, the immediate background for German sociology was the critical work of Nietzsche, Schopenhauer and Tönnies.

Although Nietzsche's relationship to the nostalgic paradigm is ambiguous and complex, he gave expression to all of these themes of the nostalgic world-view and certainly contributed to the foundations of the problem of modernity and the post-modernistic crisis (Megill, 1985). At the centre of Nietzsche's analysis of modern society is the proclamation of the death of God in *Thus Spoke Zarathustra* in 1883. The precise nature of Nietzsche's notion of the death of God has been much disputed, but clearly he intended more than simply the claim that Christian institutions had been undermined by the development of a secular industrial society. The kernel of his position was that, with the erosion of religious/moral values, the basic assumptions of western culture had collapsed, leaving a gap which could no longer be filled by the concept of God. Since this moral world had disappeared, it was no longer possible in all honesty to continue with the old project of philosophy and religion as though nothing had happened. In part Nietzsche sought to criticize contemporary philosophers and theologians for their hypocrisy, since they persisted in a language which was no longer morally sustainable. Genuine philosophy would be forced to criticize and analyse all the major assumptions and presuppositions of philosophy, religion and culture since, with the death of theological discourse nothing could be taken for granted. The consequence was a radical perspectivism; the truth of assertions depended upon the perspective from which they were seen. His critique was against nihilism and, while his philosophy had a devastating impact on traditional belief, his aim was not essentially negative. On the contrary, Nietzsche sought a revaluation of values in order to build up a new culture which would be viable in the absence of God. As part of the critique of traditional values, Nietzsche proposed a genealogical method which would unmask the pretentions of conventional and hollow values which disguised an underlying resentment against genuine power, personal autonomy and self-realization.

Nietzsche's view of history is complex and various interpretations of

33

his position are warranted. For example, while Nietzsche saw Europe in a state of crisis following the collapse of theological discourse, he also regarded this situation as full of promise and potential. Nietzsche's solution was not to substitute a new absolute position to fill the gap left by God, but rather to achieve a new form of philosophical autonomy through the revaluation of values as a method of overcoming the presence of nihilism in modern culture. Nietzsche has however been interpreted as a nostalgic thinker. A number of commentators have regarded Nietzsche as a philosopher attempting to come to terms with his own loss of faith in a society undergoing a process of secularization (E. Heller, 1961). Although Nietzsche was convinced of the importance of the death of God, he openly rejected the false optimism of nineteenth-century science, especially Darwinism and evolutionary thought.

Nietzsche thought that, by comparison with earlier periods, the world of nineteenth-century German culture was definitely one of decline (Thomas, 1983). Nietzsche's evaluation of Greek culture and society had an important place in his social perspective; Nietzsche wanted to use Greek culture as a criterion against which to measure human development. He assumed that in Greek culture there was a certain unity of art, religion and morality in which people could live their lives with a degree of completeness. He felt that the competitive struggle which characterized Greek politics and sport produced what he regarded to be healthy individuals since their interpersonal violence could be expressed in communal games. By contrast, Christianity produced a social and moral environment in which violent passions and feelings could not be adequately expressed, since they had to be disguised behind a set of rituals and beliefs which subordinated genuine passion to a false doctrine of love. Insofar as Nietzsche appears to have celebrated the aristocratic over professional values, it was because he felt that 'function' dominated professional-bourgeois culture whereas 'being' was the core of an aristocratic affirmation of joy (Mitzman, 1971).

Although Nietzsche's philosophy stands in an ambiguous relationship to the nostalgic paradigm, the dominant figures of German social theory up to the First World War were primarily nostalgic in their view of society and history. This argument applies in particular to Tönnies, Simmel and Weber. To some extent, Tönnies laid the primary basis for sociological nostalgia in his classical contrast between *Gesellschaft* and *Gemeinschaft*. There is no need to comment in great detail on the sociology of Tönnies, the elements of which are well-known (Freund, 1979). It is sufficient to note that Tönnies' sociology was based upon a contrast between organic will and reflective will; he regarded all forms of social existence as representations of will. *Gemeinschaft* is the outcome of an organic will, while *Gesellschaft* is associated with reflective will. In book one of *Gemeinschaft und Gesellschaft* he noted that community was always a response to the needs of real, organic life whereas society is a form of social relationship based upon artificial and mechanical representations of reflective will. To quote Tönnies,

all intimate, private, and exclusive living together, so we discover, is understood as life in *Gemeinschaft* (community). *Gesellschaft* (society) is public life – it is the world itself. In *Gemeinschaft* (community) with one's family, one lives from birth on bound to it in weal and woe. One goes into *Gesellschaft* (society) as one goes into a strange country (Tönnies, 1955, p. 38).

The natural and organic world of *Gemeinschaft* was gradually being eroded by the development of exchange relations and the emergence of a market society in which the relationship between individuals was dominated by external economic interest rather than by natural and local relationships. Relations between individuals would become increasingly artificial and exterior rather than natural and interior. The triumph of *Gesellschaft* over *Gemeinschaft* was the triumph of public opinion, exchange of values, cosmopolitanism and class relationships over the organic world of the village.

In order to understand Tönnies' idealization of the organic and spontaneous life of pre-industrial Germany, we should keep in mind the fact that urbanization in Germany was both late and rapid. For example, in 1871 only 5 per cent of the population lived in urban centres of more than 100, 000 people but by 1925 this proportion had expanded to 27 per cent. In the aftermath of Bismarck's reforms, German society was increasingly dominated by the state and its bureaucracy, the very essence of *Gesellschaft* relationships. The social structure and the physical environment were transformed by rapid capitalist development in the second half of the nineteenth century. Eight thousand kilometres of railway track were constructed between 1850 and 1875. The chemical industry which was dominant in Germany employed 30, 000 people in 1850; by 1913 this had expanded to 270, 000 workers. Finally, the population multiplied two and a half times between 1850 and 1913. Industrialization meant the total transformation of German society and this transformation was reflected in a basic nostalgia for the stability of pre-industrial society in German social theory in this period. These social changes were the context for a culture of despair (Ringer, 1969; Stern, 1961).

Simmel's sociology reflected the cosmopolitan world of Berlin and his formal sociology was an attempt to give expression to the new social relations of urban civilization. Although in some respects his sociology is often treated as a celebration of cosmopolitan culture, there were also strong nostalgic themes in his sociological perspective. Simmel's attitude towards contemporary German society was significantly influenced by the philosophy of Nietzsche and also by the sociological analyses of Tönnies. Although Tönnies was a critic of Simmel, there is a parallel between their approaches in that Simmel became very much the sociologist of *Gesellschaft*. Simmel's sociology was in part designed to catch the psychological anxieties and social restlessness of urban life. The anonymity of the urban world, the constant sense of change and the levelling consequences of the money economy produced a characteristically blasé attitude in the city dweller towards the world they inhabited. In this respect Simmel can be regarded as one of the first sociologists of modernity since, following Nietzsche, he recognized the essentially subjective quality of modern life in the absence of any objective security and certainty (Frisby, 1985). For Simmel it was the social consequences of money which were crucial for understanding this new culture of subjectivity (Turner, 1986a).

Simmel's nostalgic and pessimistic perspective on modern society as the product of an expanding money economy is perfectly expressed in his classic text *The Philosophy of Money*. Simmel's general argument was that there is a tragic contradiction between content and form, that is between the creative energies that go into social relations and the congealed and reified forms in which this will is expressed. In the analysis of money, Simmel expressed this 'tragedy of culture' in terms of a contradiction between the reified forms of money and the vibrant content of social interaction. The 'tragedy of culture' points to the fact that all humanly constructed forms of life must assume an independence from the human beings who originally created them in the process of sociation. Money gave expression to the reified forms of social action since money is

the reification of the pure relationship between things as expressed in their economic motion ... the activity of exchange amongst individuals is represented by money in a concrete, independent, and as it were, congealed form, in the same sense as government represents the reciprocal self regulation of the members of a community, as the palladium or the ark of the covenant represents the cohesion of the group or the military order represents its self defence ... This feature then assumes a structure of its own and the process of abstraction is brought to a conclusion when it crystallizes in a concrete formation. (Simmel, 1978, p. 176)

36

This reification of exchange in money was however simply one illustration of a more general process in which modern society is reified upon the basis of the money economy and the growing dominance of monetary exchanges.

The sociology of money for Simmel had three important components. Firstly it was the study of the historical transition from barter to a complex monetary system corresponding to a transition from *Gemeinschaft* to *Gesellschaft*. Secondly the growing dominance of money was a reflection of a prominence of impersonal social relations which found their symbolic expression in abstract money. Finally money created a certain degree of personal freedom through the extension of exchange but it also made the subjection and subordination of the individual to bureaucratic control more easy and more profound. In a sense therefore, the growth of money corresponds to the decline of innocence and in Weber's terms to the loss of grace in moral and religious discourse with the passing of charisma.

The notion of fatalism and tragedy in Weber has been explored by a variety of writers (Löwith, 1982). Although there is no settled agreement as to the central core of Weber's sociology, there is a general view that rationalization represents the focal point of his sociological enterprise (Brubaker, 1984; Schluchter, 1981). Rationalization can be seen as the more general version of Simmel's notion of the tragedy of culture, since the theme of rationalization is that our liberation from magic and superstition through the subordination of everyday life to science renders the world increasingly meaningless in moral and religious terms. The everyday world becomes, so to speak, filled up and overwhelmed by scientific knowledge and practice but, since science can never tell us what we ought to do, the world is rendered meaningless by becoming devoid of secure values. Rationalization therefore also gives expression to Nietzsche's notion of perspectivism, since the world becomes the object of a struggle between unresolved and irreconcilable paradigms. It is important to note that, when Weber wrote about rationalization, the background imagery and metaphors of his analysis are drawn from the Old Testament, specifically from the Genesis story. We have eaten from the Tree of Knowledge and discovered our nakedness which cannot be covered by the institutions of science. There is an implication in Weber's sociology that the more we know the less we understand and as a consequence we become exposed to the unresolved struggle of different value positions. As Weber said in the famous 'science as a vocation',

the fate of our times is characterised by rationalisation and intellectualisation and, above all, by the 'disenchantment of the world'. Precisely the ultimate and

37

most sublime values have retreated from public life either into the transcendental real of mystic life or into the brotherliness of direct and personal human relations (*FW*, p. 155).

The world of charismatic prophets had collapsed leaving the social realm dominated by the objective regulating force of bureaucratic authorities. In such a society, the possibility of an ethic of ultimate ends was precluded and the best chance for an intellectual commitment to reality was the modest ethic of responsibility.

The nostalgic paradigm found its most influential exponents in contemporary thought in the work of the critical theorists (especially Adorno) and in the existential and phenomenological thought of Heidegger. The impact of Nietzsche and Weber on the critical theorists has received inadequate attention (Held, 1980). It is important to recognize the strong emphasis on historical pessimism in the critical theorists in order to understand this Nietzschean legacy. Critical theory was of course damning in its view of capitalism as the final expression of instrumental rationality and the basis of modern exploitation and domination. Capitalism made it difficult for autonomous individuals to achieve their ends and to satisfy their real needs, because it depended upon not only exploitation and violence, but also on the superficial and trivial world of mass culture and consumerism. However, since the critical theorists became increasingly uncertain about the future possibilities of socialism, they were forced into a backward-looking critique of contemporary society. It is well known that writers like Marcuse became disillusioned with the politics of the working class and with other oppositional groups; the potential for liberation and social change seemed to disappear with the increasing control of capitalist administrative structures. Adorno and Horkheimer were also forced to look backwards to Greek culture, to biblical criticism and to the more positive features of the Enlightenment in order to find a purchase on reason and critical dialogue. While they saw potentialities for change in the work of Freud, the student movement, the women's movement and Black opposition to white supremacy, these provided grounds for faint hopes of change rather than for firm commitment and conviction to the imminent collapse of capitalism. The problem of critical theory was that the tradition of Enlightenment criticism appeared to have found its sinister side in the history of anti-semitism and Nazi politics. The tradition which should have maximized human liberation seemed to be associated with the maximum degree of violence and decay. The critical theorists were faced with the choice of an aesthetic position or a nostalgic critique of contemporary capitalism. This sense of pessimism, futility and nostalgia was probably most significant in the work of Adorno; it was Adorno who encapsulated the despair of critical theory and its nostalgic turn when he observed that 'to write poetry after Auschwitz is barbaric. And this corrodes even the knowledge of why it has become impossible to write poetry today' (Adorno, 1969, p. 34).

This sense of despair was even more pronounced in the work of Heidegger whose hostility to capitalism was associated with a celebration of the peasant and folk tradition of German society, albeit from the perspective of high culture. Heidegger was concerned with philosophical problems rather remote from capitalist society; however, he stood for a profound opposition to the world of industrial technology. In his philosophy of being, Heidegger was preoccupied with the problem of the loss of a sense of authenticity. Heidegger's philosophy was an attempt to identify the problem of philosophical understanding of being by examining our being in the world. The alienation and anxiety of modern people is expressed by their 'not-being-at-home' and by the 'unhomelike' character of our existence. Modern existence is characterized by this profound sense of discomfort. In his brilliant study of contemporary thought, Megill in *Prophets of Extremity* has commented at some length on Heidegger's nostalgic philosophy, pointing to the persistent themes of return, going back and rediscovering our home in Heidegger's exploration of the nature of being. While for Heidegger the philosophical quest is a significant feature of moral activity, the need for philosophy is also paradoxically an indication of our homelessness in the world. To ask philosophical questions like 'what is being?' is to suggest that we no longer know what being really is.

This ironic conception of philosophy was associated with a nostalgic view of Greek society and culture. For Heidegger, original (that is, pre-Socratic) culture was one in which there was no gap between words and things; language was not simply a system of word-signs. Plato represents both a great step forward in philosophy, but also a decline from a community in which men were at home in their language and in their being. The way back to this unified moral and social community is difficult and precarious; similarly, the philosophical task of a return to being is extremely arduous and dangerous. Surrounded by the technology and industrialization which he hated, Heidegger came to a pessimistic view of the possibility of a restoration of being. His pessimism was so profound that he argued that the concept of *Kulturpessimismus* was trivial as an account of the contemporary mood;

39

this simple observation has nothing to do with *Kulturpessimismus*, and of course it has nothing to do with any sort of optimism either; for the darkening of the world, the flight of the Gods, the destruction of the earth, transformation of men into a mass, the hatred and suspicion of everything free and creative, have assumed such proportions throughout the earth that such childish categories as pessimism and optimism have long since become absurd (Heidegger, 1959, pp. 117-25).

This expression was Heidegger's version of Adorno's claim that to write poetry after Auschwitz was sheer barbarism.

Michel Foucault and Modernism

Although the context of French social theory has been very different from that of either Germany or Britain, there are some intellectual similarities and certain common points of departure (Lemert, 1981; Kurzweil, 1980). In this comment on structuralist and post-structuralist thought, we shall be exclusively concerned with the work of Michel Foucault. The intellectual influences which have contributed to the development of Foucault's thought are clearly very diverse. However, the debt to Nietzsche is particularly obvious and extensive. Foucault has drawn heavily on Nietzsche's view of historical analysis, Nietzsche's view of language in relation to objective reality and finally on Nietzsche's critique of rationalism (Sheridan, 1980; Norris, 1982; White, 1979). Foucault's dependence on Heidegger is less obvious and has not been sufficiently discussed, although Dreyfus and Rabinow (1982) provide some useful comments on Foucault's relationship to Heidegger's hermeneutics. While Foucault was critical of Heidegger's philosophy, he was also sympathetic and his sympathy is illustrated in his introduction to Binswanger's psycho-therapy (Binswanger, 1955). The presence of Heidegger was perhaps most obvious in Foucault's *The Order of Things* where Foucault was concerned with the relationship between language and experience in chapter 9. Foucault presents the issue by noting that once language exists, there is a problem with origins, since we cannot return to a state of pre-conceptual experience. Language becomes part of a certain distance between thought and experience; that is, a naive existence is ruled out by the presence of language. There is for Foucault an unsteady and uncertain relationship between words, things and experiences. The rationalist assumption of an equation between thought and experience no longer seems tenable.

Foucault's social thought defies easy summary and there are major disagreements as to the nature and value of his work. Clearly part of his concern is with the forms of regulation, discipline and control which appear to dominate contemporary society, rendering human persons into mere objects of surveillance and control. This aspect of Foucault was particularly prominent in *Discipline and Punish*. The surveillance of populations and bodies requires a new principle of organization which following Bentham, Foucault called 'panopticism'. The regulation of bodies requires new forms of thought and new institutions which bring about a general surveillance and management of useful and docile bodies. Foucault has therefore been concerned with the relationship between power and knowledge, whereby forms of rational knowledge become the bases for the exercise of micro-politics. Modern society becomes a carceral in which a variety of institutions function through their architecture to bring about a system of virtue (Evans, 1982). The consequence of this approach is that phenomena like the body, sexuality and virtue are seen to be the effects of discourses, which constitute and construct reality implicitly and explicitly in the interests of certain institutions of power. The very existence of a biologically determined sex is itself seen to be the outcome of bureaucracy, regulation and knowledge, because one feature of contemporary bureaucratic practice is to ensure that human bodies cannot have ambiguous sexuality; that is, one is either male of female (Foucault, 1980). In a similar fashion the diseases of the body are the products of nosologic discourses (Armstrong, 1983).

While Foucault is critical of contemporary society, he refuses to offer any simple political or moral message by which we could understand or change the world in which we live. To offer a message would be to offer a discourse, which is simply another version of regulation. Because Foucault promises no easy solution to contemporary society, there is in his work an implicit search for a point of certainty or security. This implicit quest for a point of belonging introduces a certain nostalgic theme to his work. For example, in his account of madness, there is in fact a romantic account presented of the reasonableness of unreason in a world prior to the emergence of psychiatry. Foucault therefore provides a celebration of King Lear and The Fool who in their relationship present the dialectic of unreasonable reason in relation to folly (Foucault, 1967). Similarly in his study of criminality, moral priority is given to extreme passions and extreme events so that the murderer (Pierre Riviere) has a certain heroic stature in relation to his kin folk (Foucault, 1975). In his treatment of sexuality, Foucault's presentation of de Sade again reinforces this sense that Foucault is suggesting that primitive or extreme or violent emotions and passions represent a pre-conceptual state of affairs prior to language,

41

discipline and modern culture. The primitive, and especially the violent, enjoy a conceptual and possibly political superiority over refined emotion and sophisticated taste. As in Francis Bacon's famous paintings of the pope, the crisis of modernity results in a pornographic commitment to the violent and the elemental; the scream has, from the point of view of experience, a privileged status as a gesture over rational speech.

The Religo-moral Problem and the Post-modernist Crisis

The nostalgic paradigm depends upon a particular view of the relationship between society and religion, and more importantly on the character of religious decline in the modern period. We have seen that Nietzsche's prophetic pronouncement on the death of God can be taken as an event which ushers in the modern period. In simple terms, one can distinguish two broad positions with respect to secularization (Turner, 1983). First there is a sociological tradition which regards secularization as merely the social decline of religious thinking, ritual and institutions. This theory may regard the decline of religion in somewhat neutral and indifferent terms, describing secularization as merely 'the diminution in the social significance of religion' (Wilson, 1982, p. 149). Sociologists sometimes wistfully regard the loss of religious music and art as a reduction in human culture. Alternatively they regard the secularization of religion as presenting modern society with massive problems of moral coherence and moral significance. This particular version of the secularization thesis has to presuppose a golden age of religion in which there was a large degree of coherence in religious and moral perspectives.

Alternatively, sociologists like David Martin (1969) have argued that the secularization thesis has to assume a certain backward-looking view of medieval Christianity by claiming that the majority of the population were religious in a significant fashion. Martin's counter-argument is that sociologists typically exaggerate the degree of religiousness in pre-modern times, assume an 'over-secularized concept of man' and finally confuse secularization with de-Christianization. His alternative tends to suggest that no society could ever be genuinely Christian, because no group of people could sociologically embrace the full range and depth of Christian spirituality. Human beings by virtue of their very essence are secular creatures; or at least highly resistant to conversion to grace.

For Peter Berger and Thomas Luckmann (1967) all human beings require a sacred canopy of values and practices which will shield them from the potential chaos of social relations, specifically from the threat of anomie. Human beings are by their very constitution incapable of coping with chaotic social relations and meaningless cultural forms. It follows that human beings by their social construction must be religious because the threat of nihilism would be too great to bear. The ontological position of Berger and Luckmann is that human beings are creative and active in constituting their social reality, but this social reality assumes an objectivity and independence from human activity, a position which parallels the concept of tragedy in Simmel. This autonomy of the socially constructed world is an important aspect of the sacred canopy which shields people from the possibility of meaninglessness. However, their sociological view of religion draws attention to the problem in contemporary society of pluralism, diversity and differentiation.

Following the views of Alfred Schutz, Berger and Luckmann argued that we live in a world of pluralistic life-forms which emerge as a consequence of the structural differentiation of society into separate realms. This pluralization of religious culture forces human beings into a position of choice and brings into question the facticity of the religious world. The religious situation begins to approximate to that of a supermarket, where there are endless cultural commodities; these choices become bewildering and religious objects lose their authenticity as a consequence of their diversity. In addition, there is an unintended religious drive towards secularization which emerges from the Protestant emphasis on individualism, conscience and choice. In this sense, Protestantism is its own grave digger. Following the philosophical biology of Gehlen, Berger and Luckmann suggest that human beings have a biological drive for homeliness, insofar as we require cultural and symbolic security in order to function. The contemporary world of secularity is only occasionally punctured by a return of the sacred which takes the form of 'a rumour of angels' (Berger, 1969a). In the modern world the persona has become divorced from social roles and the modern individual is a free floating bundle of rights which is signified by the notion of human dignity. 'Honour' has become obsolete (Berger, 1974).

This view of the relationship between morals and roles provides a bridge with the work of MacIntyre on the historical development of moral behaviour and moral theory. MacIntyre's sociological work is remarkably unified in its purpose and character. In *A Short History of Ethics* (1967) MacIntyre criticized conventional philosophical inquiry for its failure to take sociological explanations seriously; that is, MacIntyre argued that it was philosophically impossible to hold an

43

inquiry into notions such as 'goodness' without a sociological study of the development of the concept in its social context. His argument was not simply an argument about relativism or contextualism, but rather that 'goodness' is associated in certain communities with the performance of specific social roles. 'Goodness' cannot be extracted from the society in which it is located. The other purpose of his argument was to criticize contemporary philosophical debates (especially emotivism), since MacIntyre regarded emotivism as itself a product of a particular type of society. Philosophical debates had become increasingly problematic, because of the peculiar nature of morals in contemporary society. What had made morals problematic was the transformation of the social structure by the processes of differentiation and industrialization. The decline of certain types of moral culture had made moral questions not only impossible to answer but difficult to ask. In his comparative commentary on Marxism and Christianity, he wrote that

it is not, as the Enlightenment hoped, that the great questions about God and immortality, freedom and morality, to which religion once returned answers, now receive instead a new set of secular, atheistic answers. It is rather that the questions themselves are increasingly no longer asked, that men are largely deprived of an over-all interpretation of existence. They are not atheists or humanists in any active sense; they are merely not theists (MacIntyre, 1969).

This theme was reinforced in his essay on atheism published with Ricoeur (1969) *The Religious Significance of Atheism*. MacIntyre's argument is that atheism is only a live option in a society in which it would still make sense to be a theist, but since the whole world in which religion was plausible had collapsed neither atheism nor theism represent particularly viable social positions.

MacIntyre's view of the relationship between morality and religion is somewhat unusual, going against the conventional view that moral behaviour is in some respect parasitic upon religious faith. It is conventionally argued that religious decline will lead to deviance and immorality, whereas MacIntyre wants to argue that religion is an effect of the prior existence of a coherent moral community. This argument was pursued in *Secularization and Moral Change* (1967). For MacIntyre, the pre-modern world was based upon a unified moral community, that is upon *Gemeinschaft*. In such a society, there was a natural unity between moral practice, religious belief and Christian symbolism. People lived in a world without significant cultural differentiation between religion, morality and law. Hence moral questions could be set within a broader context, where this moral unity was grounded in a

44

social structure lacking significant differentiation in terms of the division of labour and class structure; traditional societies were not challenged by the contemporary problem of pluralization. Consequently, social roles gave direct expression to social values.

This unified world has been challenged and eroded, according to MacIntyre, by the development of class relations following the emergence of industrial capitalism. The social structure has become increasingly complex resulting in differentiation of the moral system which in turn has brought about religious pluralism. In the English context, each social class came to be associated with a distinctive religious tradition, because morality had become class morality. Religion was no longer part of a unified cultural world, but instead assumed an ideological function in legitimizing the inequalities of the social structure. In England, Anglicanism articulated the social world and the ethical views of the upper class, while Methodism and other dissenting sects became the religious vehicle of the work ethic of the middle classes. Finally, the working class was attracted to the doctrines of the Labour Churches which espoused the notion of the dignity of work.

Because we live in a morally divided world, we lack the overarching moral framework within which moral debate can have any significance or authority. This pluralistic world is double-edged. While secularization through differentiation has undermined the traditional culture of modern society, this fragmentation of the social structure also means that general world views like Marxism are also limited in their social appeal. Neither Christianity nor Marxism are valid as universal belief systems in a world of fragmentation. MacIntyre's position is morally nostalgic and it is not surprising that he finds the moral view of religious thinkers like Pascal attractive as the expression of a lost world (MacIntyre, 1971).

These various approaches to the problem of the death of God are summarized in his most recent contribution to this debate which is significantly entitled *After Virtue* (1981). MacIntyre described the modern period as a catastrophe in which the moral tradition of Aristotle has largely collapsed, making it almost impossible for us to adequately describe the crisis in which we find ourselves. The disorder of our moral language is thus a direct reflection of the crisis of society. In this book most of the major schools of social theory are brought under critical attack, since for MacIntyre none of the major philosophical positions are capable of dealing with the crisis of modernity (which in essence is the gap between 'is' and 'ought'). Again he argues that emotivism is the symptom rather than the explanation of our crisis, since emotivism simply expresses the notion that all moral judgements are merely expressions of preference. It is also no accident that the world we live in is essentially Weberian, that is one characterized by administrative authority, the separation of values and science, and finally by disenchantment. Philosophically and socially we are forced to come to terms with either Aristotle or Nietzsche, since it is Nietzsche who most adequately unmasks the pretensions of modern society. It was Nietzsche who grasped the problem of perspectivism, which is part of the basis of the modern crisis. While MacIntyre praises Nietzsche as a cultural critic and commends Nietzsche's project for its unmasking of outdated moral and philosophical claims, MacIntyre in the end wants to reject Nietzsche's project as a valid basis for contemporary political and moral action. According to MacIntyre, Nietzsche's view of the supermen of morality and his account of heroic philosophy was in itself an expression of precisely the individualism, which he sought to condemn in the Germany of his time. Nietzsche's solution was too vague and incoherent as a moral framework for contemporary society; it was also too aristocratic to be valuable in a period of expanding formal democracy. MacIntyre places his hopes on the restoration and redefinition of the philosophy of Aristotle, especially the Aristotelian conception of the virtues. He wants to restate the teleological conception of morals which was the basis of Aristotelian ethics.

The Aristotelian view can provide the basis for a new conception of the good society which would tell us what the general requirements are for a good life. Aristotelian philosophy clearly avoids the problems of emotivism, while also taking into account the social and historical context of moral practice. MacIntyre's conclusion therefore is that

on the one hand we still, in spite of the ethics of three centuries of moral philosophy and one of sociology, lack any coherent rationally defensible statement of a liberal individualist point of view; and that, on the other hand, the Aristotelian tradition can be restated in a way that restores intelligibility and rationality to our moral and social attitudes and commitments (MacIntyre, 1981, p. 241).

Aristotelianism provides a perspective on the recreation of a social unity in which virtues and practices would be reconciled, in MacIntyre's view, without the false heroic elitism of Nietzsche.

MacIntyre's sociological explanation of the contemporary crisis was most forcefully stated in *Secularization and Moral Change*. Although his causal explanation is often implicit rather than explicit, it appears that the loss of moral community is an effect of industrial capitalist development, which shattered the traditional framework of morality and action by intensifying the division of labour and creating social classes with separate and fragmented moral frameworks. MacIntyre's analysis of pre-modern society appears to be distinctively nostalgic, since it posits a social unity prior to the rise of contemporary class society; his view is also nostalgic in seeking a solution for our problems through a revaluation of Aristotle.

The Critique of Nostalgia

The principal assumptions of the nostalgic paradigm – history as decline, loss of wholeness, loss of expressivity, and loss of individual autonomy – are meta-theoretical positions and as such they are not amenable to empirical criticism. Meta-theoretical assumptions are literally above theoretical scrutiny; the result is that one can only oppose one meta-theoretical assumption against another. However, the nostalgic paradigm, while based upon meta-theoretical assumptions, does of course make empirical claims about the nature of societies both past and present. The first two assumptions of nostalgic sociology have to assume some golden age of heroic virtue, moral coherence and ethical certainty; a period in which there was no gap between virtue and action, between words and things, or between function and being. Both assumptions are empirically problematic and the difficulties with this position can be very clearly illustrated from MacIntyre's account of morality and secularization. MacIntyre has to assume the absence of significant cleavage in the social structure of feudalism of either class formation or status stratification. There is now ample social and historical evidence to suggest that there were indeed major divisions in pre-capitalist society between different classes and social strata. Distinctive moral and cultural traditions existed in pre-modern society and these separate cultural traditions were organized along class lines or at least along estate lines. To consider first the questions of religious orthodoxy and adherence, much of the recent historical research shows that the mass of the rural peasantry lived completely outside the orbit of the literate, urban and orthodox ecclesiastical institutions. In terms of major religious practices such as eucharist, confession and baptism, there is clearly evidence of the great difficulty the Church had in persuading the laity of the advantages of regular and full adherence to the sacraments. Medieval Europe was not made up of a set of coherent nation-states each with its own unified morality and religion. Rather we have to imagine medieval civilization as a collection of oases

47

surrounded by a waste land of pre-literate, pre-Christian and oppositional cultural movements which were quite diverse in terms of regions and status groups. In his monumental study of medieval culture, A. J. Gurevich reminds us that the Middle Ages were a period when

points of human habitation were usually scattered here and there in the forests – lonely oases, remote from one another. Small hamlets with a limited number of farmsteads, or isolated farms, pre-dominated. Larger settlements were rarely met with, on the coast or in the fertile regions of southern Europe . . . links between settlements were very limited, consisting mainly of irregular and superficial contacts. (Gurevich, 1985, p. 42)

Given the weakness of the ideological means of transmission, we should not be surprised to discover an absence of significant moral and religious cohesion prior to the development of means of mass communication in the twentieth century. In terms of sexual ethics, there was great diversity between social groups and it was not the case that the official teaching of the Church was necessarily expressed in the practice of the majority of the population. For the dominant land-owning class, there were two systems of marriage, one conforming to the Catholic principles of chastity, virginity and marriage for life, and another lay system in which *de facto* divorce was a necessary requirement (Ariès and Béjin, 1985; Shorter, 1977). There was also widespread prostitution particularly in the second half of the fourteenth century. Throughout Europe,

the clergy and the mendicant friars had the final say, but during the 1450s there was no clash between a popular culture and a church one. The town dwellers culture was far removed from that of the peasant, while the priests and friars who were in touch with peoples' daily life were quite unaffected by the fulminations of the great preachers (Ariès and Béjin, 1985, pp. 89-90).

As a general observation we can argue that the research of French social historians (L. Febvre, M. Bloch, E. Le Roy Ladurie and F. Braudel) has shown that traditional European society had an official and an unofficial culture, significant cultural separation between rural and urban areas and finally a diverse cultural life associated with different classes and status groups (Abercrombie, Hill and Turner, 1980).

This is not to argue that the cultural world of pre-modern society was not significantly different from that of the modern world, but it is to suggest that we cannot accept a nostalgic view in which pre-modern society is seen as a moral unity, with significant cultural homogeneity or a common religious culture. Medieval theologians and moralists were perfectly aware of the diversity of morals, the indifference of the peasantry to the official culture and differences between religious traditions. For example, the problem of other religions and the contest between different truth claims has a long history; in 1312 the Church Council of Vienna decided to establish a series of professorial chairs to consider oriental cultures and languages at a number of European universities. The problem of other cultures was intensified with the development of the world system and it is possible to trace through art and literature a growing sense of the peculiarity and diversity of the world of human kind. The problem of the *pensée sauvage* can be traced back to at least the end of the sixteenth century with a series of explorations of the Dutch colonies (Bucher, 1981).

The other assumptions of the nostalgic paradigm – loss of genuine feeling and expressivity plus the loss of individual autonomy with growing state regulation – while being meta-physical assumptions nevertheless make empirical claims about history and society. There is a widespread argument in social history that prior to the emergence of mass markets and commercialization there was an expressive directness in social interaction which has been lost. For example, in Bakhtin's work (1968) there is an analysis of French society which suggests a growing sophistication of taste and culture which brought about a regulation of emotion and expression as the traditional peasant world of the festival gave way to the court of the aristocracy and then the urban world of the bourgeoisie. The history of rationalization can be seen in terms of a growing regulation of the body through dietary management, scientific exercise, gastronomy and the technology of medicine; these developments bring the body under a detailed control of the state and other institutions, precluding the possibilities of primitive experience, untutored spontaneity and unrestrained pleasures (Turner, 1982b). These developments are regarded as simply the final extension of the spirit of ascetic control which Weber had located in monasticism, army discipline and the spiritual teaching of Calvinism. A parallel development is seen to be the loss of privacy, the growing regulation of the individual and the decline of real ethical autonomy on the part of citizens. From de Tocqueville's analysis of American democracy and J. S. Mill's analysis of the problems of liberalism, the individual and privacy have been considered to be under threat from the extension of state regulation, the cultural uniformity of modern democracies, the detailed surveillance of the individual by centralized agencies (such as schools, factories, hospitals and the police), the growing documentation of the individual by bureaucratic means and the professionalization of custodial institutions. The autonomous individual is increasingly regulated by the rationalizing process of the iron cage as the system of public domination grows in relation to the private space of domestic life. Modern society is seen to be a network of disciplines which police the individual from birth to the grave (Donzelot, 1979).

Of course, moral and theoretical approaches to the individual in capitalist society are varied and often contradictory. The individual has been regarded by a number of theorists as the product of capitalist society and as the ideological consequence of liberal market values. The concepts of privacy and the autonomous individual are also regarded by critical theorists as part of bourgeois ideology, which legitimates private property through the theory of individual possessive rights. From this perspective, privacy is seen to be a conservative belief very much in line with the basic structures of capitalist society. However, we can also argue that 'civil privatism' has been to some extent undermined by the development of complex bureaucratic societies, where urban life depends upon a social infrastructure which is provided by the state. When consumer culture is seen to be a necessary facet of capitalism, it is typically argued that consumerism undermines genuine individual choice and fosters a culture of false needs and artificial wants. Within this perspective, the individual is seen to be overwhelmed by the corrosive character of consumer culture. Hence the doctrine of the autonomous individual rather than being the product of capitalist ideological systems becomes instead a point of oppositional resistance to the deadening effect of a common culture based on artificial needs.

There a number of problems with this perspective in the nostalgic paradigm. For both Marxism and mainstream sociology, capitalism is seen to produce the individual as a dominant ideology of bourgeois liberalism, but capitalist production methods and consumer culture are also seen to undermine the individual. In short, there is a tension in the analysis of capitalism which sees capitalism as both producing and undermining the individual. One problem with this theory is the inability to distinguish different forms of individualism. It is important to recognize that in western culture, as a consequence of the Christian emphasis on individual salvation, there has been for many centuries an emphasis on the individual (Abercrombie, Hill and Turner, 1986). While it would be wrong to argue that Christianity was individualistic, the subjective person was given a prominence both in doctrine and sacramental practice. The transition to Protestantism strengthened and elaborated this special feature of Christian Europe (Parsons, 1963). This emphasis on the individual as a conscious religious agent was not consequently tied in any significant way to the emergence of industrial capitalism. In addition, the doctrine of individualism which developed in the seventeenth century and came to full flower in the writings of Locke and Mill was a bourgeois liberal development which, while compatible with capitalism, again had no special relationship to capitalism. That is, the political and religious doctrines of individualism and the social structure of capitalism happen, as it were, to coincide and collide in the seventeenth and eighteenth centuries. Individualism pushed capitalism in a special direction (for example, towards private property as an exclusive right); capitalism pushed individualism in a specific direction (for example, the growing importance of possessive individualism). Individualism was an oppositional doctrine with respect to feudalism, but became increasingly compatible with market society and capitalist social and legal relationships. It is useful to further differentiate individualism from individuality which was a romantic and critical doctrine of Schopenhauer. This doctrine of individuality emphasized the uniqueness of individuals and was an elitist view of the personality.

These various meanings of the notion of the individual and individualism should be sharply differentiated from the process of individuation, that is, the bureaucratic processes by which citizens are given a specific identity for the purposes of social control, regulation and the distribution of state welfare (Turner, 1986b). When Weber and Adorno conceptualized capitalism as a system which threatens the autonomy of the individual, they were in fact referring to the process of individuation, that is the spread of administered society. Individuation is a necessary feature of contemporary capitalism, since it develops alongside the growth of urban surveillance and is associated with factory discipline and the measurement of labour power. Of course, certain forms of individuation existed long before the growth of capitalism; for example, in societies which may be referred to as 'oriental-despotic' there was significant development of bureaucratic control and regulation of slaves. Individuation therefore seems to be more closely associated with the development of large-scale regulation of populations by bureaucratic means rather than specifically and directly with modern industrial capitalism.

In short, the rise and fall of the concept of the individual, the growth of individualism as a doctrine, the evolution of methods of individuation and the elitist conception of personality in the notion of individuality have no close or determinate relationship with capitalist society. The nostalgic assumption of a loss of individual autonomy with the growth of the money economy, factory, discipline and capitalist labour relations cannot be easily supported by contemporary historical studies of the individual and individualism. The development of the notion of the subjective and sensitive individual can be traced back to the fourteenth century with the development of Courtly Love poetry, the transformation of the traditional confessional, the spread of university culture and the growing importance of an urban mercantile culture (Hepworth and Turner, 1982). Similarly, there is no clear evolution or decline in the status of women in the transition from feudalism to capitalism. For example in the Renaissance women within the court enjoyed a large measure of autonomy and were regarded as influential in the leadership of taste and culture (A. Heller, 1978). In the nineteenth century, by contrast, religious and medical opinion forced women into a domestic role which did not allow them a significant cultural role within the wider society and their individuality was somewhat undermined by the growth of Victorian sexual morality. The empirical foundations for the nostalgic paradigm appear to be flimsy and do not warrant the moral perspective assumed by writers like MacIntyre whose evaluation of the modern period has to assume a significant transformation of religious and moral values by the process of secularization and by the dominance of capitalist social relations.

Ideology, Morality and Values

Behind the nostalgic paradigm is the reconstructed history of the transition from feudalism to capitalism. In both Marxism and sociology, this transition is conventionally seen to be the crucial event of world history. This transition is in fact implicitly seen to be more profound and more crucial than the related emergence of an industrial urban society. The decline of feudalism is the event which is associated with the loss of rural community, the loss of personal expressivity and the loss of an unregulated society. Classical sociology was shaped by the legacy of the analysis of this historical reconstruction of society. The problem with the feudal imagery is not simply the questionable nature of the transition itself (Holton, 1984).

The continuing problem with Marxism and nostalgic sociology is the ontological significance and moral supremacy given to certain entities such as 'working class' and 'community'. It is at this point that we can perceive the relevance of Nietzsche's philosophy and epistemology for the debate on modernism, post-modernism and nostalgia. We have argued that Nietzsche's account of the death of God was not a nostalgic reflection upon the loss of morality and community. On the contrary,

Nietzsche opened the way for a new and progressive development, as he saw it, in ethics and political arrangements. The aim was not to look backwards to moral security but forwards to a revaluation of values. In fact, Nietzsche's main challenge was to the very foundations by which we conceptualise the world.

For Nietzsche, there could be no presuppositions and no taken-for-granted reference in moral debate in a world where God was dead. Nietzsche's challenge was to get rid of the need for God and the need to fill a gap left by God. In this respect we can see much of the sociology and philosophy that followed from Nietzsche as a departure from this challenge since sociology, Marxism and philosophy have been typically in the twentieth century in search of a Subject to fill the gap exposed by the death and departure of God as the original Subject. Durkheim's solution was to substitute a moral social order for the traditional God of the Abrahamic faiths; in the work of Marxists like Lukács it was the unfolding project of the proletariat which was to provide the secular substitute for the traditional Subject. A variety of other philosophical/sociological approaches have offered the notion of community or sacred order or rationality as that Subject to be the modern Author of the modern social environment. The ultimate answer to nostalgic memories is the rejection of any project which would assume or search for an essence. Nietzsche's position appears to be the precursor of contemporary anti-foundationalism which denies that it is possible to discover any essence or underlying foundation for values, the 'human spirit' or rationality in the modern period.

The nostalgic paradigm in sociology is not necessarily conservative. It involves a critical rejection of contemporary society along a number of dimensions. Of particular importance is the emphasis on community and the fragmentation of communal relations by the emergence of a competitive society whose principal criterion of excellence was the free functioning of the market place. Nisbet was correct in his assessment of the role of the unit ideas of sociology as critical responses to the emerging capitalism of Europe in the aftermath of the collapse of feudalism and the rise of industrial society. In short, nostalgia can function as a critique of contemporary ideologies by comparing the artificiality of organised social relations with the organic character of pre-modern society. This critical comparison was, for example, essential to Tönnies' comparison of rational and natural will in the opposition between community and association. A nostalgic world-view is, therefore, not inherently conservative, since it can provide an ideological critique of modernity from the vantage point of a theory of a golden age. In this study, we have argued that Nietzsche does not adopt a nostalgic paradigm in response to the loss of moral authority with the secularization and urbanization of modern societies under the surveillance of the state. Nietzsche's proclamation about the death of God was not a call to fundamentalism but, on the contrary, a forward-looking utopian gesture calling people to a new sense of moral crisis. His critique calls not simply for deconstruction, but the reconstruction of values, where these values will, however, not be grounded in an absolute criteria.

In his article 'Nietzsche's concept of ideology', Mark Warren (1984) provides an excellent introduction to the concept of ideology in Nietzsche's philosophy and the use of Nietzsche's principles as the basis for a critique of modern societies. Warren points out that while Nietzsche did not self-consciously and overtly use the term 'ideology', his response to contemporary society constantly involved references to idols, falsities, illusions and the meta-physics of truth. Nietzsche's approach to the problem of truth was indeed fundamentally critical and radical, since he treated all forms of human consciousness as serving particular interests, needs and necessities. Truth is a sort of mask for the relations of power. Nietzsche described truth as 'a mobile army of metaphors' in his essay 'On truth and lie in an extra-moral sense'. To present a critique of society, it is not enough, however, simply to reject all existing beliefs as mere metaphors; the result of this relativism would be in effect simply conservative as it would fall into an extreme relativist trap. Nietzsche, therefore, required a notion of truth in order to criticize existing truths and he grounded this principle of truthfulness in the notion of practical action and usage (Schacht, 1983). Truth is important and survives not because it is based upon an enduring principle, but because it is useful and relevant to the practical needs of life. Since, for Nietzsche, the notion of life is connected to the will-to-power, his discussion of truth is simply a version of his general interest in the will-to-life and the will-to-power.

Nietzsche's view of belief, truth and the relationship between being and knowledge has to be seen as part of the wider relationship between the principles of Apollo and Dionysus. For Nietzsche, that which is truthful is that which is life-affirming, giving expression to instinctual gratification and need, especially with respect to the embodiment of the agent. The negative features of life arise from a situation where individuals or groups turn the will-to-power against themselves, which in Nietzsche's perspective, is the basis for illness. The neurotic response is the negation of the will-to-power; Nietzsche saw this as reflecting the absence of genuine power by those who were incapable of transcending the limitations of their situation. The Dionysian affirmation of self-transcendence is the basis of Nietzsche's view of the genuine character of true beliefs which have withstood the tests of practical application. In presenting the problem of truth in this way, we can see once more that Nietzsche wanted to ground this debate in the practical activities of life, the reciprocity between individuals and the centrality of the body to human experience and cognition. Truth is not separate from life but rather its expression and, therefore, the intellectualization of the question of truthfulness is part of the error of modern societies.

Clearly, the application of Nietzsche's principle is difficult in practice, since his views are often expressed metaphorically and with some degree of irony. However, Nietzsche's method was to use the principle of genealogy to expose the underlying falseness of certain moral imperatives, that is to expose the levels of resentment which scientifically underline a moral viewpoint. The genealogical method exposes the operating principle of morality to be typically the expression of the subordinate, the weak and the hypocritical. In this sense, ideologies are not errors or falsities of belief but rather systematic misrepresentations of genuine feeling and action. Ideologies mask the real conditions of willing under the layer of false morality.

These notions in Nietzsche of genuine feeling presuppose a particular vision of the individual in relation to the empirical world of reciprocity and experience. In *On the Genealogy of Morals*, Nietzsche refers to 'the sovereign individual' as the rational agent, distinguishing such individuals from his notion of the overmen (*Übermensch*). When Nietzsche refers to the sovereign individual he is not discussing or reproducing Mills' notion of the individual in liberal thought as an agent standing over and above the natural world, enjoying complete autonomy and political sovereignty. For Nietzsche, to grasp the essence of one's freedom is to see oneself as part of a fundamental empirical reality which is not simply the reflection or production of one's own will or strength or imagination. Nietzsche asserted the autonomy and facticity of the everyday world and saw the recognition of this facticity as a necessary condition for the realization of the will. To regard reality as simply the product of will would be, in itself, a form of pathological nihilism.

Nietzsche, like Kierkegaard, is in a sense arguing that the usual categories of logic cannot truly express or embrace the experience of life, whether these are joy or suffering. Ofelia Schutte in *Beyond Nihilism* has aptly conceptualized Nietzsche's project; Nietzsche's aim was to relocate the elementary forms of all values in life itself and to give this conceptualization of embodiment a positive value. To ask questions about reality from the position of philosophy as traditionally conceived is an expression of nihilism, since 'existence as such does not require justification, and to raise the question of justification already shows a negation of life' (Schutte, 1984, p. 6). To return to the question of the rational character of the sovereign individual as an agent, this rationality will be manifest in the practical production of self-authenticating identity; this conception is, of course, parallel to Marx's own emphasis on praxis as the ultimate criterion of truth. Nietzsche cannot be nostalgic about the loss of community with the disappearance of God and the emergence of the utilitarian individual, since he is committed to the idea of a practical test of truth as a developing and evolving principle.

Although he considered that Nietzsche provides a powerful concept of ideology and its conditions, Warren wanted to criticize Nietzsche for remaining at an abstract level and for failing to develop an adequate understanding of social structure as reification. Nietzsche's solution is seen to be fixed at the cultural level, seeing the modern crisis as essentially a cultural crisis. To quote at some length from Warren

his desire for a hierarchical, ascriptive, neo-artistocratic society can be explained as a result of his totalization of the assumption that only a rigid division of economic and cultural labour (as in ancient Greek society) could produce a culture strong enough to overcome the crisis; he envisaged a political dominion of a few higher beings who would produce such a culture (Warren, 1984, p. 561).

Schutte also criticizes Nietzsche for failing to follow through his project of a Dionysian critique of truth on the basis of the density and facticity of everyday life and experience. Nietzsche's critical capability founders upon his elitist assumptions about the social structure and his authoritarian view of moral excellence. The issues raised by these critics are clearly problematic and complex. However, in this study we wish to argue that Nietzsche did not develop a systematic account of social structure in terms of macro-social and political relations and, in particular, he did not develop the concept of a social system in which the state would be significant as a regulating institution, precisely because he saw such reified concepts as themselves manifesting a certain alienation from the will-to-power. The abstract concepts of society and state are, in Nietzsche's thought, too vague to be useful, because they do not directly reflect the will-to-life. These concepts are reifications, not useful perspectives. In opposition to such abstract conceptualization, Nietzsche attempted to develop ideas about the body, the everyday world, exchanges of direct reciprocity and the experiences of hatred and love as the bases for a social theory, not itself reflecting the reified categories of the official world.

Concluding Unscientific Postscript

The debate over modernism and post-modernism has, in recent years, dominated intellectual argument about the character of knowledge, reason and social change in contemporary society. Any discussion of modernity must, in our view, entail some analysis of the notions of nostalgia and utopia as crucial responses to the modern moral crisis. In this chapter we have explored certain features of this issue by examining the response of social theory to certain problems raised by Nietzsche, especially in regard to the death of God. This evaluation of nostalgia has taken the form of an overview of major thinkers in contemporary social science. While it could be argued that Nietzsche embraced a type of nostalgia in terms of his celebration of pre-Socratic institutions, emotions and beliefs, we have given greater prominence to Nietzsche's moral proposal for a revaluation of values, the affirmation of positivity and the embracing of the world of everyday life as necessary components of his doctrine of *amor fati*.

The problem of nostalgia and melancholy has been endemic to western culture, especially through medical doctrines of the four humours, scholastic medicine and the theory of temperament. Melancholy had two contradictory features. In its positive form, melancholy was associated with heightened self-awareness and a number of moral virtues. Black, debilitating and bitter melancholy came to be regarded as merely a degenerate form of the uplifting sensitive and sympathetic version; positive melancholy was seen to be a moral stimulus for virtuous persons. In some seventeenth-century poetic discussions of melancholy, we can discover a tradition which placed an emphasis upon the moral value of nostalgia as an aid to heightened sensibility. In melancholy 'soft notes, sweet perfumes, dreams and landscapes mingled with darkness, solitude and even grief itself, and by this bitter-sweet contradiction served to heighten self-awareness' (Klibansky, Panofsky and Saxl, 1964, p. 230). In a literary tradition, this form of melancholy was also associated with the catharsis of suffering brought about by music as the response to individual grief. The same note of personal awareness and spiritual development was struck in John Keat's odes to melancholy and to the Grecian urn.

This ancient tradition in medicine and literature, whereby melancholy, nostalgia and self-awareness were merged into a complex sentiment of joy and sorrow was reproduced in Kant's *Observations on the Sense of the Beautiful and the Sublime*, which appeared in 1764. In this manuscript, Kant was responding to the tradition of Rousseau, and this lyrical, sympathetic fragment was wholly unlike his later more systematic and professional philosophy (Cassirer, 1981). Kant, providing an aesthetic interpretation of the traditional theory of temperaments, joined the melancholy type with the sublime on the grounds that the melancholy personality was endowed with a moral freedom, a heightened awareness and a sensibility to the dilemmas of life. Kant claimed that the melancholic was a true friend, an honest inquirer after knowledge and a person whose moral convictions could be relied upon. Such a person was melancholic precisely because they were open to the pain of our finite existence.

In this project on Nietzsche's relevance to the contemporary crisis of society, we have been critical of an unreflective nostalgia in social theory, which one-dimensionally placed a positive value on pre-modernity. By contrast, we have argued that it is important to accept the moral challenge of Nietzsche's Godless philosophy and to assume a personal responsibility for our place in this world, rather than seeking some consolation in a fairytale, rural community which never existed. However, we have also emphasized the ambiguities of the nostalgic attitude and would accept that certain elements of this traditional view of melancholy always had two potentialities, one liberating and one degenerative. Our aim is not to rationalize melancholy and to dismiss it as simply a pre-modern medical condition. In this respect, there is a certain convergence between our argument and the social theory of Arnold Gehlen (1965). Gehlen described three basic modes of action, namely rational-practical action, ritual-presentative action, and those actions which are a reversion of the orientation of a psychological drive. For Gehlen, these three forms of action were closely interlinked and highly integrated in archaic culture, and he argued that it was exactly this integration that represented the attractive quality of these types of culture. The nostalgic reference of intellectualized urban cultures towards these archaic modes of integration are therefore of special interest.

Gehlen attempted to relate these three different systems to three forms of action. The rational-experimental form of action gains its highest expression in the world-view of materialism. All meta-physics of sympathetic relations refer back to the ritual-presentative action form. These meta-physical systems find their contemporary expression in the transformation of magic into modern art. In a similar fashion, the reversion of the direction of a drive is associated with a religious vocation in the world. These three world visions, according to Gehlen, give men the potentiality for an indirect self-consciousness and self-awareness. To identify oneself with the 'non-I', with something different from humanity, and to distinguish oneself exactly within this identification process are two important conditions for a re-integration of self-conscious agents into the social world, and they form the basis for a reaffirmation of oneself through action.

Gehlen acknowledged the human condition as being essentially depressive and melancholic; this depressiveness can only be overcome through institutional systems of guidance which act towards the balancing of the anthropologically-conditioned factors of melancholy and bring about a new stability and order in human action. Gehlen himself might be taken as an example that nostalgia and melancholy are not only attitudes of cultural production in themselves, but might also lead to a strong attachment towards institutional order and the loss of individual freedom of action. Nostalgia and melancholy are not simply forms of psychic retreatism (Merton, 1964), but rather they should be seen as attitudes relevant to the construction of oppositional systems and utopias. It is obviously ritual performance within institutions which produces a relative stability and balance of performances for the individual, while reflection upon this relationship between the individual and formalized ritualism brings about a de-stabilization of the social order and a crisis of consciousness for the individual. This problem is also implied by Gehlen, who saw a necessary integration between naivety, the absence of reflexivity and submission to coercive orders and regulations.

In attempting to outline a new form of sociology based upon Nietzsche, we would draw a connection between utopianism in its astrological form and de-stabilizing nostalgia as a positive feature of anthropological melancholy. In Nietzsche's terms, some aspects of nostalgia would be pessimistic and fatalistic, locking us into a debilitating and backward-looking sentimentality. By contrast, the pessimism of strength accepts the loss of a world, but utilizes healthy nostalgia as a form of utopianism for the reconstruction of social relations. We wish to explore these radical features of nostalgia in subsequent chapters.

2

The Genealogy of Discipline

Introduction: Materialism and Nature

In this chapter, we shall consider the complex relationship between human embodiment, social reciprocity within the *habitus* of everyday reality and the institutional superstructure of regulation and restraint. We conceptualize the system of societal regulations as a form of institutionalized *ressentiment*. The aim of this discussion is to generate a general theory of the social, which will take into account the substratum of everyday experience grounded in the reality of the phenomenal body. Our assumption is that through these three dimensions (reciprocity, resentment and resistance), it is possible to elaborate a sociological perspective which is consistent with and influenced by the philosophy of Nietzsche with special reference to the doctrine of 'little things'. Within this discourse, we hope to draw upon Nietzsche's metaphors of health and sickness as criteria for the evaluation of social forms. As an approach to the sociology of the body, we use the method of indirect discussion by an historical elaboration of the problem of 'nature' in social theory. We wish to trace an analytical development within German philosophy from Karl Marx to Alfred Schutz, which we believed entailed an engagement with philosophical anthropology as an exploration of human praxis in relation to culture and nature. These developments in social philosophy in the nineteenth century were often direct responses to changes in biological theories which social theory adopted and criticized in order to generate new perspectives on human behaviour and social relations. In the twentieth century, similar developments in biological theories about the fundamental fabric of life itself have also called forth a response by social theory which has, through various theoretical developments, attempted to come to terms with the problem of life and its constitution. We can see these developments in the work of very diverse social philosophers from Talcott Parsons to Peter Berger. While many of these intellectual issues have been popularized in the form of a new positivism (namely socio-biology), the argument developed here is that a phenomenology of the body is a necessary feature of all sociological inquiry and that the concept of embodiment provides an alternative to the theoretical cul-de-sac represented by a biologizing tendency in some versions of social theory. The phenomenology of embodiment within a Nietzschean perspective offers a solution to the traditional Cartesian problem of mind and body, and generates a new perspective on the character of the agent within the conventional problem of agency-structure. It also provides the theoretical ground work for a complete theory of resistance. We suggest that modern sociology should return to the tradition linking Nietzsche to Heidegger to reconsider the ontology of 'man's place' (Harries, 1978). This chapter is therefore an attempt to rediscover the value of the concept of the will-to-power as a basis for recasting modern sociological theory.

The development of social theory in the eighteenth and nineteenth centuries was, of course, heavily dependent upon the development of medical science. Indeed, it is possible to argue that the origins of sociology are clearly located in social medicine; medical speculation about moral character significantly influenced the conception of man as simultaneously a creature of nature and a being within the spiritual world. In the French context, Cabanis' *On the Relations Between the Physical and Moral Aspects of Man* (1981) played an important part in the development of a theory of feeling based on medical ideas. In a later period, the physiology of Claud Bernard influenced the development of Durkheim's views on social organization, since Durkheim adopted much of the language of the natural sciences (Hirst, 1975). In German social thought, the impact of natural science and especially the evolutionary theories of Darwin clearly shaped the philosophical view of history and human development. Engels' *Dialectics of Nature* (1954) would be one prominent illustration.

Our argument is that, while natural science was significant in the development of Marx's views of human society, biology and related sciences were, to some extent, dismissed as merely the ideological smoke screen of bourgeois interest. The confrontation with Malthus and Darwin resulted in a dismissal of biology and the biological character of human existence in favour of economic materialism. Materialism shifted from the sensual to the economic. Although Marxism has been influenced by the materialistic tradition of Epicurus and Feuerbach, Marxism has been unable to come to terms with the

61

wider problem of materialism, because biological questions have been relegated to the category of ideology. For Marx and Engels, the struggle between the species in the evolutionary model of Darwinistic biology was a replica of the conflice of interests and the struggle between social classes in industrial capitalism (Sahlins, 1977). Similarly, Marx in *Theories of Surplus Value* (1968) condemned Malthus as an apologist for the landed classes and argued that Malthusian philosophy was a mere disguise for the interests of those who depended upon rents, sinecures and other unproductive forms of wealth (Meek, 1971).

The result was that the biological became either an effect of ideological practices or was subordinate to more fundamental processes of economic production. It is strange, therefore, that Marxist materialism never fully embraced the debate about the location of human beings within the natural world and in contemporary Marxism only Sebastiano Timpanaro in *On Materialism* (1975) has seriously addressed these issues from a theoretical and historical perspective. In twentieth-century Marxism, any concern with natural processes and the natural environment of the human species was further excluded by the philosophical interest in the classical German tradition, especially represented by Kant; the rejection of mechanistic historical explanations in vulgar Marxism by the Austro-Marxist philosophers (Bottomore and Goode, 1978) and by Karl Korsch (1972) further distanced mainstream Marxism from any debate with embodiment, biology, natural science and a conception of materialism as sensual practice.

Marx on Praxis and Nature

The debate about nature and human nature in Marxism comes down eventually to a debate about Marx's ontology. Clearly, Marx had a distinctive view of the location of human beings in nature which was elaborated in his early work, especially in the economic and philosophic manuscripts of 1844. We do not, therefore, wish to suggest that Marx had no view of human nature and the location of man in the environment of the natural world; rather we have argued that Marx's ontology was eventually submerged by the development of an economic materialism as a component within the Marxist analysis of historical change. An appreciation of Marx's understanding of human embodiment has been associated with a renewed interest in humanistic Marxism, a re-evaluation of the young Marx and a reappraisal of Marx's relation to Feuerbach. This interest in the philosophical anthropology of Marx was, of course, challenged subsequently by structuralist Marxism and in particular by the philosophical tradition represented in France by Louis Althusser. It was this structural Marxism which brought about a super-determinism in which human agency and social praxis were obliterated by so-called 'scientific Marxism'; the human agent became the mere effect of ideological and economic structures.

The re-evaluation of Marx's view of human nature, sensualism and praxis owes a great deal to the work of George Lukács (1971), Alfred Schmidt (1971) and George Markus (1978). Marx's philosophical anthropology starts with the simple premise of materialism, namely that human beings are part of nature and that labour or work is directed towards the satisfaction of needs which are generic to human beings as sentient beings. However, with the historical development of human societies, people appropriate nature and transform it through work; through this transformation and appropriation of nature, they constantly transform themselves. The transformation of the natural world by the use of tools and by the development of culture becomes an objectification of human will. Thus the basic components of Marx's ontology are included in the account of how human social beings change, transform and appropriate the natural environment through the social processes of work. Within this perspective, the natural environment is simultaneously the object and the condition of existence for human beings; the transformation of this natural environment is brought about by praxis or more generally by the conscious, practical, social activity of human groups in the satisfaction of needs. It follows from Marx's ontology that human characteristics are not fixed or static, since human biology is constantly transformed and shaped by activity itself. Furthermore, Marx did not treat the human being as an isolated agent, but based his philosophical anthropology on the premise of social relations and social activities. These social relations are historically variable and they are explained by the nature of the particular mode of production which is dominant in social relations. Therefore, the man-society-nature relationship is fundamentally historical and social.

The historical development of human society involves the expansion of human potential such that the natural boundary is constantly pushed backwards by the social development of these human abilities. Through this process, Marx argued that nature becomes 'the inorganic body' of man. This dialectical relationship between human beings, social organization and nature was expressed by Marx in the notion of the 'naturalization of man' and the 'humanization of nature'. Nature is consequently conceptualized not as a thing-in-itself, but as a social extension of human labour; however, under conditions of private

63

property, market relations and economic expropriation, social reality constantly assumes a reified character and consciousness of human agency is lost in a world dominated by fetishism.

The core of Marx's ontology was, therefore, occupied by the concept of human praxis. The importance of this idea in Marx's sociology has been lucidly outlined by Henri Lefebvre and we quote at some length from his evaluation:

The concept of praxis presupposes the rehabilitation of the world of sense, restoration of the practical-sensuous ... as Feuerbach had seen, the sensuous is the foundation of all knowledge because it [is] the foundation of Being. The sensuous is not merely rich in meaning; it is a human creation. The human world has been created by men and women in the course of their history, starting from an originary nature which is given to us already transformed by our own efforts-tools, language, concepts, signs. Wealth at once graspable and inexhaustable, the practical-sensuous shows us what praxis is ... the unity of the sensuous and the intellectual, of nature and culture, confronts us everywhere. (Lefebvre, 1968, pp. 38–9)

Marx's use of the concept of praxis also shows his dependence on the legacy of Greek philosophy, particularly the legacy of Aristotle, since it was Aristotle who used the concept of praxis to describe the activities of all animals, but insisted that, in its precise meaning, it should apply only to human beings. In Aristotlian philosophy, praxis was one of the three main activities of human beings. First, there was *theoria*, namely theoretical knowledge and secondly, *poiesis* or cultural production. In Marx's treatment of this legacy, praxis provided the fundamental definition of human beings involved in 'free conscious activity'. Praxis was also the basis of Marx's argument, which was crucial to the theses on Feuerbach, that it is social being that determines consciousness, not consciousness that determines existence. The concept of praxis also provided Marx with the basic approach to the problem of human alienation in history. While praxis or self-conscious practical activity was productive and creative, involving the activity of the free agent, the social world became, through the formation of social classes, independent of human agency and as a result the products of human labour became alienated from human agents. It was for this reason that Marx (somewhat inconsistently) often contrasted the concept of labour to that of praxis, since labour under capitalism produces commodities which are forms of alienated activity and which dominate human beings without fully satisfying their needs.

The concept of praxis in Marxism has often been criticized (Rotenstreich, 1965). One criticism centres on the problem of symbolic exchanges or more simply on communication. It is not clear where to locate signs, symbols and culture in Marx's analysis of sensuous practice. In his theory of communicative action, Jürgen Habermas has attempted to develop Marx's idea of social praxis into a more general theory of interaction (1984). Other writers, most notably Jean Baudrillard (1975), have suggested that the production of symbolic objects cannot be understood within the economic framework of Marx's analysis of use and exchange values. At this stage, we are not immediately concerned with criticisms of Marx, since we simply wish to establish the importance of the notion of creative activity and sensualism in Marx's continuing dependence on the work of Feuerbach, despite Marx's own criticisms of the Feuerbachian legacy of sensualism. The point of this exercise is to suggest important continuities between Nietzsche and Marx in terms of a theory of sensuous activity.

Nietzsche's Body

The dilemma in Marxism, and more generally in social science, is that if we treat nature as simply an effect of human activity, then we incline towards idealism. By contrast, if we treat human activity as an effect of nature, then we incline towards positivistic biology. This problem is, of course, the ancient dilemma of classical philosophy, namely to resolve the relationship between causes and reasons, between biological drives and human social action, between the moral and the natural. One solution proposed by Parsons in *The Structure of Social Action* (1937) was to treat biology as a condition of action, but this is not entirely adequate since we cannot treat the biological as simply a condition of action. We have argued that the notion of embodiment, especially in the French phenomenological tradition, offers a promising solution to this traditional dilemma. Furthermore, we have claimed that this notion of embodiment ('the lived body') can be located in the work of Nietzsche, which we have also implied is consistent with certain aspects of Marx's early work on praxis.

In *The Will to Power*, Nietzsche made various attacks on the idealism and intellectualism of modern thought which, following the legacy of Judaeo-Christian culture, had produced a hierarchy of moral orders which saw the body (the flesh) as the negation of spirituality and reason. Nietzsche wished to restore the body to its proper place in human culture and thereby, in a sense, to return to the emphasis on corporeality in Greek culture, which in competitive sport had celebrated the male body as the measure of perfection. This did not,

65

however, involve a return to any mechanical notion of the body as the product of scientific discourse. Nietzsche looked backwards towards a pre-Socratic Greece as David Levin (1985) has noted, in order to rediscover and retrieve a unified notion of sensuality and knowledge within the concept of a 'lived body'. Nietzsche, in particular, sought to develop a critique of intellectualism by denying the primacy of reason over sensual experience through embodiment. For Nietzsche, the understanding of the importance of the body was fundamental to any understanding of resistance. In Nietzsche, therefore, the discussion of the body was closely related to the whole issue of the will-to-power. The will-to-power was fundamental to all organic bodies. The will-to-power involved a universal drive to dominate, contain and overcome all other organisms and thereby add to what Nietzsche called the body's 'quanta of power':

I characterize the 'Will to Power' – that is to say, as an insatiable desire to manifest power; or the application and exercise of power as a creative instinct. There is no help for it, all movements, all 'appearances', all 'laws' must be understood as *symptoms* of an *inner* phenomenon, and the analogy of man must be used for this purpose. It is possible to trace all the instincts of an animal to the will to power; as also all the functions of organic life to this one source. (*WP*, section 619)

This expanded bodily reproduction is, in fact, the life-enhancement of the body as an ensemble of sense organs.

Because of this primary emphasis on embodiment, Nietzsche often regarded culture itself as a separation from bodily instincts, such that cultured man is a sick man. Modern medical practice contributes to the removal of our sense of the particularity of body (Johnson, 1983). This separation from being is contained in language itself, which substitutes metaphors for instinctual reality. Alternatively, this problem of embodiment and consciousness was expressed in terms of a political struggle between the higher and the lower organs.

As these instincts became blocked and redirected, the internalisation of desires produced a sickness which Nietzsche called the soul. Nietzsche, anticipating Freud's 'primal repression', argued that the growing inwardness of modern societies prevented the release of powerful instincts, so that cruelty, revenge and resentment were repressed and turned inward. This 'de-sensualization' was expressed through the idealization of western philosophyu as the legacy of Christian repression and asceticism. Within this framework, Christianity appears as the primary instance of resentment against life:

We should ascertain whether the typically *religious* man is a decadent phenomenon (the great innovators are one and all morbid and epileptic); but do not forget to include that type of the religious man who is *pagan*. Is the pagan cult not a form of gratitude for, and affirmation of, life? Ought not its most representative type be an apology and defication of life? The type of a well-constituted and ecstatically overflowing spirit! (*WP*, section 1052)

This type was represented primarily by the Dionysus of the Greeks. Resentment is, therefore, the negation of the instinct of life, the suppression of genuine will-to-power under the dominance of cultural decadence, resulting finally in nihilism and neurosis.

Nietzsche's theory of the body cannot be separated from his concern with the fictions of language. For Nietzsche, our sense of unity, continuity and self are products of the grammatical structure of language or, as he called it, the grammatical habit. The plurality of life forces which are the underlying features of embodiment are metaphorically unified under the notion of the self which is, in fact, parasitic upon organic functions. We are, according to Nietzsche, 'a plurality that has imagined itself as a unity' (*WP*, section 333). This relationship between Nietzsche's view of language and the body is well summarized in this argument from Michel Haar:

The actual 'functioning' of the Will-to-Power comes into clearest view with regard to the body understood as a multiplicity originally unintegrated but ascribing to itself for a unity. To philosophize by taking the body as the 'abiding clue' amounts to revealing the 'self' as an instrument, an expression, an interpreter of the body. It also amounts to revealing the body (in opposition to our petty faculty of reasoning, where only surface 'causes' make their appearance) as the 'grand reason' – i.e., as the totality of deeply buried causes in their mobile and contradictory diversity. Philosophy has never ceased to show disdain for the body; it has not wished to recognize that it is the body that whispers thought to the 'soul' and that consciousness is only a superficial and terminal phenomenon. Psychology has always idolized superficial unity for fear of facing the unsettling multipiicity at the depths of being. (Haar, 1977, p. 18)

This notion of multiplicity may also be associated with Nietzsche's enjoyment of the Heraclitian paradox of being and becoming, that is phenomena which have a history because they are becoming cannot be known or comprehended. Our knowledge is only of appearances which are put together because they are useful. Perspectivism is inescapable. This idea was fundamental to Nietzsche's philosophy – 'To *stamp* Becoming with the character of Being – this is the highest *will to power*' (*WP*, 617). Nietzsche argued that we lack an organ for knowing and that what we know is that which is useful in the interests of the species. In the *Twilight of the Idols*, Nietzsche argued that existence is simply an empty fiction and that the 'true' world is merely a false addition to the world of becoming and change. Furthermore, Nietzsche believed that, while many philosophers were prepared to abandon the idea of God as the perfect being, professional philosophy was still wedded to the notion that behind the changing world of appearances, there existed a higher or more perfect world of stable values, a reality against which appearances could be contrasted. Meta-physicians were still in search of the thing-in-itself. Against this background idea of becoming, Nietzsche complained that philosophers were necessarily Egyptians in that they rendered all reality into the form of a mummy by dehistoricizing it. They deny the real world of change and becoming in order to erect a false world of petrified forms, a world of the Dead. Thus in *Twilight of the Idols*, Nietzsche complained that philosophers kill the world, especially the world of senses:

Be a philosopher, be a mummy, represent monothono-theism by a grave digger-mimicry! – And away, above all, with the body, that pitiable *idée fixe* of the senses! infected with every error of logic there is, refuted, impossible even, notwithstanding its impudence enough to behave as if it actually existed! (*TI*, p. 35)

Hence, Nietzsche's enthusiasm for Heraclitus, who rejected philosophical arguments about duration and unity in favour of the evidence of the world of senses that we inhabit a reality characterized by plurality and change.

Nietzsche praised the senses above reason, commenting that the nose is a perfect instrument of observation about which no philosopher has spoken with 'respect and gratitude'. The diversion between the sacred and profane in the philosophical system of Kant, or more generally in the religious tradition of Christianity, was rejected by Nietzsche as the symptom of a declining world, that is of decadence and nihilism. Nietzsche, against this philosophical world of Kant, characteristically contrasted the tragic artist as an optimist who affirms life within the framework of Dionysian enthusiasm. Against what Nietzsche called 'the spiritualization of sensuality' as love, he argued for the creative redirection of senses, passions and emotions.

Nietzsche believed that the concept of the perfect world had a psychological function for meta-physicians. Confronted with a world of contradiction, plurality, change and falsity, philosophers like Christians sought a world beyond suffering as a compensation for pain and death

68

or, in Marxist terms, they sought an opium as a relief from the finitude of the changing world. Against the brutality of the world of becoming, philosophers and theologians posited a world of being. The world of being expresses our hatred of pain and suffering, consequent upon our embodiment. Thus Nietzsche argued that 'to imagine another, more valuable world is an expression of hatred for a world that makes one suffer: the *ressentiment* of meta-physicians against actuality is here creative' (*WP*, section 579). Intellectualization and rationalization are the revenge of philosophers on becoming.

The History of Resentment: Max Scheler

The French word *ressentiment* was used by both Nietzsche and Scheler. It has become widely accepted within the German language, although there is no full equivalent for this term in English. Derived from the French word *sentire* (to feel), the English notion of resentment indicating indignation or bitter feelings against some person or situation is not equivalent in its impact or generality to the French notion of *ressentiment*. We have suggested that the concept of *ressentiment* in Nietzsche was important as a very general critique of culture and history, which cannot be reduced to the psychological notion of indignation (Deeken, 1974). The notion of *ressentiment* had a number of important functions in Nietzsche's philosophy. Firstly, it was a very general critique of the theological development of Christianity, which posited an absolute God as the alternative, positive version of human values. Secondly, it was used as a critique of meta-physicians in *The Will to Power* where Nietzsche argued that the creation of a world of being as opposed to the world of becoming was an act of resentment, a defence mechanism for weak men. Thirdly, he treated all forms of so-called slave morality as moral systems born of *ressentiment* in, for example, *Human, All Too Human*. Nietzsche also equated the doctrine of egalitarianism with resentment and decay in the analysis of 'the order of rank' in *The Will to Power*. Nietzsche regarded such resentful moralities as a form of cultural pessimism, passing a sentence of death on existence itself and he thereby also referred to them as anti-natural moralities, because they were against the instincts of life, an argument which he developed in *Twilight of the Idols*. In short, resentment is part of a culture of the despisers of the body, and therefore an illness which is very common in modern societies; it is grounded in bad faith.

One of the most influential developments of the theory of resentment was contained in Scheler's phenomenology. While Scheler's early work

69

was dominated by theological and moral questions, as in his influential *Der Formalismus in der Ethik und die material Wertethik*, in his later works he turned more to the problems of affectivity, human existence, the body, sympathy and resentment. Of particular interest is his essay *Man's Place in Nature* (1962). We shall not pursue in detail Scheler's sociology of knowledge or his writings on ethics which have been treated fully by Alfred Schutz (1966), because we are primarily concerned with Scheler's elaboration of the theory of will and being.

Scheler was concerned to develop a phenomenology of emotions, affect and intentionality as a critique of what he regarded as Kant's moral formalism, which treated emotions as a major obstacle to the development of a rationalist theory of moral behaviour. For Kant, a moral action was one which conformed to the moral law and which was not tainted by affection, irrational emotions or by a utilitarian consideration for rewards. In order to bring the terrain of the irrational within phenomenological inspection, Scheler developed his own notion of 'the person' as the focus, not simply of rational intentions, but also of emotional commitments. Furthermore, Scheler abandoned the characteristic methodological individualism of rationalist philosophy by arguing that we can only understand the person in relation to and interaction with other persons, so that my consciousness of myself is necessarily social consciousness. This led Scheler to analyse what he called the social emotions, namely love, sympathy and shame. Scheler's phenomenology of intention was, therefore, fundamentally grounded in a philosophical anthropology and in a sociology of knowledge (Pivcevic, 1970).

In his *Man's Place in Nature*, Scheler drew upon the theoretical biology of Uexküll and Dresch (Schutz, 1966, p. 135) to explore the philosophical problem of human existence within the natural world. On the one hand, Scheler wanted to root the human species within the total complexity of organic life, but on the other hand, he wanted to identify a special world of human beings. Scheler intended to give full recognition to the natural, organic location of the human species, while also giving full recognition to the importance of Spirit (*Geist*) as the principal distinction between the animal and the human world. In order to present this argument, Scheler conceptualized life in terms of various strata or levels. The lowest level of life is the organic or vegetative existence of the plant, which, while without consciousness, is the site of elementary resistance, providing the basis for any experience of reality. The second form of life is represented by instinctual activities, which are characteristic of the animal world, representing in Scheler's view, a specialization of the life-process. While instincts often look purposeful, they are in fact fixed responses to the environment and are acquired already formed by the young animal. The third stratum of life is occupied by the associative memory of conditioned reflexes. To these reflexes, there correspond various forms of behaviour which have been developed in an infinite number of behavioural 'experiments', according to the principles made famous by Pavlov. Scheler referred to the fourth form of life in terms of 'practical intelligence' which involves the capacity to select between different courses of action. Although these activities involve consciousness, practical intelligence is also part of the animal kingdom. The principal difference between conditioned reflexes and practical intelligence is that the latter is more flexible in response to variations in the environment. This argument was, in general, important for Scheler, because he wished to argue that scientific reasoning was not the crucial difference between man and intelligent animals; by associating practical intelligence with science, Scheler wished to emphasize the idea that the difference between an intelligent animal and an intelligent scientist is one of degree rather than kind. Human beings are separated from the animal kingdom at the fifth level of life, namely the level of the Spirit, which permits us to talk about human beings as persons quite separate from animals. Human beings are not simply subject to conditioned reflexes, biological needs or practical intelligence in respect to environmental threats. We can argue that only human beings have self-consciousness, which enables them to reflect explicitly upon their biological conditions and, where necessary, to deny the satisfaction of instincts in the interests of other goals which may be cultural and spiritual.

In an argument which was quite distinct from Nietzsche, Scheler suggested that the defining characteristic of human beings is their capacity for asceticism, that is their ability to deny and detach themselves from immediate instinctual gratification. This asceticism was firmly connected with his notion of Spirit, person and action. Human beings are capable not only of reflecting upon, but also resisting their biological drives and instinctual needs. The anthropological underpinnings of Scheler's view of ethics can be explained in the following summary:

Man is a being who can 'withdraw' from the spatio-temporal world into himself and in this very act of 'withdrawal' he rediscovers the world as an object. He can 'stand back' and contemplate the world and himself with a detached mind, and only because he can do this is he able to see clearly what is essentially involved in what the existentialists call his being-in-the-world. Man can transcend the world of spatio-temporal existence, he can say 'no', and this is the foundation of his freedom. (Pivcevic, 1970, p. 101)

This no-saying behaviour is the root of all ethical life, which involves some suppression of the will-to-life, that is in Nietzsche's terms, the will-to-power.

Scheler's sympathy for and criticism of Nietzsche's theory of values and human character were both graphically illustrated in his response to the theory of resentment. In his study *Ressentiment* (1961), Scheler accepted many aspects of Nietzsche's argument, adding to Nietzsche's account a phenomenology of resentment by considering various forms of resentment in relation to diverse social roles. For example, Scheler criticized the romantic type of mind in terms of the drive for revenge and resentment. He felt that one particular illustration of this was Friedrich Schlegel's nostalgia for the world of the Middle Ages, which Scheler argued was simply a form of resentment against the modern world. However, against Nietzsche, Scheler defended the concept of Christian love as an expression of strength rather than weakness, as an effect of vitality rather than decadence. He suggested that Nietzsche had confused authentic love with Schopenhauer's version of Christian culture. As opposed to Nietzsche, Scheler regarded the culture of bourgeois society as the most profound manifestation of negative resentment. In particular, he condemned the bourgeois version of utilitarian philosophy as a perversion of true values and a subversion of genuine feeling and Christian love. For Scheler, the doctrine of the useful was the most prominent sign of moral decadence in modern capitalism.

Although Scheler disagreed sharply with many of Nietzsche's conclusions and with many of his assumptions, Scheler's phenomenology nevertheless gave a central importance to the biological and to the body in the understanding of man's place in the universe. As Schutz (1962) has noted, Scheler's views on the body played an important part in the development of his general understanding of the *alter ego* in the growth of sociality. However, while Scheler criticized previous philosophical traditions for neglecting the biological (particularly the sexual) life of humanity, he argued that it was crucial to restore the idea of the sexual act to its 'true meta-physical significance' (Scheler, 1954, p. 110). The problem of achieving an adequate analysis of sexuality was located in a dilemma which emerged within early Judaism and was subsequently reinforced by Christianity. Scheler argued that the traditional religious dilemma involved the notion that the essence of sexual activity lay in its end and that this must be either human procreation or sensual enjoyment. Scheler wanted, however, the draw a clear distinction between the instinctual roots of sexuality and the moral character of love, since whereas sexuality merely reproduces, he argued that love creates.

Although Scheler did not provide an entirely consistent or coherent phenomenology of the life-world, his attempt to analyse emotion laid some of the ground work for an adequate theory of reciprocity, resistance and resentment. Aspects of Scheler's phenomenology became important for Husserl and Merleau-Ponty in their development of the notion of the lived body and the structure of inter-subjectivity (Rabil, 1967). In this section, we are not centrally concerned with the development of French existentialism and phenomenology. Instead, we turn to an influential development of this tradition, namely to the work of Peter Berger and Thomas Luckmann, who, in elaborating an analysis of the everyday world, have followed closely the philosophical tradition of Arnold Gehlen (Berger and Kellner, 1965).

The Social Construction of Reality

Berger and Luckmann attempted to develop an innovative theory of institutions and knowledge based upon the theoretical biology and philosophical anthropology of Arnold Gehlen, A. Bolk, J. von Uexkull, A. Portmann, F. Buytendijk and Helmuth Plessner. To this biological and philosophical tradition, they sought to conjoin the analysis of life-worlds which was derived from Feuerbach, Marx, Nietzsche and Scheler. Like Scheler, they were concerned to identify the crucial differences between the animal and the human world. On the basis of developments in biological science, they argued in their early work that the human organism had an unfinished character at birth and was characterized by an 'unspecialized instinctual structure' (Berger and Kellner, 1965, p. 111). Because the human being is launched into a world from which he is, in some sense, distanced, human beings have socially to construct an environment which will provide them with the stability and coherence which they lack because of the unspecialized and unfinished character of their instinctual make-up. The evolution of social institutions represents the core of this development of cultural coherence through constant social and symbolic reproduction. Of course, the primary feature of this institutionalization of the human world is language itself, which provides a mechanism for the accumulation of knowledge over generations and the ability to structure the world in an infinitely flexible manner. By definition, language is always social, since it presupposes and requires communication and shared assumptions.

Gehlen's work was important because it had a clear view of the historical development of human societies and thereby avoided some of

73

the static assumptions concerning human essences which were characteristically a feature of nineteenth-century philosophical anthropology. In his theory of the development of social institutions, Gehlen argued that pre-modern cultures were more embracing, encompassing, integrated and taken-for-granted than is the case in contemporary industrial societies. Modern cultures are exposed to the inquiry of instrumental rationality and social differentiation which tend to shatter the normative facticity of traditional orders, exposing human beings to self-reflective anxiety. The leading characteristic of contemporary society is its 'subjectivism' at the individual level, whereby human beings are encouraged to find normative principles within their interior personal lives.

Berger and Luckmann showed how Gehlen's views on the relationship between the biological and the cultural had shaped a number of issues in contemporary German sociology. This influence was especially important in the sociology of religion and sociology of knowledge. For Helmut Schelsky (1957), the eternal truths of Christianity had rested on forms of life whose legitimacy depended upon the continuity of traditions and the stability of social structures. Modern societies have become increasingly independent from the regulation of traditional institutions; in order the adapt to the peculiar features of the modern world, the faith of Christianity can no longer continue without radical transformation. Schelsky argued that the essential feature of modern consciousness was the practice of continuous self-questioning, which rendered the stability of religious truths increasingly unstable and archaic. Modern consciousness, resting upon the prevailing rationalism, secularity and subjectivism, could no longer be contained within the traditional institutions of the Christian religion.

These themes were pursued at greater length by Luckmann in *The Invisible Religion* (1967) and by Berger in *The Social Reality of Religion* (1966). These studies in the sociology of religion have a common theme which is that, given the unfinished character of human biology, social groups create a cultural universe of meaning, which over time assumes an objective character. The authority of cultural norms rests on taken-for-granted assumptions, which in turn presuppose continuity and stability. Of course, the newly born child does not enter a cultural or social vacuum, but rather inherits the existing meaning-systems which appear to have a basic facticity;

this means that human organisms normally transcend their biological nature by internalizing a historically given universe of meaning, rather than by

74

constructing universes of meaning. This implies, further, that a human organism does not confront other human organisms; it confronts Selves. (Luckman, 1967, p. 51)

The external, objective world of cultural facts becomes an internal subjective reality of commitment and involvement via the familiar processes of socialization and internalization. While these meaning systems are of a very general character in human societies, the most significant institutionalization of these cultural systems has been through the ritual mechanisms of religion. Meaning systems become institutionally specialized in the form of religion, which is differentiated from other aspects of culture and social structure, giving rise ultimately to the universal separation discussed by Durkheim between the sacred and the profane. The differentiation and specialization of the religious system give rise to dogma and a professional stratum of religious intellectuals whose job it is to defend the authority of sacred texts (Luhmann, 1984). Both Luckmann and Berger see this religiosity as rooted in the fundamental anthropological and biological facts of human beings, namely the 'transcendence of biological nature by human organisms' (Luckmann, 1967, p. 69).

Berger and Luckmann argue that the sacred canopy of modern societies has been threatened by the pluralization of life-worlds which brings about a secularization of culture through the attrition of traditional religious institutions and belief systems. Following Gehlen, they argue that this contraction of the sacred realm brings about an increasing autonomy of the individual who becomes the main focus and carrier of contemporary religiosity. The differentiation of modern cultural systems presents the individual with the challenge of choice, whereby the absoluteness and authenticity of beliefs can no longer be simply taken for granted. The rationalization of belief, the differentiation of the social structure and the pluralism of commitment are processes which have rendered the conventional religious explanations of reality subject to massive doubt, uncertainty and indifference. In an explanation reminiscent of Weber's views on religion in modern society, Berger and Luckmann have suggested that there has been, in modern cultures, a retreat inwards towards the private sphere and the subjective as the final bastion of religious emotion, experience and belief.

These approaches to the problem of belief in modern society were extended into a general sociology of knowledge of the everyday world in *The Social Construction of Reality* (Berger and Luckmann, 1967). The theoretical and philosophical sources for this perspective on the sociology of knowledge are extremely varied and eclectic. For example, from Durkheim's sociology, they draw the argument that the moral order is experienced as a realm of social facts, which are characterized by their objectivity and externality from the human subject. From Weber, they derive an emphasis on the subjective meaning of social action from the point of view of the social actor. From Marx, they adopt an emphasis on praxis to argue that social reality is continually constructed by the repetitive activities of knowledgeable beings. They also derive the concept of resentment from Nietzsche, which they develop in connection with theories of legitimation, namely social theodicy. These sociological interpretations of the dialectical relationship between social action and moral facts are finally rooted in their view of man's biological and natural environment from the theories of Gehlen, which emphasize the 'world-openness', of the human environment. The essential core of their argument is that human beings require a normative system in order to exist and this value system structures their environment providing meaning and purpose. This normative order is based in, and depends upon, the stability of the everyday world which is essentially a taken-for-granted reality.

This somewhat eclectic theoretical apparatus is held together by an analysis of social relations in terms of three 'moments', namely externalization, objectivation and internalization. Externalization involves the praxis of active and knowledgeable human agents who, continually and necessarily, create their cultural and physical environment through collective social practices. Objectivation refers to the processes by which these humanly created products achieve an apparently objective reality, which confronts human agents as a realm of exterior facticity. Finally, internalization is the social process whereby human beings re-appropriate this exterior objective reality, transforming it into a set of structures within the subjective consciousness. Under the notion of externalization, we recognize that society is ultimately a human product; however, it is through the process of objectivation that society assumes a reality which is independent of human actions and finally, by internalization, human beings take over society once more as a product of their labour.

These three processes enable Berger and Luckmann to combine the notions of anomie, alienation and reification. Through alienation, human beings experience the social world as a natural or factual environment which provides a protective canopy against the threat of anomie and social chaos. Reification is anthropologically useful as a defence mechanism against the constant threats to the nomos. It is because human beings biologically cannot cope with the threat of cultural and moral chaos, that they require the elementary processes of reification and internalization, in order that the everyday world can be secured from ultimate collapse.

Berger and Luckmann's theory of the relationship between biology, culture and social order has been criticized on a number of grounds (Abercrombie, 1980). To some extent, they conflate two separate problems, namely the problems of order and meaning. While we might expect these to have a close relationship, they are, theoretically and empirically, somewhat separate issues. There is, of course, ample sociological and psychological evidence to suggest that disorder creates extreme anxiety, uncertainty and frustration for both the individual and social groups; human beings typically respond to these situations by structuring their environment in terms of ritual or habitual practices. Anthropological research on magic and ritual gives direct evidence that this is a common human activity in the face of uncertainty.

However, the level of disorder which human beings can tolerate is a question of empirical investigation, rather than one of theoretical stipulation. The implication of Berger and Luckmann's argument is that human beings require a total nomos which structures every detail of the life-world. This situation follows from their argument about chaos; they juxtapose an ideal typical notion of total order with an ideal typical notion of chaos. The implication of their theory is that chaos is not a sociologically viable concept. They recognize that the nomos of the contemporary world is challenged by pluralism, secularity and rapid social change. However, they have a more basic theoretical commitment to the notion that human beings cannot tolerate disorder, because they cannot survive without meaning systems. In short, Berger and Luckmann threaten us with the prospect of chaos, believing that a sacred canopy is a necessary feature of all human relationships. This problem arises in part because of their conflation of the two separate issues of meaning and order. For example, human beings could have an orderly social universe which was, nevertheless, meaningless, and alternatively they might have a meaningful universe, which was relatively disorganized. These combinations should be questions of empirical investigation rather than simply being deduced from the basic proposition concerning the openness of human instinctual life.

This problem leads to another theoretical issue which is that Berger and Luckmann define religion so broadly that no human practice or set of beliefs could fall outside the domain of religion. Religion includes all of those human practices which structure the everyday world with the effect of rendering it a factual, taken-for-granted universe. Since human beings engage in endless habitual and ritual activities, their world is essentially religious and the implication is that only religion can

77

legitimate this everyday world. Everything which 'transcends' the everyday world assumes a sacred character. Finally, their distinction between the animal world and the human world is, in practice, somewhat difficult to sustain in the terms presented by the theory. Because of the historically extensive interaction between the animal and the human world, it is not entirely clear in what sense there is a dog-world or a cat-world independent of human culture and society. Given the impact of human organization on nature, it is not self-evident that, for example, cats inhabiting contemporary New York still live in a cat-world for which their instinctual structure has uniquely equipped them to survive without ambiguity. In the modern world, cats and dogs may also need psycho-analytic investigation and therapy.

We should also note that, in many respects, Berger and Luckmann's account of the life-world is the opposite of Nietzsche's. Whereas Nietzsche developed a concept of genealogy and resentment as a far-reaching cultural critique of contemporary societies, the phenomenology of the everyday world in contemporary sociology often assumes a conservative perspective on social arrangements. The implication of phenomenology is that human beings have a biological need for religious meaning and order; Nietzsche, by contrast, saw the death of God as a historical event, liberating human beings from the regulations of asceticism and bad faith. For Nietzsche, institutionalized religion was a negation of the will-to-power.

Nietzsche versus the Phenomenologists

Nietzsche sought to criticize religion, not only as a collective illusion, but as a collective illness. However, Nietzsche fully recognized the psychological utility of bad faith, but argued that morally honest people would face up to the perspectivism of modern culture withouth self-deception. Berger and Luckmann have minimized the critical edge of German social theory by suggesting that religion is a psychological necessity and an antidote to anomic social forces. For Nietzsche, all culture (science, art and religion) is ultimately an illusion which protects us from awareness of finitude. However, Nietzsche did not seek to defend such necessities, arguing the case for a revaluation of values as the final solution to nihilism. The tragedy of modern rationalism, and hence of modern cultural systems, is that rational inquiry finally discovers its own limitations and horizons. The result is cultural pessimism.

Berger and Luckmann can be criticized for presenting a conservative version of Nietzsche's critique of contemporary culture by arguing for the positive virtues of illusions as the sacred canopy protecting the everyday world from the threat of chaos. While they promise a critical analysis of modern consciousness by showing that human agents make the world they inhabit, this potentially radical insight is undermined by the equally powerful argument that human beings need the protection of a reified cultural environment. Because human agents require social order, stability and certainty as a consequence of their biological openness and the psychological need for comfort, there is little theoretical space for de-alienation, de-institutionalization and genuine consciousness. While they stress the social character of the world as a constructed environment, their ultimate explanation of social reality involves a somewhat static, ahistorical notion of 'the constitution of man' (Berger and Luckmann, 1967, pp. 117-22; Berger and Pullberg, 1966). This essentialist, ahistorical conception of the human constitution is the mirror-image of the equally ahistorical notion of the threat of chaos. They do not provide a sociological theory of how chaos may well be sociologically constructed in the same way that the nomos is socially constructed. The consequence is a rather idealistic concept of chaos which does not allow for the facts of resistance in social life (Turner, 1977).

We can consider this problem of resistance in the phenomenology of the everyday life at two levels. First, there is the issue of ideological legitimation through the concept of theodicy in Berger and Luckmann's theory of religion and knowledge. Berger (1966, p. 59) argues that one of the major functions of religious theodicies in social groups is to explain and justify the existing patterns of inequality in terms of power and privilege. The theodicy of the unhappy and the poor functions as an opiate which legitimates misery and justifies power. By contrast, the theodicy of the rich justifies wealth and privilege, explaining the happiness and triumph of the wealthy over the poor. While this recognition of the theodicy of the poor implies the possibility of resistance, opposition and change, Berger, in fact, concentrates primarily on the cohesive functions of dominant ideologies. For example, he argues that the karma-samsara doctrine provides the most significant illustration of a theodicy which legitimates the dominance of upper caste groups over subordinate castes in the religious system of Hinduism. He does not allocate a significant function to oppositional theologies of deprivation and subordination. The theodicies of Messianic and millenarian movements offer an other-worldly solution to the problem of injustice by consolidating a resignation to this world. The implication of the analysis is that in practice all theodicies have a

79

conservative, cohesive and integrative set of consequences for both the individual and the social system. The themes of revenge and resentment, which were so prominent in the arguments of Nietzsche with respect to religion, have largely disappeared from Berger and Luckmann's phenomenology of the everyday world.

The second feature of this conservative rewriting of Nietzsche is the fact that there is no biological grounding for resistance. Berger and Luckmann, following Scheler and Gehlen, discover a biological-instinctual root for the human need for stability, order and meaning. There are natural processes which bring about a stable and conservative social order as a psychological necessity to protect individuals from the threat of social and cultural chaos. Human beings are naturally inclined towards conservatism in the literal sense of seeking a social order geared to the preservation of social stability. By contrast, Nietzsche's conception of the biological foundations of the will-to-power as a theory of the body requires the notion of resistance as a fundamental aspect of power relations. In one version of the concept of the will-to-power, Nietzsche conceived of the life-force as a quantum of resistant forces which seek to dominate and regulate the environment in which they are located. This conception of the biological grounding of action and knowledge implies a basic concept of opposition, resistance and autonomy against the invasions of social and cultural regulation. Although Nietzsche was opposed to Darwin, we could suggest, against Berger and Luckmann, that there is a Darwinistic struggle for existence which implies a biological opposition to containment, subordination and restraint. In opposition to the Berger and Luckmann version of biology, we might posit a fundamental quest for autonomy, development and resistance against the environment, namely a fundamental, biologically rooted, oppositional individualism.

Just as Berger, Luckmann, Gehlen and Scheler sought to reassert a basic Christian response to pluralism, we can argue that they subordinated any possibility of genuine oppositional beliefs against the dominant sacred canopy and the taken-for-granted facticity of the everyday world. It is difficult to locate a space within which either nostalgic critique or utopian hope could function against the overwhelming control of the sacred canopy. Karl Mannheim had envisaged a more or less unresolved conflict between ideology and utopia prior to the emergence of modern societies; Berger and Luckmann, given their basic commitment to stability and solidarity, cannot envisage a theoretical grounding or a phenomenological justification for utopian resistance to the overriding impact of the nomos; while in the short run, there may be a challenge to existing 'knowledge', in the long term normative order is always restored. The ideological thrust of their argument is, in fact, to make us comfortable within the iron cage by suggesting that cages are always biologically preferable to utopias. The consequence is a deterministic version of human life, social structure and culture.

The final problem with the phenomenology of the life-world is its lack of historical specificity in outlining the conditions whereby the life-world is produced and reproduced. The phenomenology of the life-world produces an anthropological essence of human character which is insensitive to concrete historical transformations of institutions and life-worlds. As a result, the phenomenology of the life-world suffers from the problems which Marx criticized in Feuerbach, namely an idealistic rendering of the concept of human essence as a form of consciousness. For Berger and Luckmann, the character of alienation and reification is located primarily in the misrecognition of the subjective-practical basis of reality, since the individual actor exists, as it were, in a state of social forgetfulness. However, this emphasis on consciousness is more important in their general theory of the everyday world as a world of knowledge.

Despite the emphasis on biological processes and conditions, Berger and Luckmann have provided a theory of knowledge in the everyday world, not a theory of feeling and experience. It is strange that a perspective which purports to be a phenomenological analysis of the everyday world should largely neglect everyday events, objects and practices. Berger and Luckmann, like other sociologists of religion, can be criticized for their failure to pay sufficient attention to certain basic human-social processes, such as play, sex and death (Turner, 1983). The everyday world is saturated by assumptions, by 'knowledge' and by what Schutz called typifications which structure experience, but the phenomenology of the everyday world in much contemporary sociology neglects to analyse feelings, emotions, passions and affectual behaviour. For example, much of everyday life is taken up by what we may call body maintenance, that is by washing, cleaning and preparing the body for social presentation; the everyday world is also organized around the fundamental processes of eating and sleeping, which are characteristic-ally neglected by sociology. One of the exceptions to this rule is Agnes Heller, who in *Everyday Life* (1984, p. 231) analysed the importance of what she called 'orientative feelings' such as love and hate, which direct actions in the everyday world. While such phenomena are relatively obvious as topics for sociology, we would suggest that the character, display and intensity of emotions, experience and feeling should be a matter of empirical inquiry. Such an inquiry will be concerned with more than immediate experiences. Human affectual behaviour is obviously shaped by long term historical processes of regulation and sophistication which collectively we may refer to as civilization. The analysis of these historical processes is essential for understanding modern forms of discipline.

The Civilization of Emotions: Discipline

Following Weber, we would argue that historically the roots of discipline are to be found in military organization and in the social translation and extension of monastic practices to the whole population through the impact of the Protestant Reformation. While the Catholic monastic system created a powerful form of discipline, it also created a dualistic system of ethics, one for the everyday world of the lay person and one for the religious virtuosi. Thus, Weber argued:

> The Reformation made a decisive break with this system. The dropping of the *concilia evangelica* by the Lutheran Reformation meant the disappearance of the dualistic ethics, of the distinction between a universally binding morality and a specifically advantageous code for virtuosi. The other-worldly asceticism came to an end. The stern religious characters who had previously gone into monasteries had now to practise their religion in the life of the world. (*GEH*, p. 365–6)

As a generalization of this argument, Foucault has claimed in *Discipline and Punish* that monastic practices formed part of the basis of a new system of social regulation which culminated in the development of panopticism as the model for regulating schools, prisons and asylums. For Foucault, these systems of surveillance have brought about an administration of society which is virtually total, embracing the private everyday world of the isolated citizen. Modern regulation depends upon self-regulation set within the taken-for-granted world of disciplines and habit.

Both Weber and Foucault argued that the other great source of contemporary discipline was the emergence of infantries as forms of military organization requiring detailed surveillance and regulation of large bodies of men. Weber was particularly concerned to understand the development of democracy and military rule in ancient Greece as the original location for the mass discipline of an organized infantry. This theme has been taken up recently by Michael Mann (1986) in his historical analysis of social power. In this study of the institutionalization of social power, Mann gives special emphasis to the role of violence, military power and military technology in the creation of civilized institutions. The interaction between military and other social structures is particularly important in his sociological account of the origins of Greek civilization. He suggests that Greek democracy came to depend on the effectiveness in battle of the hoplite (the heavily equipped infantry peasant carrying a heavy wooden shield) organized within the phalanx as the basic tactic of warfare. The heavy round shield employed by the hoplites meant that each fighting man was totally dependent on the heroism and commitment of his neighbour for the defence of the right side of his body. As a consequence, the military effectiveness of the phalanx required a political culture of egalitarianism and democratic participation which, in turn, presupposed the development of a politically autonomous citizenry with a vested interest in the continuity of the state. There was a significant sociological relationship between military development, the political organization of democracy and the emergence of a new culture emphasizing cohesiveness and commitment to the political system. In the long term, this system of power collapsed with the growth of the polis and the expansion of Greek colonization, which forced the political system to rely more and more on mercenary hoplites who did not, as a consequence, share the ideological commitment necessary for the political cohesion of Greek culture.

What is missing from Mann's analysis is a historical study of the relationship between military discipline and the civilization of manners, or more precisely, between the growth of civilized norms of individual conduct and the de-militarization of the aristocracy and later the populace as a whole. This aspect of cultural development has been fully analysed by Norbert Elias in *The Civilizing Process* (1978, 1982). In general historical terms, Elias was concerned to comprehend the transformation of land-owning warlords into a court elite under the control of a centralized monarchy and thereby the erosion of the life-style of this elite by the long term encroachment of professional, merchant and bourgeois status groups within the state apparatus of European societies. His analysis of civilization is, therefore, about the eventual replacement of feudal classes, the development of political absolutism from the conflicts between the forces of centralization and decentralization, and finally, the social evolution of patrimonial powers within the king's household. This analysis occupied him both in the general study of the civilizing process, but also in his analysis of *The Court Society* (1983). In more graphic terms, we can say that Elias' study as a whole is about the civilization process which converts men who fight, eat and sleep on horseback into cultivated members of the court, who are primarily concerned with individualized manners at table and with the refinement of taste within the household. In terms of artefacts, this is the study of how the table replaced the saddle and of the emergence of the fork as a symbol of personal conduct. In more subtle terms still, the civilizing process is about the transformation of crude and lusty emotions and feelings into the more refined, constrained and individualized behaviour of the aristocracy and later of the bourgeoisie. Civilization is about the transformation of savage joys, the uninhibited sexual pleasures of the aristocracy and the violent hatred for enemies and outsiders; this culture of violence gives way to the more precise, detailed and disciplined regulation of modern man. Just as people cultivate nature by subordinating it to human ends, so civilisation is the cultivation of the human body through the imposition of social manners and regulations. To civilize the body is to rationalize emotion and therefore the process of civilization identified by Elias can be seen as a special version of the rationalization process described by Weber as the master trend of modern societies. Both rationalization and civilization can be seen as a general process of the formalization of manners involving the collapse of external constraints in favour of self-restraints (Wouters, 1986).

The Ethic of World Mastery

We may further generalize the process of civilization and rationalization to regard western culture as the institutionalization of an ethic of world mastery, that is an externalization of the will-to-power. This extension of the will-to-power in the institutionalization of culture, civilization and reason can also be regarded as a colonization of the world. By 'world', we mean not only the geographical colonization of an external space, but also the colonization of the body by culture, and the colonization of mind or consciousness by reason and science. We should, therefore, conceptualize this social reality as first of all, the space or environment in which human beings are located (nature), secondly as the space of consciousness as a dimension of social reality which is an internalized space (mind), and finally as the interior environment in which the self is embodied (the body). In terms of Weber's rationalization process and Elias' civilization process, western culture is the institutionalization of the will to power in the three domains of consciousness, the human body and nature which we have conceptualized as a process of cultural and physical colonization.

84

Weber treated the development of asceticism, rationalization and the ethic of world mastery as a consequence of the tension or contradiction in the Calvinistic theology between the life of the spirit and the stubborn facts of worldliness. In Christian culture, the 'world' as a component of theology embraced a range of human issues, including pleasures, irrational passions, egoism, self-aggrandizement and the luxury of personal adornment. The central issue in this concept of the world can be seen in terms of the problem of human embodiment. That is, the problem of the world in the context of Weber's sociology of civilizations implies a fundamental sociology of the body, an issue which remained implicit in Weber's sociology as a whole. Of course, this problematic character of the body is not an issue peculiar to Weber's sociology, since the problematic features of our embodiment underline many dimensions of social theory in the European tradition.

The problematic character of human embodiment in Christian asceticism is best signified by the use of the term 'flesh'. We can, however, suggest that western culture and probably human culture as a whole, managed the problematic features of the flesh through three institutionalized orders, namely religious culture, aesthetic culture and science. These three broad institutional mechanisms mediate, present and regulate the nature of human embodiment. Religion, through a variety of ritual practices, regulates and constrains the body in the interests of spiritual existence and the coherence of social order. Religion (religio) is that which binds together and regulates the body in order to create a sacred body (corpus) of people as a moral order (nomos). The world of artistic representation is a further institutionalization of the body, by representing embodiment in the form of artistic phenomena. Art represents an appropriation of the body in cultural representation and reproduction. Finally, science, but specifically medicine, is an all-powerful and culturally diverse form of regulation, restraint and representation of the body as a problem in relation to social order. In the language of contemporary structuralism, art, religion and medicine are three great discursive formations for the rational and disciplined management of the body and populations. In Nietzsche's terms, this is a framework for the analysis of the will-to-power in art, science and religion.

The ethic of world mastery suggests that the concept of 'the world' should be taken in the broadest possible sense. In pursuing the historical dimensions of the ethic of world mastery, it is important to establish the origins of Protestant asceticism within the wider movement of bourgeois capitalist society in relation to the growth of colonies and imperialism. The notion of world mastery should, therefore, also embrace the idea of the exploration of the global environment by European capitalism. The historical sociology of the body would involve the study of the colonization of societies from the sixteenth and seventeenth centuries. This world mastery of the body is simply one dimension of a global ethic which entailed the creation of colonial dependencies. In short, we can argue that religion and art are primarily explorations of the body and the mind as terrains which have been colonized by the will-to-power and institutionalized in the form of social regulations. Science and military power combined together were the instruments for the exploration of bodies, populations and continents. Within this sense, the sociology of the body is part of a project involving the analysis of orientalism as a discourse concerned with the control, representation and management of the Orient (as a geographical Other) in the interests of power/knowledge. The Orient is a supine, feminine body under the gaze of western reason.

When Weber analysed the notion of the this-worldly ethic, he employed a theological notion of the world as alienation from God. The crucial core of this ethic was the doctrine of the seven deadly sins. These sins had their ultimate root in the fleshliness of human embodiment; Protestantism sought not simply to reject the world, but to master it through the imposition of discipline and the creation of regularities and surveillance. These disciplines were aimed at the subordination of the passions by the cultivation of consciousness, and the regularization and colonization of everyday life. Protestantism also took over the religio-medical management of the body which was handed down from medieval monastic practices as we have seen. There appears to be, as a result, an important convergence between Weber's analysis of the origins of asceticism and military discipline, Foucault's cultural analysis of disciplinary practices and Elias' account of the development of civilization. On this basis, we have argued that civilization, rationalization and colonization should be conceptualized as three moments within the broader processes of mastery and subordination of three domains (mind, body and nature).

We have argued that the development of colonial exploration and the discovery of new continents were closely associated with the emergence of a Protestant ethic of world mastery as a feature of asceticism. There are a variety of important metaphors linking the notion of opening up bodies and opening up continents. More directly, we can suggest a metaphorical relationship between the concept of opening up a continent and the development of the scientific anatomy of pathological bodies. Since medieval times, the body has been seen as the microcosm of the macrocosm. The body within western culture has been regarded as the centre of a set of relations linking the interior life of the mind, the interior environment of the body and the external universe. In the humoural theory of disease, we find an excellent illustration of how the body was directly connected to the world of the stars. The melancholic distemper of the diseased mind was linked to the stars, implying a direct relationship between knowledge, feeling and environment.

This ethic of world mastery sought firstly, the exploration and elevation of mind over the life of the senses and experience, which was rooted in bodily functions. The ethic, therefore, sought to subordinate feeling to reason, through discipline and restraint. The central challenge to this mastery of the sensual life by reason was madness itself. The emergence of the modern episteme was forced to exclude the possibility of madness in order for rational thought to remain permanently secure. Secondly, this ethic sought to subordinate the body (flesh) through religious disciplines with the aid of medicine, especially diet (Turner, 1982c). The regulation of the body by religion was eventually expanded to include a wide range of practices, namely the emergence of panopticism. The central challenge to this system of regulatory practices was the irrationality of sexuality. Thirdly, this ethic involved the exploration of space, that is the outside world as opposed to the inside world of mind and feeling. This outside space was appropriated and regulated by the emerging culture of colonialism. The central challenge to this system was that of insurrection and insubordination by local populations who were seen as an irrational eruption within a rational system of colonial powers.

These themes of body, mind and reason in relation to sexuality and irrationality were drawn together in western European cultures at the dawn of colonialism in, for example, the figure of Caliban who, in Shakespeare's *The Tempest* stands for the profound conflict between nature/flesh and nurture/spirituality represented by the figure of Miranda. Caliban is the metaphorical opposition to the authoritarian rule of Prospero representing rationality, whereby the otherness and sexuality of Caliban is a permanent threat to regulation, science and control. Caliban is the uncolonized, pre-modern embodiment of sheer energy who is the libidinous force behind the restraints of civilization on body, feeling and nature. Prospero's rationality is instrumental in ordering the island, regulating the sexuality of the young men and women, and employing the labour power of the various spirits on this new colony. The symbolism of the storm and Prospero's powers over nature and man points to the interpenetration of rationalism and colonialism. Prospero is the symbol of knowledge/power.

The Ontology of Resistance

Historical accounts of the body and civilization often assume a deterministic character and are also teleological. Even with Weber, who specifically sought to avoid teleological and evolutionary arguments, there is a certain inevitability to his account of the process of rationalization. Although Elias has also denied that his argument is evolutionary, we should note that Elias has not specifically addressed himself to the problems of what we might call de-civilization. Similar problems confront the position adopted by Foucault in the analysis of discipline. Foucault, of course, was theoretically opposed to the possibilities of concepts of progressive history and attempted to deconstruct the historical logic of science and western culture. However, Foucault's work still suggests an inevitable unfolding of disciplines through the system of panoptic control which is in sharp contrast to the thrust of his archaeological analysis. This is a very general problem in social science, namely to avoid unidimensional and teleological accounts of social change. For example, functionalism has had enormous difficulty specifying the conditions for de-differentiation.

The problem can also be seen in terms of the absence of an account of resistance and opposition in many sociological approaches to human behaviour and social organization. This is generically the problem of the so-called 'oversocialized concept of man' in contemporary sociology (Wrong, 1961). According to Wrong, contemporary sociology, especially that tradition associated with the Parsonian solution to the problem of order, has suppressed the idea of human resistance to social regulation by emphasizing the success or effectiveness of socialization and the internalization of norms. Such a position has great difficulty in explaining the persistence of deviance and deviant behaviour apart from somewhat circular arguments about inadequate socialization. In Wrong's view, the rehabilitation of the idea of opposition to social norms involved a rediscovery of the fundamental psycho-analytic views of the Freudian concept of the super-ego in opposition to the underlying forces of the id. Wrong argued, following Freud, that human beings should be regarded as social but not entirely socialized into the prevailing system of norms and values. In a subsequent version of this argument, Wrong (1977) argued that the sociological perspective would need to remedy three defects which were 'the neglect of biography, of the motivational depths and complexities of the human heart, and of the somatic, animal roots of our emotional lives' (p. 54). While we would support Wrong's contention, we would go further to

88

suggest that, since the Freudian version of the conflict between the sexual roots of life and the civilized requirements of stable social order was derived from Nietzsche, we should seek a remedy to the defects of sociological theory in the tradition of Nietzsche's philosophy, that is in the concept of the will-to-power.

We may also suggest that the problem of the oversocialized conception of human nature is, in fact, a specific instance of the more general question of agency and structure which has been a persistent issue in sociological theory. The debate about this problem in recent years has been somewhat dominated by Giddens's notion of structuration (1984). One problem with the agency/structure debate is that very few sociologists have bothered to ask the question, who or what is the agent in agency? There has been an assumption that the agent is the human person, but this is inadequate, because it fails to address the question of the phenomenology of the body and the nature of human embodiment (Smith and Turner, 1986). Often the concept of resistance in sociological theories of agency is cerebral or cognitive, while also being highly individualistic. Resistance is grounded in the actor's perception of, for example, his or her true needs or interests as against the overriding ideological impact of the dominant culture. In these theories, resistance is grounded in awareness within a rational model of social action. This position is, of course, very widespread, since Talcott Parsons' concept of the structure of social action involves an agent choosing and selecting between alternative goals and means. Similarly, Habermas conceives of action as communicative action, where communication involves knowledge, the exchange of ideas, debate and choice in an open and democratic process. These conceptions of rational choice which were rooted in the tradition of economic utilitarianism cannot provide a satisfactory account of the role of feeling, emotion and sentiment in the nature of human resistance as well as in human choice. These rational models are also highly individualistic, since it is the isolated individual who typically chooses between ends. Of course, writers like Talcott Parsons attempted to situate the unit act within a social world based upon reciprocity. However, the central emphasis is still upon the rational choice of ends or, at least, the choice of ends with reference to general values. These theories of action do not pay sufficient attention to the notion of embodiment which overcomes some of the dualistic and individualistic assumptions of classical Cartesian philosophy. By contrast, following Nietzsche, we would start with the premise that the everyday world is prior to the societal world of institutions.

This everyday world is constructed by socialized individuals who are embodied and who are involved in the ongoing world of reciprocity of symbols, feelings and objects. This is the everyday world of what Nietzsche called 'the little things', namely the world of taste, feeling, exchange, experience and becoming. We regard cognitive constructions as secondary to the world of experience or at least that the cognitive world is a reflection upon experiences, exchanges, feelings and moods. Quite literally, thinking is a rationalization of this dense everyday world of engagement and embodiment. It is the regulation of becoming by being. Therefore, following Marx, we would start with the assumption of a socialized human being as the inheriter of a world of culture, mood and organization. The notion of 'society' is an abstract rendering of the world of constant and endless reciprocities of socialized beings. We also regard this everyday world of the embodied person as a world of resistance against regulation and control.

By embodiment, we refer to a situation in which it is, in practice, impossible to separate out experiences from concepts, feelings from reasons, mind from body. To be a person is to be fundamentally bound into the body, but the body cannot be separated from the idea of conscious experiences of the world. The relation between person and body is clearly highly complex philosophically; the relationships between person, identity, social role and body are highly ambiguous. In this study, we have tried to express the idea of embodiment through a contrast between the notion of 'to have a body', 'to be a body' and 'to do embodiment'. In Cartesian philosophy, the image is one of having a body as an extension of a person, but from a phenomenological point of view this is inadequate. As Nietzsche said, there is a sense in which I am body and there is a unity of person and body which should not be divided. While I may experience my body as an alien entity during illness, human beings have an immediate sovereignty over their bodies, so that we do not normally have to think about moving our arms and legs in relation to our environment. The phenomenology of lying down illustrates the complexity of body-as-object and body-as-subject:

Even to lie motionless, which can give a strong impression of being-an-object, acquires its meaning from the purpose which is realized in this position. In the evening, I certainly do not insert myself between the sheets as an object, but I let myself be tempted by the physiognomy of the night to lie motionless . . . as soon as I take myself out of this physiognomy, and make my lying down a laying down of an object – that is as soon as I occupy myself with the object 'body' which vegetates under the blankets – my relaxed feeling is over. (van den Berg, 1966, pp. 103-4)

These experiences should not be treated in terms of isolated individuals. My experience of myself as a person is closely related to the presence of my body in interaction and the ways in which human beings respond to my embodiment in social exchanges.

In this study of Nietzsche, therefore, we will make a distinction between three levels of reality; these are the levels of individual embodiment, the everyday world of the social *habitus* and the macro-societal world of regulating institutions. We wish to argue that the institutional world of regulation is, from the point of view of Nietzsche, an institutionalization of resentment and ascetic controls translated into the form of macro-disciplines. The everyday world of the *habitus* is the world of persistent and infinite reciprocities and exchanges. The world of embodiment is the area of human resistance to regulation and control, existing in constant tension with institutionalized forms of civilization and colonization. In short, the institutionalized reality of 'society' is a superstructure emerging out of everyday reciprocities and the fundamental or elementary dimensions of human existence. We shall conceptualize the sub-structure of the *habitus* as a region with three dimensions, which are enselfment, embodiment and empowerment.

By enselfment, we are referring to the fact that human agents are knowledgeable, conscious and self-conscious actors. Their self-regulating activity presupposes consciousness and the capacity for storing information in the form of memory and autobiography. This capacity for consciousness is, of course, also bound up with their particularity and individuality as specific agents. While different cultures give a different emphasis to the individual and individualism (Marsella, Devos and Hsu, 1985), it is not possible to conceptualize the notion of a particular individual without some presupposition about the ability and capacity of human agents for consciousness, self-consciousness and knowledge of difference. To be a person is at one level to have a memory and consciousness, but also to have consciousness of difference. To be a person is to be a particular person. This argument is not falsified by the historical existence of cultures which clearly have relatively little emphasis on individual difference, placing their value on conformity to group culture, because even in societies based upon mechanical solidarity there would have to be at least some elementary capacity for awareness and self-awareness. It is, therefore, not possible for societies to exist without some development of the capacity of human agents to monitor their behaviour and actions through their consciousness of themselves as agents. As Weber emphasized in the sociology of action and the definition of social action, what is distinctive about human activities is the presence of meaningfulness, knowledge, self-awareness and self-monitoring. As the phenomenological tradition of writers like Schutz has made clear, the everyday world is a world taken-for-granted, typically as an unreflected, unreflexive world of patterned and habitual experience. The everyday world is one of practical accomplishment. However, this argument does not counteract or undermine the equally important argument that in principle all human behaviour is practical and knowledgeable. We should also note that this argument about enselfment may well look like an individualistic form of phenomenology (Alexander, 1985), but we take the social character of knowledge and interaction as a basic presupposition. Furthermore, the idea of an individual implies an 'I' which exists in interaction and in contra-distinction to 'we'.

The importance of the argument about knowledgeability is to assert that the sub-social world of individual action is one with a massive capacity for resistance. Many radical theories of ideology and interpellation (Therborn, 1980) often put an emphasis on the role of self-consciousness as the basis by which social individuals are developed, regulated and monitored by ideological structures as a result of the very subjectivity of human existence. The individual is conceptualized within social roles as simply the effect of knowledge and power. Our argument is that this human subjectivity is also a basis for opposition and resistance, because the mental functions which are necessary for following and understanding an order are also the means which are necessary for misunderstanding, disobeying and misconduct. In short, knowledge is always pliable and ambiguous, being the basis for simultaneously following orders and disobeying orders. To follow a rule presupposes the capacity for not following rules, and indeed, the very nature of a rule or an order is that it would be possible for a knowledgeable actor to disobey it. By a parallel argument, the consciousness necessary for obeying an ideological demand also produces the capacity or ability for avoiding or misinterpreting such forms of cultural domination. The capacity for interpellation within social systems thereby implies the presence of dis-interpellation as a basis for resistance. This argument is somewhat like the argument about normative order in Durkheim's theory of cultural control; the presence of a normative order implies its opposite, namely deviance and opposition.

Our argument is that conscious enselfment is a basic element of the notion of a human being as an agent, a fundamental aspect of resistance to ideological control and an element within all utopian opposition to ideological constraints. The importance of this emphasis on knowledge-ability and enselfment is to lay the ground work for an alternative to the over-socialized concept of man, an alternative which flows from Nietzsche's account of the will-to-power.

The second dimension to human agency, as we have argued, is the importance of human embodiment. We do not need here to repeat arguments about the problems of a Cartesian model of mind and body as separate dimensions or entities, of the body as an extension. We have emphasized the importance of embodiment, following Nietzsche's views on thinking and rationalization, in order to give greater prominence to experiential phenomena and, in particular, to give an emphasis to feeling and emotion. We have suggested throughout that the sociological definition of agent and agency is too intellectualized in the sense of giving too much prominence to cognitive decision-making over the taken-for-granted reality of the world, over habit and over the importance of experience and feeling. Another aspect of this cognitive dimension is that conventional sociology often takes over a number of cultural assumptions about the body as a form of enslavement. It is typical for sociologists to criticize consumerism, for example, on the grounds that this false satisfaction of needs is a modern form of social enslavement. The idea is that need makes us dependent on institutional regulation and hence subject to control. However, we have suggested, following Marx and Nietzsche, that the individuality of this sensual embodiment is fundamental to the traditional importance of praxis and it would be impossible to develop an adequate theory of agent and agency without some reference to sensual praxis which, in our view, depends upon a theory of embodiment. In contemporary sociology, the way in which the human agent is presented and described often suggests a form of dis-embodiment, since we as sociologists, characteristically talk about the actor in terms of pure choices with reference to norms and values which are evaluated from a solely cognitive and rational dimension. This is the sociological version of economic man as rational actor.

Finally, the concept of praxis or practical-conscious activities also presupposes the notion of human empowerment, that is the capacity for doing, for action, for choosing and for bringing about desirable states of affairs. This conception of empowerment is fundamental to a number of traditions in sociology, including Marx's idea of praxis, Feuerbach's notion of sensual action, Parsons' concept of voluntarism in the theory of action and finally, Giddens' view of structuration. As Giddens has emphasized, the idea of 'action' is not simply a one-off event but on the contrary, a continuous flow of activities, interventions and behaviours of embodied persons in the everyday world. This notion of practical activity as a stream of interventions is an important position to develop within a sociology of the body, since it provides a major alternative to those theoretical traditions in sociology which provide too great a prevalence for coercive, determining and restrictive social institutions. Nietzsche observed that 'The will to power can manifest itself only against *obstacles*; it therefore goes in search of what resists it' (*WP*, 656). The notion of praxis provides an alternative to structural determinism, which in both Marxism and sociology, precludes practical, sensual resistance to social structures; however, the notion of practical activity on the part of conscious embodied agents is also fundamental to the notion of power as resources which enable social actors to bring about desirable goals.

The concept of empowerment is not inherently methodologically individualist, since empowerment would apply to social groups and collectivities as much as it would to isolated individual actors. We start, however, with the ontology of power in order to provide a basis for more elaborate notions concerning the habitus or institutional forms of power. The notion of empowerment, furthermore, does not involve or entail a view that all actions are intended and are the outcomes of conscious interventions. On the contrary, the idea of empowerment and practical action is perfectly compatible with the notion of unintended consequences and with the idea that the unintended consequences of actions may well be restraining and stand in a negative relationship to human agency (Turner, 1981). The idea of empowerment, in our view, is furthermore embedded in Nietzsche's view of the will-to-power, as a quantum of forces of resistance. The notion of empowerment and enablement, therefore, appears basic to the very concept of life and indeed, to social life.

This treatment of praxis in terms of the three dimensions of knowledge, body and power is an attempt to provide an ontological basis for certain theoretical arguments against the idea of ideological incorporation and subordination, which was implied at least in the critique of dominant ideologies (Abercrombie, Hill and Turner, 1980). Since, following Marx, we may argue that it is social being which determines consciousness, not consciousness that determines social being, we need to start an analysis of social forms with an interpretation of the notion of 'social being'. It is too narrow an interpretation to regard the concept of 'social being' as ultimately or exclusively grounded in the idea of labour and furthermore, that the idea of labour can only be understood in terms of the social relations following from the mode of production. To render 'social being' as a primarily economic category is to misunderstand the ultimate roots of Marx's notion of praxis via Feuerbach through to Aristotle's idea of practical agency. Consciousness is clearly shaped by the practical problems of economic relations and production (that is, by the dull compulsion of economic forces), but social being is also fundamental to the notion of embodiment and it is the total practical conscious activity of sensuous agents which determines the content and form of consciousness which is ultimately based upon the ongoing character of the everyday habitus. The roots of resistance, therefore, are not simply grounded in the struggle over the relations of production or more generally, over economic forms, but include a multidimensionality of human endeavours and actions including their struggle over biological reality.

We have argued that social relations and social activities may be conceptualized at three levels. There is the world of empowered, embodied and conscious beings involved in the never-ending stream of actions which are necessary for their life. Secondly, there is the *habitus* of dense reciprocities between such social beings. This everyday world is the bedrock on which social institutions rest and the stability of this *habitus* is, in the last analysis, the stability of total social systems. Finally, the everyday world is, in turn, structured by and organized around three primary institutional relations which are the economic, political and cultural. In our view of social relations, we have argued that these three structures correspond to the three dimensions of the praxis of social beings. Human beings have needs, interests and goals which are satisfied in the economic realm; corresponding to embodiment there is the world of production and consumption in the economic sphere. The empowerment of human agents corresponds to the structure of political relations or macro-social power and finally, the conscious enselfment of persons corresponds to the cultural or ideological system. Our argument is that there is both reciprocal exchange between *habitus* and societal institutions, but also conflict, tension and ambiguity between the everyday world of embodied agents and the reified, historically continuous and overarching system of social disciplines and regulations. The macro-social world of the state is, as it were, the perverted mirror-image of the world of reciprocities in the everyday life of embodied persons. The recurrent features of reciprocity are reproduced at the societal level in terms of recurring institutions and institutionalization.

This version of the agency/structure problem could be seen as a reflection upon the theory of structuration (Giddens, 1984). However, we would suggest that the theory of three levels of social relations is derived ultimately from Nietzsche's account of the will-to-power and that this rendering of the traditional problems of social forms, social content and agency has the following specific characteristics. First, it is based upon the notion of the essential and ineluctable presence of resistance in all human life and social interaction, following the character of human agents as embodiments of the will-to-power. Resistance in this perspective is not second order or accidental, but a necessary feature of social life. Secondly, we place particular emphasis on the reciprocity of agents within the everyday world of 'little things', thereby giving a primacy to experiential exchanges within the *habitus*, rather than giving primacy to the notion of the cognitive agent choosing hypothetical or future goals of action. Third, this perspective from Nietzsche regards society and social forms as parasitic upon the stability and solidarity of the everyday world; society is ultimately a fictional discourse for the ordering and regulation of patterns of exchange. Fourthly, we have emphasized the notion that the growth of disciplines regulating embodied persons and social reciprocities are the historical outcome of a long process of rationalization. The paradox which lies at the centre of Nietzsche's social philosophy is that the will-to-power is a colonization of reality which creates social structures which are inimical to the realization of the will-to-power. This was the tragedy of culture outlined by Simmel, developed in the work of Scheler, and elaborated by Berger and Luckmann in their analysis of the social construction of the everyday world. The domination of discipline is an effect of instrumental reason as a manifestation of the will-to-power in its institutionalized form as science.

Science, Domination and Nature: Conclusion

Nietzsche's problem with scientific knowledge laid the basis for Weber's pessimism concerning rationalism and the iron cage. Nietzsche saw the domination of nature by reason as an effect of the will-to-power and therefore as a consequence of the ordering of reality by thought and action. In this chapter, we have spoken of the ethic of world mastery as a project of colonization, that is as an occupation of being, mind and nature. Nietzsche's critique of science as the domination of men and nature by forces which have become alienated from human purposes was adopted on the one hand by Heidegger and on the other by the critical theorists of the Frankfurt School. Although the name of Nietzsche occurs on only three occasions in *Being and Time*, Heidegger's project was dominated by issues contained in Nietzsche and in Nietzsche's legacy (Krell, 1975). This critique of domination in the form of science was also developed by Herbert Marcuse in *Negations* (1968) and in *One Dimensional Man* (1964).

96

These various interpretations of the domination of nature (Leiss, 1972) have, therefore, a common root in Nietzsche's critique of science as a reified form of human willing, turned in against man as a negation of life, just as resentment turned in against man is a neurosis of the body. Nietzsche's position was complex, involving the notion of knowledge as useful, knowledge/power as domination and science as an illusion, alongside religion and art, for the comfort of conscious beings in their ordering and willing of reality. The core of Nietzsche's position was that

Knowledge works as a tool of power ... in order for a particular species to maintain itself and increase its power, its conception of reality must comprehend enough of the calculable and constant for it to base a scheme of behaviour on it. The utility of preservation ... stands as the motive behind the development of the organs of knowledge – they develop in such a way that their observation suffices for our preservation. In other words: the measure of the desire for knowledge depends upon the measure to which the will to power grows in a species: a species grasps a certain amount of reality in order to become master of it, in order to press it into service. (*WP*, section 480)

This outline of the character of rational knowledge as power, enablement and constraint laid the ground work for contemporary critical theory and its response to capitalism as institutionalized rationalism, that is as the organization of the ethic of world mastery as vengeance against man. The Frankfurt School owed more to Nietzsche than to Marx.

3

The Priest is a Beefsteak Eater – Rationalization and Cultural Control in Weber

Introduction

Although there is no broad agreement about the central questions of Weber's sociology (Hennis, 1983; Tenbruck, 1980), there is some agreement as to the general intellectual and social forces which shaped and dominated Weber's sociological perspective. These general conditions include the problem of the relativity of values and the question of ethical responsibility in a world without absolute moral agreement. This problem of value relativity was particularly prominent in Weber's essays on politics and science as vocations, but it also influenced his general approach to the question of value freedom in sociology. This issue of moral incoherence was also significant in his personal moral dilemmas and these problems of ethical perspectivism shaped his world-view. This is evident from Marianne Weber's biography of her husband (M. Weber, 1975; Kent, 1985).

The second general influence on Weber's sociology follows from this, namely the problem of providing an adequate legitimation for the objective and focus of sociological inquiry; that is, if we live in a world of moral incoherence, could there be an agreement about the project of sociology itself? If we live in a world where the collapse of values makes the project of modernism impossible, then the 'grand narratives' of sociology also become impossible. Sociology is merely a fragment within a discursive event. Although Weber was overtly committed to the notion of value neutrality in professional sociology, he was also committed to the idea of value relevance in research. Weber, however, constantly abandoned this formal separation of fact and values in his empirical research; this feature of his sociology was especially evident in his arguments on economic policy and the role of the state in Germany (Mommsen, 1985; Tribe, 1983). When Weber was writing about foreign policy with respect to the protection of German economic interests, he simply assumed that sociology would be developed in the interests of the formation of a strong state. Similarly, Weber's commentaries on the ethnic character of the German labour force also brought out the centrality of political value commitments in his agrarian sociology, but Weberian sociology has difficulty in providing a rational justification for these positions, or at least a justification which is compatible with its premises.

The third component of Weber's sociology was, consequently, grounded in the political context of Germany in the late nineteenth century. We can only fully understand Weber's attitude towards the state bureaucracy and political leadership within the framework of German social and political development, where in Weber's view there was the absence of genuine political leadership to direct German society in a context of international competition (Giddens, 1972; Mommsen, 1974; Ringer, 1969). By drawing these components together, it can be argued that Weber's sociology is grounded in a series of tensions between morality and political force, and morality and utilitarian economics. Although the question of political domination has been frequently acknowledged in the literature on Weber as representing a leading theme of Weberian sociology (Parkin, 1982; Eden, 1984), the problem of ethics and economics in Weber's sociology has received insufficient attention. It is important to note that the contradictions between utilitarian economic self-interest and the moral framework of society were a central theme of nineteenth-century sociology generally, being prominent in the work of writers like Durkheim and Tönnies. The importance of this issue was recognised by Talcott Parsons (1937) but the general ramifications of this issue have not been fully explored in the sociological literature (Holton and Turner, 1986).

The notion that Weber's sociology was orientated towards a number of tensions or contradictions has been an important feature of recent interpretations of his work. These antinomies are well known: charisma versus bureaucracy; intention versus consequence; religion versus economics; action versus structure. These theoretic oppositions can be summarized under the notion of the fatalism of Weber's sociology where human intention is seen to be denied by the iron cage of modern society (Turner, 1981). A number of sociologists have attempted to minimize these apparent contradictions and tensions in Weberian sociology by locating a unifying theme in his work, especially around the idea of ethical responsibility (Roth and Schluchter, 1979; Scaff, 1984; Thomas, 1984). These liberal interpretations of Weber could be regarded as an attempt to domesticate the problems of Weberian

99

sociology within an empirical framework which neutralizes the moral uncertainty of Weber's world. The central paradox of Weber's view of history is that all that is virtuous (reason, imagination and moral altruism) results in a world which stands in opposition to human creativity, because instrumental rationality lays the foundations of an administered society and the iron cage. The central lesson of Weber's sociology is that whatever set of circumstances went into making rational capitalism, there is a fateful logic to this combination of intellectual rationalization and capitalist enterprise. Once instrumental rationality had combined with the forces giving rise to capitalist methods of production and regulation, then modern developments took an inexorable direction. Weber's view of history is thus full of ironies about the long term consequences of the Reformation, the emergence of science and the development of economic individualism.

Of course, Weber's pessimism in this respect was shared with writers like Simmel, especially in his view of the tragedy of culture and the impact of money on the rationalization of the modern world (Simmel, 1978; Turner, 1986a). Indeed this theme of the tragic combination of reason and economic change was common to German social thought generally, being particularly evident in the work of Tönnies who in *Gemeinschaft und Gesellschaft* outlined the general problem of the transformation of communities into rational institutions where individual initiative was denied by the very growth of objective institutions (Freund, 1979).

These antinomies in Weber's thought can be understood as an attempt by Weber to come to terms with the legacy of Nietzsche. From Nietzsche, Weber inherited the debate about the problem of action in a world of moral devaluation and social decadence, but this legacy was not adequately acknowledged by Weber and in subsequent interpretations of Weber's sociology Nietzsche's problem has not been fully explored. There are of course a number of commentaries on the relationship between Nietzsche and Weber (Aron, 1971; Fleischmann, 1964; Kent, 1983; MacRae, 1974; Robertson, 1978; Turner, 1981; Turner, 1982a). These diverse commentaries on the relationship between Nietzsche and Weber are in a number of respects inadequate, since they fail to grasp the full range of these interconnections, and they also fail to comment on Weber's suppression, exclusion and transformation of Nietzsche within sociology. The principal exception to this claim can be found in Wilhelm Hennis's *Max Weber's Fragestellung* (1987) where there is an extensive discussion of the Nietzsche legacy. Despite recent re-evaluation of Nietzsche, we argue that Nietzsche is the unrecognized presence in Weber's sociology which gave his sociology a central theme around the problem of morals in relation to rationality.

Of course Weber once said that 'one can measure the honesty of a contemporary scholar and above all of a contemporary philosopher in his posture towards Nietzsche and Marx' (Mitzman, 1971, p. 182). The development of Weber's knowledge of Nietzsche is outlined with almost philological precision by Hennis (1986; 1987). Weber's own posture towards Nietzsche was self-evident in the discussion of resentment in the sociology of religion and also in the discussion of moral values in relation to political actions in a world of value relativism. We can also detect certain superficial relations between Weber's sociology and Nietzsche's philosophy in respect of charismatic leadership, and the problem of state power. In this discussion, however, we wish to suggest that these relationships are less important than the more general presuppositions of Weberian sociology which in many respects denied or suppressed Nietzsche rather than elaborated his philosophy in an open confrontation. To use modern jargon, we wish to suggest that Nietzsche is the absent centre of Weberian sociology and this argument could be extended to modern social science as a whole where, as we have suggested, Nietzsche's themes of language, morality and reason form the framework for modern analysis of the character of modernism and post-modernism.

The Nietzsche Legacy

Martin Heidegger once observed that the confrontation with Nietzsche had not yet begun nor had the pre-requisite for such a confrontation been established. Over a long period Nietzsche has been celebrated or has become reviled and his contribution to western culture, according to Heidegger, is still too threatening and problematic to receive adequate resolution. We are not concerned with the problem of exploiting or celebrating Nietzsche; rather we wish to establish some features of the relationship between Nietzsche and Weber's construction of social theory as a basis for eventually recasting contemporary social thought. Furthermore, we are not concerned with Weber's secret appropriation of Nietzsche, but rather with the type of treatment Weber gave to some ultimate moral questions which were originally posed by Nietzsche. This chapter is, therefore, merely an exercise in tracing some questions relating to Weber's theory of action and in examining modern solutions of these ethical dilemmas.

The principal problem facing Weber from Nietzsche was the

101

question of political and personal action in a world where common values were no longer possible. Weber thought that given the collapse of traditional morality, an ethic of ultimate ends was no longer possible and that an ethic of responsibility had to be constituted as a realistic response to the crisis of social relations in German capitalism and more broadly in a world dominated by formal or instrumental reason. We can see Weber's sociology (and much subsequent sociology) as an attempt to come to terms with Nietzsche's discovery that God was dead, that is how to live in a world without clear moral guidelines.

With the death of God, it is morality itself that becomes a problem. The problem of morality arises within the discovery that in the absence of God the institution of revenge and reconciliation is missing. It is the discovery of God's death that enables us to transform morality into a profane object of science and hence the project of sociology becomes possible as a science of morals, that is the reduction of moral intention to quantifiable social relations. Nietzsche linked the emergence of sociology therefore with the collapse of traditional forms of moral authenticity and regarded sociology itself as part of the development of a profane and secular world. Weber's attempt to construct a sociology of meaning for action and to understand the intentions which lie behind such actions can therefore be seen as part of this secularization of culture where morality becomes simultaneously a problem and an object of inquiry.

We should point out, however, that Nietzsche and Weber took very different positions with respect to the death of God and the collapse of values. Nietzsche treated this event, along with the emergence of nihilism, as a challenge to the development of a new authenticity in moral life, without the hypocrisy and shallowness which characterized bourgeois German culture. Nietzsche did not, therefore, lament the end of a divine authority in morality, but saw this transformation of culture as an opportunity for establishing a new base for morals. Nietzsche argued against the possibility of a monopolistic authority in moral affairs, especially where that monopoly was institutionalized in a repressive apparatus such as the traditional Church. Nietzsche saw the growth of moral diversity in a positive light (as a challenge) and on occasion welcomed polytheism as a liberating cultural condition. For example, Nietzsche argued that:

The invention of Gods, heroes and supermen of all kinds, together with that of fictitious fellow men and sub-men, of dwarfs, fairies, centaurs, satyrs, demons and devils, was the invaluable preparatory exercise for the justification of the selfishness and autocracy of the individual: the freedom one accorded the God in relation to other Gods at last gave oneself in relation to laws and customs and neighbours. Monotheism, on the other hand, that rigid consequence of the teaching of a standard human being – therefore the belief in a standard God beside whom other Gods were no more than false and fraudulent – has been perhaps the greatest danger facing mankind hitherto: mankind was threatened with that premature inertia which, as far as we can see, other species of animals reached long ago (*GS*, section 143).

Nietzsche saw polytheism as a form of theological reasoning which prefigured the development of individual differences, freedom and autonomy. He saw what he termed 'multi-spiritedness' as the counterpart of a multiplicity of norms which was associated with the rights of autonomous, morally genuine, individuals. By contrast, Weber regarded the polytheism of modern society in terms of a relativity of values which made coherent moral actions increasingly impossible. In speaking about the vocations of science and politics, Weber used Nietzsche's critique of modernity to characterize the modern problem of values and facts in terms of a conflict of perspectives (Kronman, 1983). This struggle of values made genuine moral commitment increasingly difficult and, in Weber's terms, it inhibited the autonomy of personality rather than making its development possible. Perspectivism ruled out the possibility of a coherent life-plan.

We can also see that this problem of secularization and moral relativism lay behind the whole issue of legitimacy and legitimate action in Weber's sociological studies of action, institutions and power. Although Weber was often treated as the principal sociologist of legitimate authority, his political sociology was actually grounded in an empirical analysis of coercion, domination and force. Weber believed, in a way which was similar to Nietzsche's position, that with the collapse of natural law, the state would emerge simply as an institution which exercised the monopoly of violence in a given territory. Weber's view of the state as mere power was also related to his perspective on law as command backed up by threats of physical and symbolic violence from the state. Just as Weber viewed the state as the fountain of pure physical force, so he saw the Church as an institution enjoying the monopoly of spiritual power. In this situation capitalist society was conceptualized as an arena of conflict between the working class making demands for substantive justice and the capitalist class appealing to the rule of law as the mainstay of formal legality which served their interests. Weber, rather than regarding capitalism as an organized set of institutions based upon legal rational authority, conceptualized capitalism as a space of naked power conflict between interest groups attempting to realize their ends through a variety of political and social strategies. This form of society and this type of state power were closely connected with a moral system which had declined into nihilism. Legitimacy could no longer be established through the sanctifying power of God, or through God's instrument in the natural law system or through God's institutionalized power in the form of the Church as the treasury of merit, or through heroic men as prophets of God.

Weber nevertheless retained a sociological commitment to the possibility of charisma as a guiding force in political affairs, despite the overall trend towards a secular bureaucratic form of political management. Weber complained that Germany had not come to terms with the disappearance of the system of leadership created by Bismarck (1815-98). Weber thought that Germany was exposed to the superior economic force of Britain and America in a context where imperial struggles for territory were at a premium. He recognized that German bureaucracy lacked distinctive direction and finally he argued that in the First World War the German army had been betrayed by weak and ineffectual leadership. While he recognized the growing power of administrative institutions in the realm of politics, Weber looked towards a future political leadership which would be authoritative if not authoritarian; Weber's hostility towards democratic, bureaucratic political organizations is well known and much discussed within the literature. While there is clearly a relationship between Nietzsche's views on the superman and Weber's politics of charisma, we should note that Nietzsche's critique of nationalism, German folk philosophy and objections to the dominating state was remote from Weber's political interests and perspective (Thomas, 1983; Mommsen, 1985).

In more general terms we can argue that in Weber's sociology the Nietzschean problem of how to be morally authentic in the contemporary world was transformed into the sociological issue of how to root institutions in some form of legitimizing power without the social support of a common morality or a natural law. Within a wider context, this was the problem of how to maintain the order of civilization against the threat of nihilism and how to preserve a moral stand without genuine values of a common or ultimate character. It was also the problem of finding a set of values for public polity in a society divided by class and status politics. The answer given to these problems by Weber was never fully developed, but involved some plea for an ethic of responsibility and a moral strategy organized around the notion of a calling in the world with respect to political and intellectual leadership. This answer was incoherent, because Weber simultaneously admired the ethics of professionalism and authoritarian leadership, while expressing abhorrence about mindless professionalism and people of merely economic calling within an administered bureaucratic society.

The Oversocialized Conception of Man

Western social philosophy has often seen sociability itself in a negative fashion. The negative sociability of humankind is an act of self-denial and in modern social thought this perspective is typically expressed in so-called philosophical anthropology. This type of perspective is particularly prominent in the work of writers like Helmunt Plessner and Arnold Gehlen whose recent followers (Berger and Luckmann, 1967) have converted this denial of the will-to-power into a theory of institutional rationality. The subordination of interest and biological necessity are compensated for in the creation of enduring social relations, but these relations must of necessity produce human alienation as the antidote to anomie. Berger and Luckmann saw the social in terms of three moments, whereby human beings culturally create the world they have to inhabit, forget through an act of alienation their self-creativity and finally experience the world as a reified reality as a consequence of their collective forgetfulness. This reified world is a necessary protection (a sacred canopy) against the forces of chaos and destruction; a condition of reification is an essential feature of all human society as such. Human self-denial must be legitimated through the threat of anomic conditions which are allegedly endemic to social relations, although in reality they are simply socially constructed as legitimations of this original denial. In the work of Berger, this doctrine is converted into a theory which sees human beings as biologically unfinished, requiring the constraints of culture and institutions which bring about social and individual contentment, but they are still seen to be forms of alienation. For those writers who oppose human nature and institutions, the world must always appear as a form of necessary denial, whereby we sacrifice our 'real' natures for a modicum of contentment. Berger and Luckmann produce a highly conservative social theory as a result of their lyrical stress on the virtues of order and their theoretcal focus on the constants of human nature (Abercrombie, 1980, p. 163).

For Nietzsche, instincts, the will for existence and social institutions cannot be reconciled. The repetitive forces entailed in the will-to-power are the forces of ultimate order and this is the lesson of understanding; the mechanisms of self-denial do not hold together as a consistent system (and they indeed lead to their own destruction in the

105

killing of God). Thus we have (according to traditional wisdom) to submit and humankind can only be reconciled with civilization through a profound process of the revaluation of morals (even when in the last instance this involves seeing themselves as beings without value). This revaluation of morality for Nietzsche is only possible by means of 'an extra moral' morality and a non-intentional display of intentions.

In these two issues of revaluation and the eternal return, Nietzsche posed a variety of ultimate issues which Weber could not reconcile with his ethic of responsibility, the history of asceticism and the philosophy of social science. For Weber, the rise of nihilism coincides with the unfolding of an institutional totality bringing constraints on the freedom of individual action. Unlike the anthropological philosophers, Weber saw a complimentary relationship between social being and institutions. The iron cage is the historical outcome of the ascetic shaping of the world and the regulation of social life by the forces of rationalization and intellectualism.

These contradictory relations between instincts and institutions, emotion and reason, and structure and action were also expressed in Weber's view of the importance of charisma in history. With the concept of charisma, Weber responded to the problem of the will to power as an instrument for the re-orientation of institutions through extra-moral mechanisms. The establishment of charisma in leadership and in philosophy was to be seen as a form of social therapy or medicine to preserve the healthy quality of institutions and to establish the groundwork for the free competition of thought and political will. The role of charisma at the empirical level was to bring politics and science back into the orbit of communal action from where they had departed as a consequence of the historical process of rationalization.

Individuality, Subjectivity and Modernity

Both Nietzsche and Weber were concerned with the problem of individuality and individualism in the context of the social conditions of modern life, which are increasingly dominated by the bureaucracy of the state. For Nietzsche, the 'man of belief' was to be seen as the dependent man proper, a man who cannot place or regard himself as an end, that is as a moral being. Every type of belief for Nietzsche was in itself an expression of self-denial and of self-alienation. Furthermore, Nietzsche argued that for most people a regulative or alienating force (as a means of coercion) was necessary for survival. It is here that the modern man rises as a man of conviction, as the antagonist of truth, not to see many things, to be prejudiced in all issues and to have rigid and necessary optics in all values. Nietzsche distinguished between the individualism of the disinterested and the individualism of the noble life. To some extent this division resembled that made by Alexis de Tocqueville's elaboration of the old and the new individualism in American society (Eden, 1983). It is worth remembering that Nietzsche was an avid reader of de Tocqueville and was clearly influenced and impressed by his discussion of individualism in the context of the equalizing forces of American democracy and popular culture. The problem of the individual and individuation was a continuous theme of Nietzsche's thought. In *Beyond Good and Evil*, Nietzsche spoke of the uniform social levelling of individuals as the 'animalization of man' which would subdue the noble man to the values of a faceless herd. The same criticism appeared in *The Birth of Tragedy* where individuation is an aspect of Apolline culture with the loss of wholeness. The issue was also part of his rejection of Kant in the later works on morality and religion.

Weber's ideal of the individualism of responsibility was created to counteract the negative elements arising from this new regulated individualism in industrial capitalism. The fact that Weber so persistently and forcefully evoked the ideal of responsibility underlined his concern for the maintenance of institutions, while both Nietzsche and de Tocqueville saw this new individualism as fully linked with the state of modern institutions and the comfort given to individuals by this social democracy. Weber's denial of the nihilism of the project of modernity itself and his insistence on the meaningfulness of modern institutions against the threat of nihilism reconstructed individualism as an ultimate comfort which can only be achieved through the ascetic work of vocational tasks. It is exactly here that Weber's will to the life of ultimate reconciliation was a construction of social theory which was written simultaneously with and against Nietzsche. This was part of an implicit strategy of reversing Nietzsche's philosophy which was most evident in Weber's *Economy and Society*. The construction of the iron cage, which will survive long after both fascism and socialism, has to be seen as the construction of a sociality which is grounded in the foundations of the individualism of responsibility through the individualism of disinterestedness. Weber allied with Kant as opposed to Nietzsche.

The strains and contradictions within Weber's sociology are especially evident in *Economy and Society* where he distinguished four types of social action. These were instrumental-rational action, value-rational action, affectual action and finally traditional action. As Weber argued, affectual and traditional action are on the borderline between meaningfully orientated action and mere behaviour. From this distinction, we can see that Weber sought to reserve the notion of action for activities which are relatively self-conscious, orientated towards specific goals, involving human subjectivity and the ascription of meaning. Action is essentially purposeful action, involving knowledge and intention. Traditional action for Weber is action which involves what he called 'ingrained habituation' (*ES*, vol. 1, p. 25). In a similar way, affectual behaviour which involves emotionally charged activity is also on the margin of genuine purposeful action, that is, lying on the borderline between unreflecting behaviour and self-conscious intentionality. The oddity of this position is that, as Weber himself argued, actions in the everyday world involve activity which is generally habitual, routine, regulative and unreflecting. The relationship between behaviour, action, interaction and meaning in Weber's interpretative sociology of action have been the focus of much philosophical discussion and critique (Habermas, 1984; Schutz, 1971). Our argument is that Weber's definition of rational action precludes an analysis of the everyday world.

On Weber's own definition, therefore, the everyday world to some extent lies outside the interests of a sociology of action, and everyday life is an arena in which interpretative sociology has little relevance. Weber's stringent view of meaning in and for action as the activity of a moral agent equipped with rationality thus leaves everyday life as a phenomenon more suitable to the approach of behaviouralism. The everyday world of ordinary people is a space dominated largely by habit, tradition and emotion, whereas Weber's notion of action and interpretative sociology would apply to a rather limited range of human agents, that is agents who had, as it were, lifted themselves out of the mire of unreflecting everyday habituation. The world of everyday affect and habit, the common world of ordinary behaviour charged with emotion and feeling is thus beyond the pale of rationality and agency.

By contrast, Nietzsche attempted to write from the standpoint of what he called 'the little things', that is from the perspective of the practical sensuality of the everyday world of the *habitus*. This position reflected his distrust of the rationality of thought characteristic of the professional man in an age which he regarded as Alexandrian in its commitment to knowledge. Furthermore, Nietzsche was critical of the Kantian assumptions of the moral framework of individual choice, partly on the grounds that Kant's philosophy was a form of disguised Christianity. In more general terms, Nietzsche regarded the elaborate development of the notions of rationality, intentionality and individual choice as a consequence of intellectual alienation and as a feature of a false individualism. Nietzsche tended therefore to see Kantian moral philosophy in the same light that he regarded Christianity, namely as a denial of genuine moral autonomy and as an expression of inverted resentment. Nietzsche, in particular, regarded the central concepts of Christianity as we have seen as illusionary or epiphenomenal forms. The conventional concepts of Christianity and moral philosophy existed on an imaginary plane. Nietzsche characteristically argued that Christianity had no real grounding in the everyday world of real moral choices:

Nothing but imaginary *causes*, ('God', 'soul', 'ego', 'spirit', 'free-will' or 'unfree-will'): nothing but imaginary *effects* ('sin', 'redemption', 'grace', 'punishment', 'forgiveness of sins'). A traffic between *imaginary beings* ('God', 'spirits', 'souls'): an imaginary *natural* science (anthropocentric; complete lack of the concept of natural causes); an imaginary *psychology* (nothing but self-misunderstanding, interpretations of pleasant or unpleasant general feelings, for example the condition of the *nervus sympathicus*, with the aid of the sign-language of the religio-moral idiosyncracy – 'repentence', 'sting of conscience', 'temptation by the devil', 'the proximity of God'); an imaginary *teleology* ('the kingdom of God', 'the Last Judgement', 'eternal life'). (*AC*, section 15)

While Weber saw the project of a moral life in the conventional sense as still desirable despite the relativity of values in industrial society, Nietzsche was sceptical of moral claims seeing both conventional morality and philosophy as a rationalization and denial of life. The dominance of professional intellectuals was part of the sickness of modern society, where instrumentalism denied the wholeness of instincts. At best, philosophy was parasitic on the life-process.

For sociologists, Weber had provided the basic set of principles and concepts for understanding modern society. We have been taught that rationalization is the logic, the inner path and the underlying pattern of modern social evolution (Brubaker, 1984; Löwith, 1982). In *The Protestant Ethic and the Spirit of Capitalism*, Weber connected these processes of western rationalization and intellectualism with a particular type of asceticism (that is inner-worldly asceticism) which is primarily orientated to the regulation and reproduction of the very foundations of everyday life. Inner-worldly asceticism links the practical necessities of this everyday order with the religious needs of salvation. Self-control is seen to be the foundation logic of human control. In comparing these different sets of asceticism in relation to the needs of the everyday world and of salvation, Weber developed the notion of economic ethics and, through a number of comparative studies of world religions, he attempted to show how specific types of economic ethics were related to different forms and routes of rationalization. In this chapter, we do not enter into a debate about the relation between religion in classical civilizations, economics and social change in Nietzsche or Weber (Müller, 1986). These debates in Weber with respect to economic ethics and the rationalization of the everyday world were the sociological products of Nietzsche's critique of utilitarianism in morals and his discovery of the morals resentment.

In *The Genealogy of Morals*, Nietzsche stated that the continuity of ritualized everyday morals through history was a necessary part of social existence. Ritualization of the life-world is linked with the whole nature of utilitarian thought; there is a need for repetition, even cyclical repetition, in the actions of the life-world in order to satisfy the pure necessities of human survival. The prominent position of repetition and rule in a very practical and even biological sense in Nietzsche's theory of knowledge becomes most apparent in *The Will to Power* (*WP*, section 480). Non-egoistic action is connected to these necessities for basic survival. Non-egoism, however, becomes dangerous for human survival where it is transformed into an overwhelming pattern or focus of morality (as in the case of Christianity in Nietzsche's critique of the Antichrist). For Nietzsche, Kant's categorical imperative is nothing other than a Konigsberger version of Christianity. Everyday morals and their non-egoistic features have always served as the morals of the people; why should they now with modernization be converted into ruling morals? It is this conversion of what Nietzsche called the morality of the lowest instincts into the logic of modern society in which we find the counter-argument to culture (the nihilism of European civilization) where the highest values became devalued by the herd. It is exactly this development from the common instincts of necessity to the morals of impersonal duty which Nietzsche called, in a critical and ironic sense, the revaluation of all values as the final process of the rebellion of slavery in morals. The success of the moral rebellion of slavery is unthinkable without what Nietzsche referred to as the morals of resentment.

Resentment for Nietzsche is a sentiment that is basically created through self-restraint which arises in its broadest form in Christianity where the basic attributes of beauty, wealth, enjoyment and generosity are turned into attributes of evil. In the first rebellion of slavery in morality, this resentment becomes the moral expression of a priesthood that turns itself into a ruling class. It is through this process that resentment becomes a creative cultural force in history in transforming the most evil and weak ideals into tools of cultural formation. This is the 'scandal of history' which Nietzsche lamented in which the instincts of resentment, of non-egoism, of mediocrity and the instincts of the disinterested became the reasons of every culture. It was on this level of the mechanism of these transformations and transfigurations of the instincts of resentment created in Judaism and elaborated and refined in Christianity into a system of rule, that morality and cruelty become interchangeable and indistinguishable.

Within this framework, it is possible to see utilitarianism as a form of inner-worldly asceticism. Like Nietzsche, Weber in the sociology of religion located the foundations of the modern world in Judaism and Christianity. As a modification of this assertion, we have to keep in view Nietzsche's great interest in the contribution of pre-Socratic culture to history (Silk and Stern, 1981). Like Nietzsche, Weber referred to Buddhism and Islam in order to formulate a source of alternative illustrations for this relationship between morality and economics. This was the project of orientalism (Turner, 1978). Nietzsche's argument was that the utilitarian aspect of morality came to its final realization in contemporary Christianity, but Weber turned the notion of moral nihilism simply into an understanding of the modern foundations of contemporary society. Weber converted Nietzsche's cultural-historical critique into a shallow social psychology of Jewish and Christian resentment by subordinates against superior strata. Weber reinterpreted Nietzsche's critique of Judeo-Christian culture and re-analysed history on the grounds of this new reinterpretation. Weber's question was simply: which type of religious ethic fostered economic utilitarianism? Weber elaborated the category of inner-worldly asceticism and this category of ethical and religious activity (directed to the utilitarian rationality and finally into economic actions) was identified solely with Christianity rather than with Judaism. Weber dismissed Judaism as a significant basis for modern rationality on the grounds that Judaism was a particularistic religion tied to antique dietary rules and personal regulations. Nietzsche's critical approach to utilitarianism as such disappeared in Weber's economic sociology. This disappearance of morality in modern economic behaviour through the development of utilitarianism is simply taken for granted in Weber's economic sociology. For Nietzsche, utilitarianism in morals constituted the termination of morality. By contrast, it was Weber who developed a sociology of utilitarian discipline and rationality as the origins of modernity. It was in this concersion (from a critique of utilitarianism in morals to the establishment of economic ethics as a category of the universal foundation for morals) that Weber completed the process of the revaluation of morality. This is why the notion of resentment (so

111

central in Nietzsche's critique of modernity) was relegated to a marginal theoretical position in Weberian sociology. By contrast, the utilitarian aspect of economic ethics and actions was transformed into the positive notion of inner-worldly asceticism and it was this notion which became the basis of Weber's whole sociology.

Resentment and Modernity

For Nietzsche, the morals of resentment were developed to their highest level in Christianity. While Judaism was acknowledged as the religion which originally underwent the revaluation process by means of a need for revenge against powerful overlords through the medium of powerless and deprived priests, Nietzsche looked towards Christianity as the appropriate carrier of this Jewish legacy. Judaism, although revaluing the low as the good, still preached immediate revenge; Christianity developed a more subtle, a higher, a more indirect and culturally more productive form of revenge in the doctrine of spiritual love. In Christianity, there was a transfer of love into the highest value from a tool of the lowest interest. Weber, however, denied the subtlety of this second stage of revaluation, which in Nietzsche was fully elaborated in *The Genealogy of Morals*, and separated Judaism (the religion of revenge) from Christianity (the religion of asceticism).

Weber said that the factor of resentment as first outlined by Nietzsche had a double importance in the Jewish form of ethical salvation, although it had been completely absent in all magical and caste religions (*ES*, vol. 1, p. 492). Weber transformed Nietzsche's concept of resentment through a positivistic reductionism and separated the concept from its psycho-anthropological roots. The concept became merely a concomitant of the notion of an ethic of disprivilege with respect to a variety of world religions. The concept of resentment lost its dynamic philosophical and anthropological purchase by being transformed into a notion of the theodicy of disprivileged social strata. These theodicies became simply a compensation for revenge. Furthermore, Weber almost exclusively identified this resentment morality with Judaism in its first struggle against Roman occupation and later against Gentile subordination; that is, the concept became associated merely with the notion of a revengeful God in a specific cultural context. Weber, therefore, implicitly protected Christianity and its drive for salvation against the argument in Nietzsche that the highest religious ethic is the outcome of resentment in morals, and he also protected Christianity by simply identifying resentment with a class of the disprivileged. His idea of a drive for salvation in Christianity became associated with intellectualism as the powerful source of the need for a sense of personal salvation. Intellectualism as 'another source besides the social condition of the disprivileged' is related more particularly to 'the meta-physical needs of the human mind as it is driven to reflect on ethical and religious questions, driven not by material need but by an inner compulsion to understand the world as a meaningful cosmos and to take up a position towards it' (*ES*, vol. 1, p. 499). Both medieval and modern Christianity are taken as powerful examples of this intellectualism as the root of modern forms of the quest for salvation. The problem for Weber was to protect these intellectual needs against the needs of everyday life and the realm of necessity. Priesthood, professionalism and intellectualism are separated from any notion of a drive for pure revenge. In a very general way, Weber gave Christianity a privileged position within the hierarchy of world religions, since Christianity had become the most spiritual and intellectual form of opposition to the world, that is to the everyday life of feeling, emotion, sensitivity and practice. This privileged position was, therefore, given to a religion of denial which stood against the natural world, that is the actual world.

While Weber attempted to locate the modern drive for salvation in an intellectual quest for meaning, Nietzsche was quite convinced of the importance of the everyday world and material needs in the development of intellectualism. Against Weber's idealistic assumptions, we can contrast Nietzsche's concern with the practical and material dimensions of the everday world and its construction of routine tasks. For example, Nietzsche wrote:

these little things – nutriment, place, climate, recreation, the whole casuistry of selfishness – are beyond all conception of greater importance than anything that has been considered of importance hitherto. It is precisely here that one has to begin to *learn anew*. Those things which mankind has hitherto pondered seriously are not even realities, merely imaginings more strictly speaking lies from the bad instincts of sick, in the profoundest sense injurious natures – all the concepts of 'God', 'soul', 'virtue', 'sin', 'the Beyond', 'truth', 'external life'. (*EH*, p. 66)

This affirmation of the everyday world follows in the text immediately from his condemnation of professional academic life as a denial of genuine reality. Nietzsche saw intellectualism as the construction of an imaginary world over and against the everyday world in order to deny the reality of the little things.

While Nietzsche was concerned with the material base of interests in

113

the everyday world, we should note that his concept of resentment was not exclusively explained by reference to the deprivation of material needs. The notion of resentment in Nietzsche was the negation of desire and affect in all the various aspects of social relations. Sickness is ultimately resentment turned against the self via the sufferings of the body. In a wider sense, it is the envy of self-restraint which turns into a type of general or abstract love with the envied. It is in fact this meaning of the concept of resentment that Weber so publicly tried to eradicate or at least to move to one side as merely an aspect of psychology. This move can be best illustrated in his critique of Nietzsche's application of resentment to Buddhism:

The limited significance of the factor of *resentiment* and the dubiousness of applying the conceptual schema of 'repression' almost universally, appear most clearly when Nietzsche mistakenly applies his scheme to the altogether inappropriate example of Buddhism. Constituting the most radical antithesis to every type of *resentiment* morality, Buddhism clearly arose as the salvation doctrine of an intellectual stratum, originally recruited almost entirely from the privileged castes, especially the warrior caste, which proudly and aristocratically rejected the illusions of life both here and hereafter. (*ES*, vol. 1, p. 499)

Again Weber followed this observation by stressing the importance of intellectualism in a genuine salvation religion where it was Protestant Christianity which had most fully elaborated this intellectual and spiritual rejection of the everyday world and the bases of resentment.

Weber's interpretation of Nietzsche's concept of resentment with respect to Buddhism is peculiar in this context. In the relevant aphorisms of *The Genealogy of Morals* to which Weber referred in his discussion of resentment with respect to Buddhism, Nietzsche simply attacked the 'hysteria of the ascetic ideals', the 'meta-physics of priesthood', 'their self-hypnotization in the way of fakirs' and 'their satiety which they had to cure radically with its negation (or with God – the want for a *unio mystica* with God, this is the want of the Buddhists for negation, Nirvana – and nothing more.)' We need to inquire here why for Weber the privileged strata, and specifically the privileged priesthood in both medieval and modern Christianity, could not develop a resentment morality? Weber's topic in searching for the logic of the transition to modernity was not resentment, but rather what he called 'inner-worldly asceticism'. The contribution in particular of Calvinistic asceticism was the development of a disciplined and orderly life-style, specifically around the notion of self-control over passion and organic impulses, and their subordination to a rational and methodical plan. Although it was Calvinism which formed the pure illustration of such a calling, Weber was also interested in the contributions of, for example the Quakers, the Baptists and the Methodists. Although the ascetic ethic of Methodism was watered down by its emotionalism, the very title of the Methodist societies indicated their interest for Weber, namely their commitment to a methodical style of life.

Although these salvation movements in Christianity were not seen to be a necessary precondition for modernity, they were certainly directly linked with it in the form of an elective affinity. Again Weber separated this intellectual form of rational control in the Protestant sects from the discipline characteristic of Judaism. He wrote that 'when one compares Judaism with other salvation religions, one finds that in Judaism the doctrine of religious resentment has an idiosyncratic quality and plays a unique role not found among the disprivileged classes of any other religion' (*ES*, vol. 1, p. 496). In his sociology of religion, Weber related resentment to the Jewish religious community, but in some passages of *Economy and Society* he also connected resentment with the social revolutionary ethics and proletarian instincts of the subordinate working classes. However, the influence of such ethics and instincts in Christianity was not thought to be entirely significant. Instead, Weber saw salvation religions as fundamentally influenced by the intellectualism of the priesthood as a separate and distinctive profession. Although in Weber's own terms Buddhism would count as an intellectualized religion of a privileged stratum and thus have the characteristics of an aristocratic ethic which rejected the necessities of the mundane world, Weber developed the argument that the intellectualized salvation of medieval and modern Christianity was the product of the priesthood as an intellectual class far removed from the mundane realities of the everyday world and thus also removed from a basic resentment. This intellectual class of priests developed various forms of ascetic life-styles in realizing their rejection of the illusions of life.

Although Weber appeared to be content to describe Jewish ethics as the outcome of resentment, in general he wanted to disassociate the higher religions from mere 'interest situations' and to distinguish himself from Marx who on occasion regarded religion as simply an 'opium of the people' and also from Nietzsche who saw morals as simply an effect of the will-to-power of the weak. The ambiguity of Weber's position with respect to Nietzsche is clear in *Economy and Society*, in the author's introduction to the Protestant Ethic thesis, and also in the essay on the work ethic of world religions. Weber tended to regard Nietzsche's theory of resentment as simply a theory of class determination. Weber suggested that a notion of the class determination of religious ethics 'might be deduced from the theory of resentment known since Friedrich Nietzsche's brilliant essay and since then spiritually tested by psychologists' (*FW*, P. 270). For Weber, the theory of resentment is related to both class analysis and to psychological determination, but both aspects have a very limited bearing for Weber on the understanding of social ethics. While Weber recognized that bureaucrats might be motivated by a sense of resentment against the lordly stratum who lived free of duties, he argued that the rationalization of life conduct as such and the development of moral standards had 'nothing whatsoever to do with resentment' (*FW*, p. 271).

This use of Nietzsche by Weber, however, completely obscured the critical cutting edge of Nietzsche's sharp critique of altruism as a form of self-alienation, self-humiliation and denial. It also obscured Nietzsche's attempt to analyse the sanctification of low instincts in Christianity by treating Christianity as an intellectualized theology and theodicy of a privileged stratum. By restricting the problem of resentment to the question of class and psychology, Weber tried implicitly at least to protect Christianity and intellectualism from Nietzsche's critique. This denial that resentment could have anything to do with the different forms of ethical rationalization of life conduct resulted instead in an analysis of the theme of suffering in religious ethics, where Weber elaborated the analysis of suffering as a condition for the need for religious salvation. In his study of the importance of suffering for theodicy, Weber admitted that these theodicies could be 'coloured by resentment' and that suffering and resentment were 'significant as one factor, amongst others, in influencing the religiously determined rationalism of socially disadvantaged strata' (*FW*, p. 276).

Then Weber surprisingly admitted that 'there can be no doubt that the prophets and priests through intentional and unintentional propaganda have taken the resentment of the masses into their service' (*FW*, p. 277). In general, Weber wanted to argue that the prophets as charismatic leaders were separate from the mass of the population and that their following was largely restricted to a small group of devoted disciples (Zeitlin, 1984). Weber's perception of the Old Testament prophet was a person who rejected popular acclaim in the interests of a religious message. However, Weber also needed to recognize that a successful prophet with a discipleship and social influence had to be in tune with and in touch with more popular strata within society. Weber consequently saw the prophet caught between a religious calling and the need for popular influence. It may be that, in attempting to reconcile this theory of pure charisma with that of social leadership, Weber had to admit that the prophets needed to respond to and incorporate the resentment of the masses within their message. In addition of course, Weber saw Judaism generally and the Jewish prophets in particular as very much motivated by resentment. This analysis of suffering, resentment and intellectual leadership was set within a comparative sociology of the relationship between religion as a doctrine of love and the state as an institution of violence; Weber sought to analyse the various forms of accommodation of religion to the necessities of state violence (Turner, 1985b).

Intellectuals and the Meaningful Cosmos

The development of intellectualism was for Weber a crucial feature of the rationalization of the world and as we have seen he identified some aspects of this intellectualism with the emergence of a Calvinistic calling in the world. Weber had to see this intellectualism as a denial of everyday mundane interests. In *The Sociology of Religion*, Weber noted that 'the most elementary forms of behaviour motivated by religious or magical factors are oriented to this world' (*SR*, p. 1). Weber saw the development of a separate priestly stratum as an essential requirement for the intellectualization of this 'religious' instinct away from the mundane requirements of everyday life. The priesthood subsequently provided the model for the development of other professional groups offering intellectual and social services for a clientele in terms of an ethic of disinterestedness. The development of a separate and professionally trained group of lawyers was crucial to the development of legal rationalism and more generally the growth of bureaucracy depended on the development of men of calling who were separated from the realities and necessities of the mundane world. The rationalization of intellectualism involved a form of alienation from the everyday world, but also from the control of the bureaucratic apparatus. One of the defining features of these men of calling was the fact that they did not own the bureaucratic apparatus, the legal machinery or the scientific laboratory. Again Weber's sociology of the professions illustrated the tensions which are characteristic of his whole sociology. In this case the tension was between the ideal of intellectual leadership and personal charisma versus the deadening consequences of the bureaucratic context within which intellectuals are forced to work. On the one hand, Weber welcomed intellectualism as a control of the passion and the irrational forces of instinct, but on the other hand he saw it as part of a general disenchantment of reality. The domination of reality by this intellectualism was simply another feature of the growth

117

of the iron cage with the result that there was a contradiction between science as a vocation and science as merely the mechanical application of knowledge within a bureaucratic context of jobs and specifications. University academics could not function as genuine thinkers because they were subordinated to the dull routine of bureaucracy; they had become experts and specialists; they were mere functionaries without souls.

We also know that this intellectualism created a paradox since in the lecture on science as vocation Weber noted that science eventually renders the world meaningless and thus devoid of moral guidelines for professionals, intellectuals and other privileged strata. The very growth of science undermined the ability to make sense of the world, while at the same time giving greater control over it. Rather than producing personal enlightenment and development, science had become a central component of the ethic of world mastery. The result was to leave the world more exposed to competing values and moral systems which Weber imagined in terms of a conflict between a pantheon of gods where there was no central value system capable of adjudicating this cosmic struggle for meaning. Some aspects of Weber's view • of the intellectuals were dependent upon Nietzsche's treatment of the history of philosophy in respect to the growth of men of professions. Nietzsche, of course, rejected professional intellectualism on the grounds that it was the illness which purported to be the cure for the decay of modern society. In his rejection of the professional academic life, Nietzsche shared much in common with Schopenhauer as he made clear in *The Untimely Meditations* (McGill, 1931). It was only by liberating themselves from the worship of the idol of the state that intellectuals, more specifically philosophers, could come to pay a critical and radical role in modern society in the development of new values.

Economic Ethics and Civil Strata

Protestant Christianity's contribution to modernization, or more specifically to modernity, was the provision of a disciplined life-style, an intellectualization of rationality, the founding of morality in guilt and the development of a scientific orientation towards nature. In the course of this inquiry into modernity through and against Nietzsche, Weber came also to identify utilitarian morals as a third root of modernism. As with resentment and intellectualism, Weber again associated utilitarianism with the rise of a certain class, namely 'artisans, traders, entrepreneurs engaged in cottage industry and their derivatives established only in the modern occident' (*FW*, p. 284). It was within this intermediary class of petty bourgeoisie, which Weber called the 'civic strata', that the rational and individual pursuit of salvation was most firmly located within the urban environment of western societies. Weber regarded this intermediate urban group as the primary bearer of Christian rationality and discipline; he detected an elective affinity between life-styles and rationalism:

The tendency towards a classical rationalism in conduct is common to all civic strata; it is conditioned by the nature of their way of life, which is greatly detached from economic bonds to nature. Their whole existence has been based upon technological and economic calculations and upon the mastery of nature and of men, however primitive the means at their disposal. (*FW*, p. 284)

Whereas Weber treated the warrior as the typical carrier of Islam and the mendicant monk as the bearer of Buddhism, it was this urban, rational, artisan class which was the primary location for Christianity and ultimately the central audience for Protestant Reformism. It was also among these groups that intellectualism became one way of rationalizing everyday conduct where 'science contributes to the technology of control in life by calculating external objects as well as man's activity' (*EW*, p. 150). We should note Weber regarded the emotionalism of the Methodist sect in England as a deviation from this bourgeois rationalism, characteristic of the older dissenting groups such as the Quakers and the Baptists.

Weber regarded these Protestant men of calling as bearers of world mastery involving a denial of irrational passions. Their lives were committed to an ethic of control to subordinate such deviant emotions. Alongside these religious figures, Weber also placed the professional and the scientist as men of calling, whose lives were organized by a rational plan in the interests of their personal achievement of status, but also as the method for establishing personality (in the sense of a unified life project towards empirical goals). Their religious calling drove them beyond what was necessary for the satisfaction of everyday needs, wants and requirements; this was the irrationality of utilitarian rationality. However, this striving for mastery, particularly in science, brought a new form of disillusionment and moral anxiety, insofar as science renders the world increasingly meaningless. Therefore Weber was forced to ask:

who – aside from certain big children who are indeed found in the natural sciences – still believes that the findings of astronomy, biology, physics or chemistry could teach us anything about the meaning of the world? (*FW*, p. 142)

Weber argued that the fate of our times is characterized by an increasing rationalization and intellectualization of the everyday world which leads ultimately to disenchantment. These processes of rationalization and disenchantment have often focused on the problem of the control of the body as the source of irrational drives and passions, since it is the organic life which needs ultimately to be managed by administration, science and specialized disciplines (Turner, 1984). Western history can be seen, from Weber's perspective, as the diffusion of the body-disciplines of the monastery and army to the whole society via the factory and the school. The problem then is how to escape this fate and how to overcome the means of this disenchantment.

Although there has been much debate as to the relevance of Weber's ethic of responsibility as a solution to the ultimate problems of modern society, our argument is that Weber in fact offered no significant solution to the fate of our times, but merely provided some descriptions in 'science as a vocation' of somewhat distinctive orientations to the modern world. The first was described in the following terms:

The only thing that is strange is the method that is now followed: the spheres of the irrational, the only spheres that intellectualism has not yet touched, are now raised into consciousness and put under its lens. For in practice this is where the modern intellectualist form of romantic irrationalism leads. This method of emancipation from intellectualism may well bring about the very opposite of what those who take it conceive as its goal. (*FW*, p. 143)

Weber regarded this quest for experience within the romantic and the irrational as an illustration of what Nietzsche had referred to as the quest of the 'last men' who 'invented happiness'. Weber despised this orientation to the modern world, rejecting it as a merely childish quest. The second solution could be seen in the following terms:

Precisely the ultimate and most sublime values have retreated from public life either into the transcendental realm of mystic life or into the brotherliness of direct and personal human relations. It is not accidental that our greatest art is intimate and not monumental. (*FW*. p. 155)

Weber argued that this approach to the problem of rationalism involved a return to the intimate personal human situations where direct experience became possible. He regarded this as a life-style which could be described in terms of the musical notion of *pianissimo* but he viewed this orientation to the crisis of meaning as a defeat. It was essentially a withdrawal from engagement and commitment, a withdrawal from the asceticism of the man of calling.

120

Finally, Weber saw religion in the modern world as an 'intellectual sacrifice' (*FW*, p. 155) in favour of an unconditional religious devotion. Weber recognized that the traditional Church was still available as an option even in a world of unrelenting secularization, but this orientation lacked the seriousness and the commitment which he felt was required by the crisis of the times. Weber rejected these options because they were not sufficient as vocations and therefore he turned to the idea of intellectual integrity in politics as one partial solution to the dilemma of moral relativism and the crisis of intellectualism. In summary, Weber regarded modern movements to solve the great crisis of our time as either romantic irrationalism or the personal solution of intimate relations or finally the sacrifice of the mind to religious faith. His own solution at best was a realistic evaluation of one's situation through the medium of science or politics, but this is no solution even in Weber's own terms, since it cannot tell us which goals to follow, but only provides as it were short term adjustments to immediacy.

Weber's Departure from Nietzsche

We have seen that Weber drew significantly from Nietzsche's moral critique of modern society and that they shared a number of concepts and also to some extent a perspective on the centrality of value struggle and conflict in the shaping of the modern world. We know from biographical and textual evidence that Nietzsche's influence on Weber was a long term and profound one (Hennis, 1987). In this chapter, we have not been concerned merely to repeat this evidence; our aim is more to change the direction of sociology through an encounter with Nietzsche. Weber, as we have seen, regarded Nietzsche as one of the major thinkers of the modern period. There was a common interest in the question of resentment with respect to religion, but Weber narrowed and restricted Nietzsche's view of resentment by converting it into a form of psychological theory. By contrast, Nietzsche had employed the notion of resentment as a far-ranging cultural critique, seeing resentment as much more than a psychology of revenge on the part of the disprivileged. In particular, Nietzsche felt that resentment was a crucial dynamic to thought itself. In a similar fashion, we could superficially say that both Weber and Nietzsche had a commitment to individualism or more precisely to individuality, but Nietzsche was also highly critical of the notion of the individual and individualism as mere social constructions of bourgeois culture. As we have seen, Nietzsche was more likely to argue that it is the 'it' which thinks and that the

121

notion of the 'I' is a mere presumption. Nietzsche saw the problem of desire and need as the fundamental roots of experience rather than an intellectual orientation to experience. In this regard, Nietzsche's philosophy represented a fundamental divergence from the German tradition of both Hegel and Kant; Nietzsche had more in common with Kierkegaard and Kierkegaard's critique of Hegel than with Weber and Weber's rejection of the systematization of thought in Marx (Thulstrup, 1980). Nietzsche, like Kierkegaard, tended to regard intellectualism and rationalism as a false reconstruction of experience and Nietzsche criticized the arrogance and presumption of thought on the grounds that rational thinking is essentially metaphorical, but denies its metaphoricality by regarding itself as a direct representation of reality. This critique of the intellectual rationalization of the world was also connected with Nietzsche's critique of the professional, professionalism and professional thinking in academic life, as in Germany academics had become merely agents of the state. Although Nietzsche had abandoned his own academic career partly on grounds of illness, he also had a strong moral and intellectual objection to the very idea of routinized thought. In a joke against intellectuals and intellectualism, Nietzsche suggested that dancing might be a more appropriate mode than thinking. These critical objections and the distance between Weber and Nietzsche go back to Nietzsche's commitment to the centrality of what he called 'the little things', namely the *habitus* of the everyday world in which we are embodied and engaged.

4

The Return of Freud – Religion, Sex and Civilization

Introduction: Great Thoughts

Within a relativistic perspective, we can always regard great thinking as merely a social construction brought about by the availability of audiences and the market for published works, but this is unsatisfactory as a characterization of significant contributions to human culture. In more fundamentalistic terms, we can argue that great thinking embodies the contradictions of the period in which it is set, exhibits massive self-reflexivity with respect to these conditions, provides some transcendence of the limitations of existing patterns of thought and finally creates an anticipation of transformation and resolution of contradictions. In this sense, great thinking is not confined within a nostalgic paradigm. That is, we would not wish to argue that significant thinking entirely transcends* and departs from current modes of analysis, but rather great thinking exhibits and manifests these limitations, while also indicating future reconciliations. This way of expressing greatness in thinking corresponds to some extent to the notion of *Aufhebung* where the concept embraces the notions of abolition, overcoming and preservation within a dialectical framework. Great thought knows its region, but also, by identifying its horizon, points forward to a new formation of the character of thinking itself (Heidegger, 1966). Rational thought must in Nietzsche's terms be tragic as a consequence of knowing its limit. The greatness of a thinker may well reside in his or her rootedness in the concrete and specific problems of their time; their relevance to these issues does not exclusively signal the limitations of their thought, but precisely their ability to express and exhibit the character of their time.

The issue of relevance and transcendence may be an important issue with respect to the consistency of thought and the inherent contradiction of theoretical systems. Most so-called great thinkers are typically assumed to have a young and a mature phase whereby the aberrations of their youth are resolved in the calmness of their old age. We thus speak about the young Marx and the mature Marx by noting the existence of an epistemological rupture in thought (Althusser, 1969). In a similar fashion it has been argued that in the work of Talcott Parsons a break occurs between the early emphasis on voluntary action and the later concern with the systemic character of social structure (Hamilton, 1983). The question of coherence and consistency however is deeply problematic, since within an author-centred interpretation, one presupposes that the author had from the foundation of his or her work a project, whereas if we are mainly concerned with the character of texts, then the problem of coherence may well turn out to be one which is entirely constructed. There is however an even deeper problem, namely in what would coherence consist? This question in turn brings into focus the issue of whether an author is responsible for his work.

In this study of Nietzsche, we have not been primarily concerned with the question of exegesis, since our argument is that interpretation is typically a second order activity. We are concerned to identify certain themes in Nietzsche's work – embodiment, reciprocity and resistance – as the basis for a project in sociology. In the case of Nietzsche however, this question of coherence and consistency is crucially important, since Nietzsche appears to be an anti-system thinker, on the grounds that all systems involve the standardization of the unique and the incomparable. A system implies the imposition of a rule on creative experience. It is the specific merit of J. P. Stern to have noted Nietzsche's greatness in terms of the openness and autonomy of his thinking (Stern, 1978; Stern, 1979).

Nietzsche's personality was necessarily important for the character of his work and when interpreting Nietzsche it is impossible to separate out the question of his personal authority and the authoritative nature of his text; Nietzsche's works exhibit the quest for freedom and individual authenticity in a way which has hardly been matched. Writing of this aspect of Nietzsche's work, Stern makes the following observations:

He chooses to be as free from the obligations of society (of family, class, nation, profession) as a man can be – a man who retains a deep longing for friendship, for a public, and for disciples, too. He forces the circumstances – including his health, his temperament, the failure of his professional prospects, to force the choice on him. This is his *amor fati*, the experience of life he chooses his philosophizing to reflect. And since this experience has provided him with amazingly little insight into any form of institutionalization – political, social or national – how can the arguments of his thoughts be other than unsystematic, unspecialized and unconfined, a unique free venture? (1978, p. 21)

This involves the dance-like qualities of Nietzsche's thought. This quest for autonomy partly explains the stylistic qualities of Nietzsche's work, especially their playfulness and their wilfullness. In addition, Nietzsche felt that, since the world was fragmented, literary style would also have a fragmented and aphoristic character. The ambiguity of his work is a fundamental feature of its very modernity.

Freud's Thought

In this chapter we examine the relationship between Freud and Nietzsche with special reference to their views on religion, morality and civilization. We have chosen Freud partly because of his contemporary significance, but also because Freud adopted and adapted much of Nietzsche's moral philosophy to the problems of psycho-analysis (although as we have noted previously Freud systematically denied this influence). Both Freud and Nietzsche can be considered to be great thinkers in terms of our definition, since in their work we find the problems of relevance and transcendence in a critical conjunction. Freud was a great thinker, not in the superficial and narrow sense of being widely recognized, but in the more important meaning of embodying and pointing beyond the contradictions of his time. In the last analysis however, our argument is that Freud failed to carry out to its ultimate implication the radical starting point of psycho-analysis; in this sense Freud's radical journey was incomplete (Breger, 1981).

Freud is often dismissed out of hand on the grounds that his psycho-analytic theories express misguidedly the subordination of women, especially women within the patriarchal bourgeois family. This particular interpretation of Freud is superficial (Mitchell, 1974) and the psycho-analysis of women with respect to female autonomy, art and pornography raises a range of issues which have yet to be entirely resolved in a fashion which is theoretically powerful (Carter, 1979; Faust, 1982; Sontag, 1969). Although these particular dismissals of Freud have been brought into question, Freud's thought is characteristically seen to be the expression of the contradictions of European capitalism at a certain conjuncture and in particular of the crises of Viennese society and its Jewish community at the turn of the century.

We can examine Freudianism in terms of a series of contradictions between duty and desire, civilization and instinct; these polarities in Freudian psycho-analysis express the crisis of the patriarchal family at the point of its demise.

Freudian theory has often been perceived in terms of somewhat rigid dichotomies between the ego and the id, the life and the death instincts and between male and female principles; these fixed oppositions represent a somewhat narrow conceptualization of the range of human possibilities, where this narrowness expresses the remnants of a formal moral system which was in a state of crisis. It is often mistakenly assumed that the contrast between id and super-ego corresponds to Nietzsche's contrast between Dionysus and Apollo; we shall argue that this misrepresents Nietzsche who was in fact a critic of Socratic rationalism not Apollonian culture. The dualism of Freud's theory was typical of the nineteenth century; the notion of homo duplex was fundamental to sociology itself. For example, Durkheim's theory of suicide was grounded in a vision of homo duplex, that is of individuals caught in the pressure of social forces and instinctual drives. Durkheimian sociology embraced these two principles that social forces exercise an external constraint over the individuals who constitute society and that these individuals were themselves hierarchically structured by the effect of these social forces (Gane, 1983). Freud's social theory, like Durkheim's view of suicide, often assumed that women were organized by the forces of instinct rather than culture, whereas male behaviour was more significantly the outcome of socialization into a rational culture of the public sphere. While Freud's social theory exhibited these traditional nineteenth-century assumptions with respect to sexuality, some aspects of Freud's work were also structured by Darwinistic assumptions about mechanical evolutionism. Although Freud's theory was in many respects revolutionary, it also gave expression to quite conservative principles, whether by intention or by effect. For example, there is the assumption in Freudianism that the characteristics of human nature are fixed and that historical change is somewhat irrelevant to the basic forces of hatred and revenge; therefore attempts to reorganize human nature through a process of social restructuring are either naive or irrelevant (Brown, 1961).

Turning more specifically to a consideration of the contradictions of Freud's thought, we may first consider the general relationship between conservative and radical elements in Freudianism. Freud by focusing upon the sexual bases of human behaviour, especially within children, had broken with some basic Victorian principles of silence concerning this dimension of human existence. In *The History of Sexuality*, Foucault (1979) argued that ironically the silence regarding sex produced an ever-present discourse of sexual deviance. Freud's characterization of sex was both an important departure from existing assumptions and practices and a reproduction of its discourse. Freud radicalized sex by making it more prominent and all pervasive. Freudianism was also revolutionary in bringing the language of sexuality rather than the physiology of sex to the centre of his theoretical speculations. This radical feature of Freud was particularly evident in the treatment of hysteria where he rejected the conventional wisdom that hysterical behaviour had its origins in sexual malfunction and specifically in physiology (*SE*, vol. 2). By arguing that hysterics suffered from reminiscences, Freud was able to reject the conventional notion that hysteria was an exclusively female problem. This particular viewpoint was at the time regarded as an absurdity. In Freudianism, the metaphors of hysteria are problems in language, not in the reproductive problems of the womb.

Despite these radical features, Freud's theory of sexuality remained fundamentally ambiguous. It contained within it the notion that the stories of sexual seduction in children were real and also that they were the expression of a sexual wish; this ambiguity was often resolved by an implicit commitment in Freudianism to the figures of authority, that is to men as heads of households. Freud vacillated between regarding the sexual instinct as corrosive and destructive of social relations, and regarding sexuality as the source of energy and vitality in culture. The neurotic suffering of the victim was the expression of the power of society on the one hand, but this suffering was also regarded as the fault of sexual drives themselves (Breger, 1981, p. 79). It was along these lines that Fromm (1973, p. 47) criticized Freud's homo sexualis as merely a new version of the classical homo economicus on the grounds that Freudianism was the perfect psychology of bourgeois political economy. Freudianism was seen to be a defense of force, authority and control in bourgeois society, because it was simply a legitimatization of parental authority within the capitalist household.

These contradictions in Freud's thought were fundamentally related to an ambiguity in his view of science and consequently in his perspective on therapy. This contradiction is well known. While Freud's project pointed towards a philosophical social psychology in which language and imagination would be given a certain autonomy, he also retained a deep commitment to positivistic science in which neuroses could be explained in mechanistic terms where the brain is seen to function in terms of a biochemical system (Levin, 1978). In describing the unconscious as a sort of place, Freud adhered to a Cartesian map of the mind as a distinct realm in which ideas are entities which bounce against each other. That is, while Freud's theory pointed towards a hermeneutic interpretation of the unconscious as a language, his commitment to a positivistic version of science compelled him to describe the unconscious in the terminology of mechanics on the assumption that ultimately only observables have a legitimate place in science (MacIntyre, 1958). Freud's psycho-analysis suggested a liberating, emancipatory and reflexive practice which would enable patients to gain an insight into the social constraints which limited their lives, but his commitment to a positivistic model of dream analysis and therapy inhibited the realization of this emancipatory dynamic (Bernstein, 1976). Nietzsche by contrast, having exposed the violent roots of civilization, rejected science itself as merely a comforting illusion.

Given this ambiguity in Freud's stance, we can understand why contemporary interpretations of Freudianism have often given a special significance to the role of language in Freudian theory and practice. By seeing the problem of the unconscious as a problem of language, it is possible to avoid the nineteenth-century implications of Freud's positivistic view of science. Once the problem of the patient is conceived as a problem of language, we can more fully appreciate the special significance of Freud's lay confessional, in which the semantic dilemmas of the patient are allowed to unfold in a way which becomes constructive. Reading the problem of the patient becomes analogous to reading a text: that is, the illness has to be decoded (Lacan, 1977). Traditional medical practice involves the reading of signs and symptoms which disclose the story of a disease. Illness is a discourse and the role of the psycho-analyst is to comprehend the message which is hidden within the discursive character of symptoms. For example, anorexia may be interpreted not only as a refusal of food, but as a refusal of words. Maud Mannoni, a follower of Lacan, writes of the symptom and the word:

the reality of the 'illness' is never underestimated in psycho-analysis but an attempt is made to pinpoint just how the real situation is lived in by the child and his family. It is then that the symbolic value that the subject attaches to the situation, re-echoing a given family history takes on a meaning. For the child it is the words spoken by those around him about his 'illness' that assume importance. These words or the absence of them, create the dimension of the lived experience in him. This attempt to regain the radical dimension of Freud therefore involves a return to the theory of semiotics and furthermore to the idea that language is fundamentally a metaphorical activity since the nature of things depends upon the structure of discourse. (1973, p. 61)

The contention of this chapter is that the recovery of language in the radical features of Freudianism involves the rediscovery of one aspect of the Nietzsche problematic behind psycho-analysis. This recovery was the basis for Lacan's practice which rejected cure (mental health and mental hygiene) as a goal of psycho-analysis; to be cured is to be dead. The aim of Lacanian practice was the verbalization of the unconscious (Schneiderman, 1983). The official character of Freudianism has thereby masked the underlying threat of Nietzsche. In particular, we argue that psycho-analysis is an analysis of the language of drama which is structured by the figures of Apollo, Dionysus and Socrates.

Freud and the Social Sciences

Before turning to a study of the importance of *The Birth of Tragedy* in Nietzsche's analysis of dramatic myth in social evolution, we wish to place Nietzsche's confrontation with the Dionysian principle in the context of the sociological analysis of the non-rational. This digression creates the scene in which we can see Freudianism as a rationalist treatment of drama. It is possible to interpret the rise of sociology in the second half of the nineteenth century as a response to the problem of rational action and rational thought. The problem which sociology addressed was how to locate theoretically the role of values, symbols and cultural facts in relation to economic behaviour and political processes. Specifically, sociology addressed itself to the moral realm in relation to economic utility. Sociology involved a critique of the dominant models of economic reasoning (specifically utilitarian demand and supply models), but it also responded to the behaviouralist assumptions of psychology, penology and criminology. It is possible to speak of a 're-orientation of European social thought' (Hughes, 1959) between the period 1890 and 1930 when sociology attempted to provide a theoretical space for the role of non-rational and irrational forces in human society. In German sociology, this problem was expressed in terms of the contradiction between the will-to-life and the cultural forms of social action.

It is interesting to take note of the fact that the major figures in this European re-orientation were all born and died within a remarkably short time span: Durkheim (1858–1917), Weber (1864–1920), Simmel (1858–1918), Mead (1863–1931), Pareto (1848–1923) and Freud (1856–1938). Although Nietzsche is rather infrequently included in this list, it is clear that Nietzsche's own attempt to examine the problem of rational thought in a post-theological age (with special reference to the forces of resentment and power in social life) was part of a broader sweep of social analysis of the non-rational. Both Nietzsche and Freud can be regarded as theorists who retrieved the importance of the non-rational and the irrational in individual and social life; furthermore, they both addressed this theoretical issue in terms of a discussion concerning the place of religion and myth in social life. However, Nietzsche's contribution to the development of the sociology of religion has been neglected by mainstream sociology.

The paradigm which Nietzsche established, especially the concern for myth and ritual in tragedy, had close parallels to aspects of the thought of Durkheim and we should note the obvious fact that Durkheim's attempt to come to terms with the role of the non-rational, the symbolic and the poetic was conducted in terms of an anthropological study of religion and an analysis of public ritual in social drama. Here again the convergence between Durkheim, Freud, Weber and Nietzsche is striking (Anderson, 1980; Parsons, 1937; Scharf, 1970). Durkheim offered a sociological account of the relationship between passion and duty as against Freud's bio-psychological treatment of human behaviour (Lukes, 1975, p. 188); Durkheim developed this theory with special reference to the problem of totemism as a language of social relationships. The contrast between sacred and profane reality is in fact a consequence of the structure of language as the fabric of collective culture. While both Nietzsche and Freud were clearly relevant to the sociological analysis of the role of the non-rational in society, the main debate about magic, ritual and religion has been largely dominated by the work of Malinowski, Durkheim and Mauss (Wilson, 1970). Freud and Nietzsche therefore had relatively little overt and official influence on classical sociology in the period 1880–1914. Weber, while aware of the work of Freud, was scathing in his rejection of Freudianism as a form of mental hygiene. Pareto, while developing a theory of the non-rational, did not refer to the work of Freud. There is no evidence apparently that Durkheim was aware of Freud's analyses of religion and the neurotic (Lukes, 1975, p. 433). Freud and Nietzsche consequently had little direct involvement in the sociological confrontation with the problem of the irrational in the classical founding generation of sociologists in the 1890s.

The Americanization of Freud

The contradictory features of Freud's social theory were reflected in his reception in social science, namely that the radical and conservative implications of psycho-analysis were both adopted by different types of sociology under somewhat different sets of circumstances. For example, in the American context Freud entered contemporary social theory through the channel of Talcott Parsons' views on socialization as expressed through the theory of social systems (Parsons, 1951), through the analysis of the 'sick role', and through the notion of the interaction process (Parsons, Bales and Shils, 1953). Parsons used Freud largely as the basis for a theory of socialization which provided the linkage between the concepts of the personality and the social system. Freud was introduced into American social theory as a conservative theorist of the necessary relationship between individual satisfactions and social requirements. Whereas both Nietzsche and Freud saw the relationship between social requirements and individual autonomy as conflictual and contradictory, in much of Parsons' theory of socialization this essential tension was diminished or jettisoned. In Parsons' early analysis of the social system, the needs of the individual and the requirements of the social system were simultaneously satisfied via a system of socialization where social gratification became the basis for the incorporation of the individual (Menzies, 1976). The stability of social systems (the classical problem of social order) was eventually solved by the notion that the need-dispositions of individuals become perfectly consistent with the requirements of the social system through the merger of these dispositions with value-patterns from the cultural system; Parsons adopted Freudian theory by suggesting that childhood socialization produces a stable personality which over time finds fulfilment through meeting system requirements (Parsons and Shils, 1951). In this theory of internalization, Freud's distinction between the id and the ego was reduced to merely a difference between affectivity and discipline. It was on this basis that Parsons and functionalism generally were accused of developing an 'oversocialized conception of man' in contemporary sociological theory, a conception which ruled out any notion of change and conflict resulting from the disparity of individual needs and system requirements (Wrong, 1961; Wrong, 1963). In Parsonian sociology the critical edge of Freud's view of an incompatibility between civilization and the instinctual bases of behaviour was lost or subordinated in the theory of system requirements. However, in defence of Parsons, we can note that his analysis of Freudianism, biology and cybernetics in his final works was a more sophisticated development of his first encounter with Freud. It remains the case, however, that the original formulation of functionalism lacked a valid analysis of conflict and strains in social systems (Alexander, 1985).

In early social anthropology, there was a significant debate with

Freud (although the debate was frequently indirect), because Freud's theory implied a fixed character to human personality in terms of an eternal struggle between the id and the super-ego. The findings of social anthropology called into question the alleged universality of Freudian psycho-analytic theory. Anthropologists through their field-work provided evidence to suggest that human personality and hence human sexuality were extremely variable across cultures. The variability of human personality and behaviour was particularly important in relation to comparative studies of sexuality. For example, Malinowski on the basis of his own fieldwork described Trobiand society as a sexual utopia in which there was relatively little inter-generational conflict and wide tolerance of sexual deviance and sexual exploration between the sexes (Malinowski, 1927). In a similar fashion, the research of Margaret Mead, Clyde Kluckhon and Ralph Linton pointed to the existence of extreme variation in sexual roles and sexual personality, so that in certain societies the biological men performed traditionally female roles, while biological females often assumed roles which required leadership, public authority and the exercise of force. In short, it became important to distinguish between biological sex, sex-type roles, gender and gender-personality. Mead's research became a crucial factor in the development of feminist theory, since it pointed to the cultural limitations of Freud's Eurocentric view of sexuality.

While this social anthropology suggested that the conflict between discipline and affectivity could be resolved in a variety of institutional ways, cultural anthropology also had a certain conservative implication. The cultural relativism of anthropology suggested that, while the concept of the non-rational was appropriate to much human behaviour, the idea that human behaviour, institutions and values could be irrational was abandoned. All behaviour which on the surface appears bizzare can be shown to be functionally valid once located in an appropriate context. Anthropology began to interpret 'functionally valid' as equivalent to 'rational'. Since no behaviour could be regarded as bizzare, non-utilitarian or irrational, anthropology was unable to criticize any society. Because all apparently bizzare behaviours are in fact functionally relevant, anthropology was cast in a conservative and descriptive role as the mere observer of cultural fact. This was the basis of the classical debate with the philosophy of Peter Winch, who following Wittgenstein, argued that the role of social science was merely to interpret social action, thereby leaving everything as it is (Winch, 1958). The animality of desire had been domesticated by a functional framework in which all behaviour has beneficial consequences.

At the core of Malinowski's cultural anthropology was the notion that

132

all human beings are *qua* human beings necessarily rational, sensible and consistent (Leach, 1957). This is a morally persuasive position since it protects aboriginal societies from a colonial cultural critique, but the implications of the theory were ultimately conservative, since by extension it followed that social science could never be critical of society or the individuals within social relations. The capacity for criticism involves some notion of consistent rational behaviour against which we could measure irrational and affectual forms of conduct. Alternatively, it involves some commitment to a universal value whereby the constraints of a particular historical society can be scrutinized and evaluated. It was this appeal to the role of a universalistic critique which formed the basis of contemporary critical theory and the Frankfurt School.

Freud and Critical Theory

It is well known that the critical theorists made extensive use of Freud's psycho-analytic theory as a way of extending and amplifying the critical tradition which they had inherited from Marx and Marxism. However, Freud was also used to fill certain gaps left in this legacy. In particular Marx's neglect of the dynamics of personality was felt to be an area of weakness in traditional Marxism which had become dominated by mechanistic models of behaviour. Freud's theory was attractive because in its radical version it had a dynamic conception of personality as the constant struggle between contradictory forces. It was possible to graft Freudianism onto Marxism without massive redefinition and elaboration. Freud's picture of the individual, as the contradictory resolution of certain personality forces, matched Marx's view of civil society in capitalism as a system of never-ending conflict and contradiction. In this respect, Freud's treatment of personality offered Marxism a solution to the relationship between biological phenomena, the person and social relations. We should note however that neither Marxism nor critical theory have produced a coherent account of the realtionship between biology, society and history (Timpanaro, 1975).

Freudianism entered critical theory in particular via the analysis of capitalism as renunciation, especially in the *Dialectic of Enlightenment* where Adorno and Horkheimer used both Freud and Nietzsche to understand the contradictory logic of discipline and desire. More specifically, Freud provided an important basis for Marcuse's critique of capitalism as the negation of Eros and the triumph of superfluous regulation (Marcuse, 1955). Freud's theories and the psycho-analytic method were also part of the rejection of anti-semitism and fascism in the political development of modern capitalism. Freud's account of the non-rational and the unconscious provided a basis for the analysis of Nazi Germany via an understanding of symbolic and ritual activity. The critique of fascism under the influence of Freud found its expression in the theory of the authoritarian personality and in the critique of mass society (Reich, 1975). However, the attitude of the critical theorists to Freud and Nietzsche remained highly ambiguous, since Nietzsche called into question many of the assumptions of rational criticism which provided the basis for the Frankfurt School itself.

The ambiguities of the Freudian legacy in social science can be further illustrated by reference to the work of Philip Reiff who employed Freud's notion of the super-ego to restate the theory of religion by arguing the necessity of some sacred canopy as a protective device in social relations. Reiff (1966) argued that all traditional cultures had been based upon a complex balance between moral demand and expressive release which had made possible the conditions for social stability and individual commitment. Rieff claimed that all moral cultures were organized in terms of two main functions, namely the organization of moral demands and the organization of expressive remissions. Traditional cultures were cultures of commitment, where commandments had an authoritative origin, namely in some supernatural assumption. He argued that contemporary cultures are cultures of therapy in which the internal restraints upon individuals had been diminished in favour of an expressive revolution. Commitments no longer have any authority and it is difficult to legitimize the demands which are still necessary for individuals to survive in society.

In this context, the emergence of psycho-analysis played an important part in replacing the language of faith with the language of compensation and recovery. Psycho-analysis was an effect of social changes and it was psycho-analysis which made possible the re-adjustment of individuals in a world without authoritative regulations and in which there is, as it were, a surplus of remissive components. Reiff felt that Weber's notions of rationalization and disenchantment were no longer particularly relevant in cultures which had taken a definitely remissive direction and where the old law of economic scarcity no longer necessarily prevailed. The contrast between denial in the workplace and hedonism in consumption has become a central feature of the contradictions of capitalism (Bell, 1976). The old symbols lose their significance and efficacy; the traditional cultural elite which gave expression to this symboic reality had declined and was being replaced by an elite of therapy and welfare; this new elite could not give expression to viable community myths. There is a correspond-ing decline of what Rieff referred to as 'compassionate' communities which are replaced by agencies of ethical accommodation through the new systems of therapy. For Rieff therefore, the Freudian analysis of religion had shown the importance of religious controls in limiting desire in the interests of discipline, but Freudianism had made commitment increasingly impossible since it contained a secular critique of religious commandments. Freud offered analysis, not faith. It was for this reason that Rieff found Jung more congenial, since Jungian psycho-analysis had sought to discover in myth an alternative to the Christian God in an age of secularity. It is interesting that Rieff rarely quotes Nietzsche and his attack on Freud owes more to Jung than to the original theorist of the problem of the death of God. Rieff attempted to develop a humanistic analysis of contemporary society and sought to discover functional alternatives to God in the notion of some authoritative and genuine community.

In contemporary sociology, there is considerable interest in Freud's contribution to social theory (Badcock, 1980; Bocock, 1983; Wollheim, 1971). However, as we have attempted to show, the reception of Freud has often been somewhat superficial; furthermore, this reception has demonstrated the ambiguities of Freudianism as both a conservative critique of sexuality and as a radical recognition of its role in the structuring of human society and history. We have also argued that behind Freud there stood Nietzsche and Nietzsche's contribution to psycho-analysis and sociology has been inadequately explored, despite the growing interest in Nietzsche in both France and Germany (Stephens, 1986). Nietzsche provided not merely a sociology of religion, but a critique of modern cultures through his analysis of the roots of our dilemma in terms of a genealogy of myth, ritual and drama. In order to pursue this issue in more detail, we turn now to a comparison of Nietzsche and Freud on the role of religion in the history of civilization.

Society and the Death of God

Nietzsche's relationship with religion and to Christianity in particular is complex and problematic. Given the complexity of his perspective, it has often been thought that in many respects Nietzsche's final philosophical position was in fact compatible with the moral thrust of Christianity as a plea for a genuine spirituality against the hyprocrisy of bourgeois culture in the nineteenth century. Rather than repudiating

135

Christ, Nietzsche merely offered a critique of the ascetic ethic of Christianity which, rather than dealing with desire, simply denied it (Kaufmann, 1974). Nietzsche like Kierkegaard appears to be merely a critic of the Christian system rather than the essence of Christianity as such. Nietzsche's real critique therefore is against the hypocrisy and cant of the formal Church. Nietzsche's critique is often as a result seen as an objection to specific forms of Protestantism as a religious version of nihilism. Protestantism celebrated individualism, rationality and asceticism; it was the antithesis of unreflective spontaneity. Nietzsche's aim was to produce a moral code which would be suitable for someone of passion who had nevertheless gained control and direction over emotion; in this respect Nietzsche's writing on resentment becomes clear, since he is against a moral system which would disguise the real nature of power and passion behind a creed of insipid moral regulations; he was opposed to aesthetic Socratism. It is for this reason that the prophet 'laughed at the weaklings who thought themselves good because they had no claws' (*Z*, part II, section 13). In a similar fashion, Nietzsche felt great contempt for such virtues as 'neighbourly love' and 'pity' on the grounds that these were weak virtues; instead Nietzsche had a great respect for the essential quality of friendship between those who were strong.

In summary, within this perspective, Nietzsche's criticisms amount to a rejection of organized Christianity as an institution grounded necessarily in untruth, but his philosophy has also been treated as a defence of Christ who can be regarded as the first and the last of all Christians.

Nietzsche's view of Christ is particularly unstable and unresolved. Dionysus (as an affirmation of life) is both opposed to Christ and equated with Christ in *The Birth of Tragedy*. In addition, Christianity is regarded as part of the Dionysiac impulse against the rationalism of Socrates (Silk and Stern, 1981, p. 121). A similar interpretation of Nietzsche is also adopted by Stern (1978) who perceives Nietzsche as a philosopher attempting to come to terms with the problem of a post-Christian era, but nevertheless retaining much of the message of Christ. For example, Stern suggests that, far from being incompatible with Christianity as a religious outlook, Nietzsche's philosophy was actually the product of Christian thinking, because one aspect of Christianity emphasized the importance of truthfulness as a moral position. In a similar vein, Hollingdale (1973) argued that Nietzsche's critique of religion was aimed against the false institutionalization of the Christian message in the repressive moral apparatus of the official Church; however, Nietzsche had a great deal of sympathy with

'Christianness' where Christ's teaching can be seen to be a life affirmative doctrine. Here again Hollingdale sides with the view that the core of Nietzsche's philosophy is a rejection of all life-denying traditions in favour of an affirmation of passion and its individual and biological roots. Finally, we might note the interpretation of Eric Heller (1961) who regarded Nietzsche as a philosopher who, having lost his faith in Christianity, sought to discover a tenable position in modern society which would be in some respects a re-writing of the Christian moral position as the antedote to nihilism. In these re-interpretations of Nietzsche's anti-religious critique, there is the implication that Nietzsche offered, along with Kierkegaard, an existential response to the loss of faith, the death of God and the cultural crisis of modernity. Nietzsche, Kierkegaard and Schopenhauer are anti-Hegelian critics of the falsity of the State and Church. Although these are sympathetic and intelligent interpretations of Nietzsche, they have the effect of domesticating his thought and making it compatible with a humanistic, comfortable view of the world. They make, in a metaphor which Nietzsche would have approved, dangerous ideas edible for human consumption.

In interpreting Nietzsche's thought we should give some central recognition to his violent and dangerous thoughts on the relationship between religion, society and the individual. Let us start by reminding ourselves of the extent of Nietzsche's rejection of Christianity: 'I call Christianity the *one* great curse, the *one* great intrinsic depravity, the *one* great instinct for revenge for which no expedient is sufficiently poisonous, secret, subterranean, *petty* – I call it the *one* immortal blemish of mankind' (*AC*, section 62). Unlike many nineteenth-century thinkers who adopted an implicit orientalism, Nietzsche looked towards Islam as the carrier of fundamental passions which were compatible with man as a being of feeling and strength. Nietzsche accused Christianity of destroying the harvest of the classical world and through the crusades of destroying Islamic virtues. He wrote that:

The wonderful Moorish cultural world of Spain, more closely related to *us* at bottom, speaking more directly to our senses and taste, than Greece and Rome was *trampled* down . . . why? Because it was noble, because it owed its origins to manly instincts, because it said Yes to life even in the rare and exquisite treasures of Moorish life (*AC*, section 60).

Nietzsche's sympathy with Islam is a vehicle for expressing this commitment to affirmation, but we should not interpret this as Nietzsche's substitute for traditional faith. Nietzsche used Islam and

137

Buddhism as a stick with which to beat religion as the neurosis of life.

The death of God for Nietzsche was an intellectual and moral challenge which, in bringing to an end the false authority of a previous set of institutions, liberated moral agents for a new and dangerous adventure. The existence of this gap was a hopeful challenge to people of steel nerves and Nietzsche did not look towards the substitution of God for some new absolute. Unlike contemporary secular theologians, Nietzsche did not promote love or community or situational ethics as a solution. He did not hope that a new set of rituals would produce a catharsis in the weak Aristotelian sense. The death of God did not induce in Nietzsche a nostalgia for the past, but announced the need for a total revaluation of values. Although Nietzsche is often seen therefore as a theorist of existentialism, we should remember that Nietzsche had great difficulty in reconciling himself to the notion of the 'I'. In Nietzsche's philosophy the 'I' is the product of language and the assumption that 'I' refers to some consistent entity in reality is deeply problematic. Those philosophers who wish to assimilate Nietzsche to atheistic Christianity or to the existential individualism or to moral humanism should remember the importance of language in Nietzsche's analysis of philosophical issues. For Nietzsche, the discourse of moral systems is based on an army of metaphors. Whatever comfort we have in the world will not be the product of philosophical or religious wisdom. Comfort cannot come from reflection.

For Nietzsche the structure of the universe was dependent upon the structure of grammar. We think in terms of subject and predicate so that in this grammar it makes sense to say I do, I feel and so forth. For Nietzsche the notion of 'God-world' was simply another version of 'subject-predicate'. Once the world had been relativized or at least seen to be the product of language, Nietzsche turned towards the everyday world, physiological need, embodiment, feeling, and reciprocity as a source of experience and value. It was partly for this reason that in *Zarathustra* that Nietzsche complained of 'the despisers of the body', and welcomed the naive attitude that the person is in fact thoroughly embodied so that the self is simply the name for something in the body. From this framework, we can see why Nietzsche felt that the denial of the flesh in Christianity was its weakest point from the view of authenticity and why the spiritual rejection of the body merely produced a sublimation of passion which had dangerous if not disastrous consequences for both the individual and society. Nietzsche attempted to develop a psychology which would not deny desire, but direct passions towards beneficial outcomes, especially in the world of art and cultural creativity. The way out of nihilism was through a life-affirming philosophy which would reconcile morality and art through the expressivity of needs which had their origins in the fundamental fact of our embodiment. Once seen in this perspective, the important overlap between Nietzsche and Freud on religion becomes obvious and significant.

Religion in Freud's Theory

Freud wrote extensively on religious topics and his major works included *Totem and Taboo* in 1913 (*SE*, vol. 13, 1955), *The Future of an Illusion* in 1927 (*SE*, vol. 21, 1961). *Civilization and its Discontents* in 1930 (*SE*, vol. 21, 1961) and *Moses and Monotheism* in 1939 (*SE*, vol. 23, 1964). Freud's analysis of religion covered a variety of topics, concerning the religious life of individuals, the history of religion and the relationship between religion and society. At the individual level, Freud was concerned with both the phylogenetic and the ontogenetic development of religion, but here we are mainly concerned with Freud's view of the specific functions of religion in terms of the life of the individual and social organization (Pruyser, 1973).

In *Totem and Taboo* Freud argued that the taboo on sexual intercourse between close kin was the first imposition of discipline over instinctual drives and that the taboo on unlimited sexual activity was the first index of the development of civilization as a set of norms over nature. The regulation of natural instincts was thus the first act of society. Freud like Durkheim turned to anthropological studies of the Australian aborigines to draw his evidence together concerning the connections between the prohibitions on incest, exogamy, systems of descent, the totemic classification of food and the limitations on the breaking of ritual norms. The role of the totemic myth was to provide the symbolic connections between these various social institutions (Fox, 1966). In this study, Freud brought together his other studies of neurotic behaviour, by noting a similarity between religious taboos and the obsessional restrictions which some neurotics developed with respect to certain objects or actions. There was a close relationship between ritual activity in religion generally and the ritualistic activity of obsessional neurotics. Following Nietzsche, Freud also turned to Greek mythology and religion as illustrative of the fundamental conflict between nature and norm. Freud's analysis of the tragedy of *Oedipus Rex* was a major step in the development of his theory of sexual relations within the family.

Freud's argument was that the prohibition on the eating of the totem animal and the prohibition on sexual relations with women of the same totem clan were in fact the same prohibition which expressed the ambiguity of emotion surrounding the relationship between father and sons. The totemic myth is a substitute for the real history of the killing of the father within the primal horde. Within the context of a patriarchal society, the brothers band together to kill the father in order to have access to women within the group. This mythological/historical event provides the basis for the origin of the sacrificial meal within the totemic clan and according to Freud is the creation event of social organizations, moral ideas and of religion itself. Religion is closely bound up with guilt concerning secret deeds, involves ritualistic activity of an obsessional variety and has the social consequence of binding the group together insofar as all members share a common mythological history and participate in a common totemic meal. The religious rituals of contemporary practice have the effect of, as it were, keeping alive the memory of the original deed and the paradox of ritual is that it both generates the sense of guilt and copes with it. It was on this level that Freud recognized a parallel in terms of the psychology of abreaction of confession in Catholicism and in psycho-analysis (Hepworth and Turner, 1982).

In *The Future of an Illusion*, Freud made a distinction between two functions of civilization, namely the control and exploitation of nature in order to satisfy human needs, and secondly the function of regulation and discipline which was necessary to manage social relations in the interests of social order. It is interesting that in a passage very reminiscent of Weber's Protestant Ethic thesis, Freud argued that human beings were not spontaneously interested in work for its own sake and that some element of dull compulsion was necessary to force people to labour to satisfy needs. Freud noticed a contradictory relationship between civilization and need in that a certain degree of denial is necessary for the demands of cultivated existence. Although these denials and regulations are necessary and experienced as restrictive, there are personal compensations which follow from social commitment and involvement, such as some degree of protection from external violence from enemies and from deprivation. Freud argued that it was religion which was the crucial institution for the training of individuals into an acceptance of the renunciation of sexual passion and desire in the interests of social order. It was this dilemma which was communicated in the myth of *Oedipus Rex*. Although it is possible to study religion rationally (as in the sociology of religion) religion itself is not based upon reason but upon emotion, experience and tradition. Religious ideas are basically illusions, but they are necessary for social continuity. Freud felt that the illusion of religion would not survive long in a period of secular rationalism and that it was possible to organize society on the basis of rational arguments. Through rationalism, it was possible to discover alternatives to the prohibitions which religion had defended in terms of faith and experience.

In both *Totem and Taboo* and *The Future of an Illusion*, we see Freud adopting a method which was familiar to Nietzsche, namely a genealogy of culture which was critical of existing beliefs and institutions. By uncovering the past it was possible to show the real foundations upon which contemporary institutions are based. The foundations of civilization turn out to be horrific and terrifying: civilization is rooted in murder, sexual lust, betrayal and conflict. However, civilization functions by obscuring these roots of morality by various cultural devices which cope with individual and collective guilt (Carroll, 1985). In Freud's analysis we also see that the cost of civilization is very high and has the consequence of bringing about various forms of illness which are associated with guilt feelings.

It was this issue of the cost of civilization which was the theme of *Civilization and Its Discontent*. Freud in this study took up the themes of his earlier work, namely the role of frustration and sublimation in the development of civilization, but Freud now added a new dimension to the issue in the death instinct whose outward manifestation was aggression. The development of civilization for Freud now became the struggle between Eros and Death, that is between the instincts of life and of destruction (*SE*, vol. 21, p. 122). The problem for civilization now became specifically the management of aggression. Freud thought that various institutions had emerged to cope with this problem, such as the intensification of communal feeling, aggression towards outsiders, internalization and finally rational criticism. These social responses to aggression are always partial and the ethic of brotherly love (love thy neighbour as thyself) is always threatened by the fact that according to Freud instinctual passions are always stronger than reason. In this text therefore, Freud saw the greatest threat to civilized life in terms of aggression as the expression of the death principle rather than sexual attraction as a manifestation of Eros. Freud as a result came to perceive society as the struggle between these two principles, that is a struggle over life itself. There is a strong parallel here between Nietzsche's notion of the will-to-power and the conflict between the principles of death and creation, although Freud in his published works rarely made any direct reference to these parallels.

Freud's final publications were written in the context of growing anti-semitism in Europe and one of Freud's final contributions to the psychology of religion was *Moses and Monotheism*. In this work Freud considered the history of two parricides. In the first, Freud argued that the Jews had originally killed an Egyptian Moses but had suppressed the memory by developing Christianity as a movement within Judaism. In this new religious movement, a Son was offered to a divine Father to compensate for the memory of a guilt carried out under Egyptian conditions. The book is also concerned with the problem of the continuity of Judaism over a long period of human history. However, the study is more interesting possibly for its argument that every advance of intellectuality requires the suppression of an instinct. While Freud wanted to claim that in general the suppression of desire is always painful and that discipline is maintained at a cost, in *Moses and Monotheism* he argued that the rewards for suppression were also substantial. He noted that intellectuality had become particularly prominent in Judaism which was characterized by 'the omnipotence of thoughts' (*SE*, vol. 23, p. 113). In Judaism this growing intellectualism was associated with a very literate religiosity directed towards the book and with the injunction that God should not be represented by an image. This transformation of cultural ethos was associated with a social order switching from matriarchy to patriarchy. This intellectuality combined with patriarchy was part of the secret of the long survival of Judaism as a separate social group:

All such advances in intellectuality have as their consequence that the individual's self-esteem is increased, that he is made proud – so that he feels superior to other people who have remained under the spell of sensuality. Moses, as we know, conveyed to the Jews an exulted sense of being a chosen people. The dematerialization of God brought a fresh and valuable contribution to this secret treasure. The Jews retained their inclination to intellectual interests. The nation's political misfortune taught it to value at its true worth the one possession that remained to it – its literature. (*SE*, vol. 23, p. 115)

This view of Judaism represents of course a sharp departure from the position adopted by Nietzsche, for whom the stability and continuity of Judaism depended upon its institutionalization of resentment rather than anxiety and guilt. It is also worth bearing in mind that Weber's account of Judaism also placed an important emphasis on the role of the prophets, the conception of a high God with whom a contract had been made, the development of a book religion encouraging intellect-ualism and the adoption of dietary practices as a form of group membership. In Freud's account the peculiarity of the Jews was their successful renunciation of instincts through the development of an ethical code which bound the people together as a separate group. This peculiarity found its ritual symbol in the rights of circumcision, which stood in place of an act of real castration. The symbolic substitute pointed to an act of obedience on the part of the people to their Father's will. The great burden of renunciation came therefore to be borne collectively and ritualistically.

Nietzsche and Freud on Religion and Art

We can summarize Freud's position by saying that Freudian psycho-analysis conceptualized religion as a form of sublimation of instinctual desires and pleasures, but this sublimation was only partially successful. Freud remained critical of religion; for example, he associated psycho-pathology with religious vocations. His clinical and historical investigations had uncovered hysterical deliria in religious persons, widespread evidence of witchcraft and demonic possession, and extensive evidence of hallucinations among young women. Although historically religion had contributed to the development of civilization, morals and intellect, the cost of this development was considerable and, since sublimation was only partial, neurotic behaviour would be manifest in religious cultures. The final answer to the dilemma of social existence was to be found in the scientific attitude itself, of which psycho-analysis was a leading example. In the scientific attitude, the individual submits 'resignedly to death and to the other necessities of nature' (*SE*, vol. 13, p. 88). This orientation of Freud was remarkably similar to that adopted by Weber in the ethic of responsibility. Since the old myths had lost their power, serious people would accept their fate, and commit themselves to a scientific disposition which would approach the world in a realistic and responsible fashion. With the end of religious calling, the scientific vocation became the only plausible perspective which remained open to a person of serious intentions. The rationalism of Freud and Weber was realistic, but not optimistic; it represented an adjustment or accommodation to the 'facts of life'. Of course Freud also recognized that art was a sublimation of instinct, but art lacked the seriousness of purpose which Freud associated with the intellectual activity of the scientist. His analysis of Leonardo da Vinci (*SE*, vol. 11) attempted to demonstrate that the artistic creations of Leonardo were the consequence of a conversion of passion into a thirst for knowledge. However, the unresolved violence of Leonardo's work was manifest in a certain displacement of affect onto the everyday world. Freud attempted to show that Leonardo's obsession for detail and trivial lists

143

of everyday activity were both repressions and displacements of unconscious activity.

As we have seen there are important points of agreement between Nietzsche and Freud with respect to the nature of religion. Nietzsche treated religion generally as a renunciation of passions and a denial of life itself. This denial was related to resentment and guilt, and Nietzsche therefore rejected the religious orientation to reality, since it inevitably involved a negative philosophy of life. However, Nietzsche could not accept a scientific profession as an alternative calling to religion, since Nietzsche's theory of language made the claim of science deeply questionable. The model of the mind which flows from Freudian psycho-analysis was itself merely a metaphor, an effect of the grammar of language. Nietzsche's challenge is that all such constructs require de-construction and that we cannot take the claims of science simply for granted. The scientific orientation to reality adopted by both Weber and Freud is in Nietzsche's philosophy also an illusion. Nietzsche's reflexivity challenged the notion that science was a serious orientation to the world, since for Nietzsche science is yet another sublimation of culture alongside religion. By contrast, Nietzsche's evaluation of art took a different direction.

Nietzsche saw nineteenth-century science as a new illusion to replace the illusion of religion. Following the death of God, it was not Nietzsche's intention to substitute the authority of religion with the authority of science. Nietzsche could not have agreed with Weber's view of science and politics as a calling anymore than he would have agreed with Freud's final commitment to the rationality of science. Nietzsche championed the artist and art, because art represented essential creativity. The strength and well-being of the artist transforms reality and gives expression to the life-affirming activity of individuals. The artist recreates myth and transforms experience through the metaphors of representation. Art is not a denial or a suppression but an affirmation of reality in which human beings experience again their genuine creativity and unity with life. They become re-absorbed in action; reason as thinking about thinking is neurotic procrastination. In Nietzsche's final works, the Dionysian mode stands for a direct impulse for participation in the world of experience against the mediation of Socratic rationalism. The Socratic or scientific perspective is a mediation or in Nietzsche's terms a stepping back from reality to contemplation (Megill, 1985). In order to understand the relationship between Freudian psycho-analysis as a science of behaviour and Nietzsche's cultural critique, we must turn finally to Nietzsche's analysis of tragedy.

Tragedy and the Pessimism of Strength

As Nietzsche recognized in *The Untimely Meditations* and *The Case of Wagner* his personal and philosophical development depended, especially during his early career, on Schopenhauer's *Die Welt als Wille und Vorstellung* (1859), on the Schopenhauerian theory of music and on Wagner's music as the basis for the cultural reform of Germany. In Schopenhauer's pessimistic treatment of the human dilemma, external reality is merely an illusion; the universe is full of the blind will-to-exist. The escape from this meaningless veil of illusion is through a Buddhist rejection of the world in terms of a doctrine of nirvana or through the transformative experience of art, especially music and drama. The value of drama in Schopenhauer's aesthetics was that first it presents in a striking fashion the pointless quality of human life (thereby making our renunciation more complete) and secondly it provides an opportunity for catharsis. Of the various forms of art, Schopenhauer argued that music penetrates most completely to the core of meta-physical truth. In his hierarchy of artistic forms, Schopenhauer placed architecture (and other practical arts) on the lowest level; the apex of his system was occupied by music. Whereas the plastic arts merely describe and evaluate the ordinary world in terms of the assumptions of mundane discourse, music provides an insight (a non-representational experience) into the ground of being. Therefore, music is a universal language and represents pure creativity with a capacity for transcendence. Because it represents primordial energy, Nietzsche called music the Dionysiac art. Although Nietzsche came eventually to revise his views on the significance of both Schopenhauer and Wagner, his evaluation of the personal and cultural importance of art was a constant and continuous feature of Nietzsche's world-view.

Nietzsche's *The Birth of Tragedy* provides a systematic statement of his analysis of the origins of tragedy in Greek culture, his conception of the transformative nature of music and his evaluation of the modern crisis. Our argument is that, through a study of Nietzsche's view of Greek myth, we can come to a fuller evaluation of the relationship between Freud and Nietzsche. More importantly, his study of tragedy provides a major understanding of his response to the relativity of values. Both Nietzsche and Freud were steeped in Hellenism. We should take particular notice of the centrality of the *Oedipus Rex* myth in the development of Freud's theory of civilization and Nietzsche's rejection of the conventional view of Greek culture as a confident, serene and optimistic expression of reason. For Nietzsche, the origins of Greek culture were violent, archaic, destructive and pessimistic (Silk and Stern, 1981).

The Birth of Tragedy begins with a discussion of the relationship between Apolline and Dionysiac influences on art and culture. Apollo was associated with form and structure, being a god of civilization through his association with medicine. The pure artistic expression of the Apolline principle is sculpture. By contrast, the Dionysiac dimension was associated with energy, sexuality, fertility and nature. The pure Dionysiac art was music. Whereas the Apolline experience is found in the dream, the Dionysiac experience is characteristically that of intoxication. The dream has a form (the image); intoxication is by definition formless. While these two principles are often found in opposition, in the highest instances of artistic creation they are brought together. For Nietzsche, it was Greek tragedy which represented the classical synthesis of these two principles.

Nietzsche argued that the outward optimism and serenity of the Olympian religion masked an underside which was the Dionysiac truth that our lives are a painful subjection to death. The Olympian religions of the Apolline culture made pain tolerable by the sublimation of suffering into art. The problem of pain and suffering was made worse by the individuation and separation of human beings into competitive individuals. Against this 'curse of individuation', the Dionysiac cults pulled these individuals back into a basic unity through the power of orgiastic intoxication. The original form of Greek tragedy was, therefore, to be found in the ecstacies of the worshippers of Dionysus who, as a consequence of their transformative experience, saw themselves returned to nature as the satyrs of the god Dionysus. Intoxication was the antidote to individuation. It is art which makes our existence in the world bearable because, following Schopenhauer, the only justification for the world is an aesthetic one.

Greek drama emerged out of tragedy when the sufferings of Dionysus were represented by an actor bearing a mask. The stage was set for a division between the worshippers and the audience. The dialogue of the Homeric epic was now expressed through the Apolline emphasis on form and regularity. These Apolline dialogues make life acceptable by presenting it in philosophical terms. However, these Apolline forms still disguised the underlying pessimism and violence of the Dionysiac cults. For example, in *Oedipus Rex* the conceptual solution to the riddle presented by the Sphinx shows that a noble man may triumph finally over suffering and sin. The optimism of Sophocles's message is set within a myth where Oedipus must kill his father and marry his mother. The plays of the classical Greek tradition present a tragic account of the loss of unity through individuation and the promise of art as a solution to our existential suffering.

In Nietzsche's treatment of classical Greek culture, the decline of tragedy and epic drama was brought about by the obliteration of Dionysiac forces in favour of a more restrained and reasonable representation of natural processes. This elimination was brought about by Euripides in drama and by Socrates in philosophy. Socrates repudiated tragedy and conveyed an optimistic message that the riddles of the world can be eventually solved by reason with the aid of logic. Socrates provided western culture with a new hero – theoretical man, whose knowledge rests on the serene mastery of emotions. The problem of modern cultural systems is that heroic rationalism eventually discovers its own limits; the rationalist quest is necessarily tragic, since it must falter with the discovery of its own horizon. This tragic vision was a fundamental aspect of Weber's ambiguity towards the claims of *Wissenschaft* with respect to the social sciences. Reason cannot tell us what is valuable, but, since escapism is not acceptable, we must adopt a position of active resignation. By contrast, Freud found it profoundly difficult to countenance the notion that reason (for example psycho-analysis) was ultimately a futile gesture. Freud's was the response of the theoretical man.

As a conclusion to his genealogy of tragedy, Nietzsche identified three great and necessary illusions which make life bearable. Human culture at its articulate and higher levels is structured by three elements: the Socratic commitment to knowledge and reason; the Apolline appreciation of the beauty of art; and finally a Dionysiac faith in the ultimate indestructability of life. These three cultural illusions make human existence tolerable by offering it a meaning. Correspond-ing to these three principles or illusions, we find three different cultural systems through human history: Alexandrian (Socratic systems), Hellenic artistic systems) and Buddhistic (tragic systems). The modern world is Alexandrian because it has elevated theoretical man as the model of excellence in human endeavour. Theoretical man is isolated, competitive and contemplative. The cultural production of the theoretical hero is dependent on education rather than on aristocratic birth. This culture is secular and optimistic, but it is also in crisis. First the survival of such a system requires a slave class, but its optimistic ideology pretends that no such class is required. Secondly, its leading figures (Kant and Schopenhauer) have used reason to show the limits of reason. As a result, the Socratic optimism is beginning to evaporate and the disease of modern society is revealed in its art which is superficial, eclectic, scholarly and parasitic. Nietzsche's solution in *The Birth of Tragedy* to the crisis of modernity was aesthetic – a revival of genuine Hellenic values through tragic music.

Although Nietzsche's account of ancient Greece was in part a reflection of the importance of Hellenism in nineteenth-century Germany, his emphasis on the historical and cultural significance of the Dionysiac culture has not been overturned by more recent scholarship (Dodds, 1951; O'Flaherty, Sellner and Helm, 1976; Lloyd-Jones, 1971). However, the historical accuracy of *The Birth of Tragedy* is not immediately of interest, since we take the study to be a document of the problem of modern not classical cultures. For the student of Nietzsche, his analysis of tragedy is an important guide to his response to the threat of nihilism. In order to understand Nietzsche's position, we need to emphasize the fact that the Dionysiac and Apolline themes are not contradictions; they are ultimately fused in great art. It is therefore too simplistic to conceptualize an opposition between Dionysus (sexuality, desire, nature) and Apollo (discipline, restraint, culture). The problem of human society is not ultimately the contradiction between sexuality and taboo (between gratification and control). What Nietzsche expressed in these two principles was the idea that a genuine moral response to life involves a realistic acceptance of limitation and an ecstatic overcoming and transcendence of our limitations. The dialectic of Apollo (limitation) and Dionysus (rapture) is the defining characteristic of the 'pessimism of strength'.

The importance of this concept became even more prominent in the *Self-Criticism* of 1886. In this re-evaluation of his relationship to tragedy and pessimism, Nietzsche once more rejected the Schopenhauerian solution (a Buddhist negation of will) in favour of an Hellenistic pessimism of strength. Nietzsche accepts pessimism because he cannot accept the Socratic assumption that the riddle of life can have a cognitive solution. However, this position is not a passive pessimism because Nietzsche argues for an active acceptance of life based on a Dionysiac joy in its indestructability. This joy was eventually expressed in his views on the eternal return. This attitude was eventually defined by Nietzsche in terms of *amor fati*, namely a dialectical relationship between Apollonian serenity and Dionysiac suffering. Such an attitude enables a moral person to face the most terrible truths of death and pain with resolution.

Once more Weber's notion of 'a vocation' (a resolute commitment to face reality without the false supports of conventional religion) appears to have a source in Nietzsche's concept of the pessimism of strength. However, from a Nietzsche perspective, Weber's solution would be too

Socratic, namely a rationalist approach to tragedy. Nietzsche repeats the theme constantly (in section 15 of *The Birth of Tragedy*) against the rationalism of Weber and Freud that reason must be self-destructive and self-defeating. The rationalist premise (that by thought an individual could know reality and even change it) is merely a comforting illusion. The quest for reliable knowledge must discover the limits of knowledge. At this point, reason must become tragic and pessimistic the solution offered in *The Birth of Tragedy* is that a pessimism of strength involves an artistic but active response to our being and to reality. Of course, Weber discovered the limits of reason, because science can never tell us whether life or knowledge are worthwhile. Weber rejects Nietzsche's Hellenistic programme in favour of science and politics as vocations and Freud in a similar fashion discovered the unconscious as the libidinal root of reason, but retained a commitment to the rationalist project. While psycho-analysis cannot make us happy and does not promise to make the world valuable, it does pretent to make the world intelligible. Whereas Freud praised Judaism for retaining an 'inclination to intellectual interests', Nietzsche looked towards Greek tragedy as the basis of a yes-saying philosophy. It was this attitude towards suffering which permitted the Greeks to 'live resolutely in wholeness and fullness' (*BT*, p. 18).

Conclusion

Within Freudian psycho-analysis, the great myths of the general culture are worked out in the minor tragedies of the neurotic patient. Freud implicitly adopted the Nietzsche contrast between the life-energy of Dionysus and the requirements of civilization (formalization of constraints). Psycho-therapy is a resolution of these tensions because the patient is offered both insight into their dilemma and the catharsis of affect through speech. They perform their own minor tragedy through the verbalization of the unconscious wish. The parallels between Freudianism and Nietzsche's aesthetics are relatively obvious. However, Nietzsche argued that the problem of modern culture was not the conflict between Dionysus (desire) and Apollo (discipline), but between the synthesis of Dionysus and Apollo in higher tragedy and the synthesis of Euripedes and Socrates in optimistic rationalism. It was on this basis that Freud rejected the idea that Nietzsche (the artist) could achieve a direct and superior insight into the psyche without the labour of science. In addition, Freud argued that the primitive functions of religion and myth could be replaced by science (especially by psycho-analysis). By contrast, Nietzsche assumed that the major solution to the crisis of reason in modern cultures was a rebirth of tragedy through great art. Music produces a cartharsis which permits us to affirm suffering in life and to face the darkest truth.

5

The Joy of God – Self-affirmation against Reciprocity in Adorno

Introduction

With the theoretical and political crisis of organized Marxism in the late twentieth century, radical thinkers have turned to alternative sources for critique and practice in modern societies. In this respect, the critical theorists of the Frankfurt School have been particularly important in providing an alternative framework to conventional Marxism which, while drawing upon the work of Marx himself, introduced new elements of critical thought into the mainstream of contemporary social science. It is well known, for example, that the critical theory of personality in relation to the authoritative structures of modern industrial capitalism. We can argue, following Rolf Wiggershaus (1987, p. 10), that the Frankfurt School attempted to create a new paradigm which, in combining philosophy and social science, developed a range of issues within psycho-analysis. In creating a critical stance, the critical theorists also adopted ideas from the 'life-philosophers' (Schopenhauer, Nietzsche and Klages) who were suspicious of the claims of rationalism and meta-physics. It is only in recent years that the impact of Nietzsche on the early critical theorists, especially Horkheimer and Adorno, has been recognized (Dews, 1986; Held, 1980; Jay, 1973). While the impact of Nietzsche on the critical theorists has remained somewhat disguised, in retrospect the convergence of Horkheimer and Adorno on the philosophy of Nietzsche appears to be relatively obvious and direct. In the 1930s, writers like Horkheimer were quick to appreciate Nietzsche's critique of the epistemological assumptions of positivism; Horkheimer took direct notice of Nietzsche's recognition of the relationship between positivistic knowledge and state power as it was emerging in the new Reich of unified Germany. In addition, Nietzsche's perception of the history of rationalization as the domination of nature and of man was obviously compatible with the underlying attitude towards enlightenment on the part of critical theorists. Nietzsche's critique of Christianity and, more specifically, his observations on asceticism laid the foundation for subsequent critical theoretical reflection upon psychological oppression and the requirements of capitalism. In short, Nietzsche's approach to the problem of nihilism in contemporary cultures provided a perspective for the emergence of a critical theory approach to modern industrial societies, especially in the area of cultural critique (Goudsblom, 1980). Finally, unlike other critics of Nietzsche, Horkheimer at least recognized that Nietzsche was somewhat separate from the romantic rejection of industrial capitalism which had developed amongst the cultural elite of German society. While there was some recognition of Nietzsche's contribution, the Nietzschean underpinnings of critical theory have, as we have noted, only recently emerged partly through the revival of Nietzsche in France and partly as a consequence of the post-modernist crisis of contemporary cultures.

In this chapter, we are concerned to identify certain aspects of the convergence between Nietzsche, Horkeimer and Adorno. These points of convergence are explored in terms of epistemology, the critique of ideology and the perception of rationalization among the critical theorists. This overview then provides the basis for some reflections on Habermas's intervention into the debate in recent years. The conclusion of this chapter is to defend Nietzsche as a theorist with perspectives which go far beyond the specific concerns of critical theory. We argue that critical theory has not entirely broken through the conventional rationalist framework and that Nietzsche's interest in the body, senses, the everyday life and in his affirmation of 'reality' provides an alternative basis for the revaluation of values within a nihilistic culture.

Adorno – Cultural Criticism and Society

While Weber approached the twentieth century as a man of the 'ethic of responsibility' in terms of which he attempted to bridge the gap between individual fate and professional function, between utilitarian interest and freedom of knowledge, between individualism and bureaucratic domination, the philosophers of the critical school appear to have remained in a position of critical distance towards all attempts to link the interest of the individual with institutional power. In this respect, Adorno's early discovery of the social determination of subjectivity in *Negative Dialectics* remains a central issue. For example, the self-reflective tension with which Adorno re-interprets the constitutive power of subjectivity back into the world of the object signifies the historically unbridgeable distance between the 'nature' of the social world and, to use an expression from the preface of the *Negative Dialectics*, 'the strength of the subject to break through the fallacy of constitutive subjectivity' (*ND*, p. XX). While Weber's moral concern remained tied to a belief in certain basic institutions of modern society and the values through which they were once created and maintained, Adorno raised again the question of the obvious contradiction between a society based on a concept of the subject and the social mechanism, which promises to eradicate individual difference. In this contradictory situation, Adorno continued to be concerned with the problem of how 'to trust his own mental impulses' (*ND*, ibid.). In other words, against Weber's attitude of self-affirmation towards Nietzsche's critique of occidental civilization, Adorno himself re-erects Nietzsche's critical stand. Thus – as Maurer (1981/2: 34) puts it – the critical theory of the Frankfurt School remains only 'one . . . among at least two of them'. In tracing the basic sociological issues in the relation between Nietzsche's critique and the critical school, perhaps we may discover, in a true Durkheimian sense, some fields of intensity in which the essential issues of a critique (a joyful social theory) could be based.

Although critical theory has enjoyed and still holds a prominent position in modern social theory, not only in Germany but even more in England and America, the writings of the Frankfurtians have become increasingly influential (Jay, 1973; Rose, 1978; McCarthey, 1978; Jay, 1985; Roderick, 1986); it is not surprising therefore that some reference and attention has been given to the origin of the Frankfurt School and its roots in the spirit of time of the pre-fascist period of German thought (Jay, 1973; Slater, 1977).

This mixed admiration that Nietzsche enjoyed among the critical theorists has remained virtually unexplored. For example, Jay mentions how Horkheimer 'was impressed by Nietzsche's critique of the masochistic quality of traditional western morality'. He had been the first to note, Horkheimer approvingly commented (1934, p. 36), how misery could be transformed into a social norm, as in the case of asceticism, and how that norm permeated western culture through the 'slave morality' of Christian ethics (Jay, 1973, p. 50). However, the overwhelming influence of Nietzsche on Adorno has remained somewhat neglected in the interpretation of the development of critical theory. Adorno's early writing on Kierkegaard in 1933 suggested rather that Kierkegaard was the dominant figure of spiritual influence on his own work (Wiggershaus, 1987, p. 109).

153

The long shadow thrown on Adorno and Horkheimer by Nietzsche's philosophy remained for a long time disguised in most of their writings. In the contemporary re-evaluation of Nietzsche, this connection between the early work of the critical school (especially Adorno) and the cultural critique of modern nihilism by Nietzsche has become a central issue of debate (Dews, 1986). However, one of the most important, if not the most important book of the two authors, the *Dialectic of Enlightenment*, must be mentioned here as an exception. In re-integrating the basic thoughts developed by its two authors in the 1920s and 1930s, and also in setting the theoretical foundations for the debates, in which the authors were subsequently engaged in the 1950s and 1960s, the *Dialectic of Enlightenment* of Horkheimer and Adorno is the fundamental text of the critical school; it is also the only text in which Nietzsche is quoted extensively. Although the way in which Nietzsche is discussed in the *Dialectic of Enlightenment* might be regarded as ambiguous and peculiar, the influence of Nietzsche is less suppressed than in most of their other writings (Pütz, 1973).

This generally disguised position of Nietzsche in the works of the critical theorists might also explain why until recently little reference has been given to the significance of Nietzsche's critique of modernity within critical theory. One important exception is the analysis of Adorno and Nietzsche by Gillian Rose (1978). What has been written on the relation between Nietzsche and the Frankfurt School remains hitherto somewhat insignificant (Pütz, 1974; Maurer, 1981; for marginal comments see also Baier, 1981/2; Holzkamp, 1968; Miller, 1979; Odnev, 1977; Held, 1980; Kilminster, 1979). However, the general relationship between literature (in the work of Nietzsche, George, Rilke and Klages) and sociology in German social theory has been thoroughly researched by Wolf Lepenies (1985).

As in a note on Wagner, both Adorno and Horkheimer generally refer to Nietzsche as a witness of western culture who 'expressed the humane in a world in which humanity had become a shame' and comment on his life as a 'unique demonstration of the repressive character of occidental culture' (Jay, 1973, p. 311). However, these references to Nietzsche rather disguised his real place within the growth of the new school of social theory. Nietzsche's key position, as the critic of modernity among those who insisted on critique as the key world to modernity, has yet to be discovered and fully evaluated.

There are certain antinomies which Lukács once pointed to in his work as the 'position of taking up residence' in the 'Grand Hotel Abyss'. These issues may be considered, for example, in the preface to the second edition of *The Theory of the Novel*. Lukács' understanding of these antinomies reflected the contradictions associated with an anti-communism grounded in intellectual leftism, which lacked any practical political orientation. In this respect, Hans Jugen Krahl's critique of Adorno's 'Objective Contradiction' which 'made the socialist students into political adversaries of their philosophical teacher' (Krahl, 1984, p. 308) continues to be a document of historical significance. However, what is more striking in Frankfurtian thought is its obviously ambiguous position towards consumerism, defending western civilization as the project of modernity which turns into a critique of mass culture as a culture of commodity fetishism. For the Frankfurtians, and more specifically for Adorno, living at the edge of the abyss was meant to include the tension of the vital experience of the social contradictions entailed in modern civilization.

Like Weber, the Frankfurtians first addressed the project of morality and a moral stand in modern society. Like Weber, they were aware that this stand was fundamentally threatened by Nietzsche's discovery of the death of God. However, they gave a different answer to the problem of nihilism and modern culture, namely to continue the project of enlightenment as the only basis for opposition to political reaction and the alienation of capitalist consumerism. With the background experience of fascism, Stalinism and – no less threatening for a sensitive apologetic of culture in modernity – mass culture and the culture-industry, Nietzsche's idea of the sensual apparatus as a source of interpretation must have appeared as a major tool of criticism to the critical theorists who, in most of their work, followed the principle outlined in *Aspects of Sociology* (1973, p. VII) 'to establish that relationship between the informative element and critical self-awareness (*Selbstbesinnung*), which the science of sociology as such demands, just as thus the consciousness of those who occupy themselves with it'. The answer was to insist on the practical experience of the self as a source of the critique of ideology, but also they sought to maintain and to recreate the historical categories which were seen to resurrect the cause of humanity and the achievement of culture against the nihilism of both instrumental and subjectivist empiricism. Here again critical thought assumed a rather ambiguous position between idealism and the ontological thought of the life-philosophers. While they analysed and predicted the destruction of identity by both instrumental and perspectivist ideologies, they insisted on a rather idealistic concept of the 'notion'. For them, it was 'the notion' that had to be thrown against 'the thing' in order to recreate its identity. Consequently, it is from this perspective that we understand the Frankfurtian attempts to base the intellectualism of enlightenment in the historical forms of intellectualism of myth and religion, as a critique of Weberian and neo-Kantian approaches to establishing intellectualism as instrumental reason and value-free reflection of the logic of the cosmos.

In the period before the First World War, to understand the real threat of Nietzsche's concept of resentment morals to the intellectuals, one would fail in pointing only to Weber's personal crisis in the early years of the century as an exceptional or unusual case (Lepenies, 1985, p. 299). We should instead quote Lukács here who gives a full account of Nietzsche's influence:

if the speech comes to something bad, I have to turn to Nietzsche. Nietzsche for example has discovered, that the whole class consciousness of the proletarian is a resentment of slaves. And this ideology – that I knew from my youth – has many well thinking intellectuals prevented from taking the side of the working class. Because for their consciousness, they could by a noble and moral person not tolerate resentments and no support of resentments. (Lukács, 1967, p. 72)

However, Horkheimer, and more specifically Adorno, shared their intellectual youth with a post-war generation. In fact, none of the inner circle of the Frankfurt School is reported to have been profoundly threatened by Nietzsche's genealogy. Unlike Weber and Simmel, they were not personally or directly influenced by Nietzsche and thus for the Frankfurtians Nietzsche remained what he was for most of their generation – a symbolic figure, through the writings of whom, the basic features of their own cultural criticism were re-experienced.

Although Kant, Hegel and Marx are generally considered to be the primary influences upon Horkheimer and Adorno, Nietzsche's life-story and his attitudes towards art and culture seem to have been more influential on Benjamin and Adorno and their post First World War generation of young intellectuals (Putz, 1973, pp. 175ff). Nietzsche's critique of the *Bildungsphilister* (the cultural philistinist) remained particularly significant. The new Reich when it was created in 1871 offered money, positions and status for the celebration of its culture and its new high esteem as the nation-state. In that context, revolutionary romanticism, with which the German 'Revolution' of 1848 found its end, was transformed into a reactionary state ideology. It was this whole new class of *Staatsbürger* and *Bildungsbürger* which thus came under attack. Nietzsche, the lonely dreamer of antiquity, hated the purified taste and the false Christian morals of this class of intellectuals who suddenly appeared in state posts as spokesmen of an official culture. We should remind ourselves that it was exactly the advent of this class that was so prominently defended by Weber in his post-war lectures, who once felt so badly damaged by Nietzsche's cultural attack. Nietzsche's profound objections to the *Bildungsphilister* (with which he attacked David Friedrich Strauss, the theologian of the new Reich, and Richard Wagner, its ascending musician) continued to provide a critical reference point for a young, post-war generation of intellectuals against the remnants of the previously dominant class of the old regime. For the surviving youth, the bankruptcy of this class was symbolized (or rather concretized) in the nihilism of the lunar landscape of Verdun and the Somme. In this post-war situation, cultural criticism, as Adorno expressed it in his reply to Karl Mannheim in *Prisms*, had clearly changed its function and purpose. Reconstructing the old struggles in the Frankfurt Institute in the 1920s, Adorno attacked Mannheim as a 'cultural philistine' who 'has long ceased to be the man of progress, the figure with which Nietzsche identified David Friedrich Strauss. Instead he has learned profundity and pessimism. In their name he denies the humanity which has become incompatible with his present interests, and his venerable impulse to destruction turns against the products of the culture whose decline he sentimentally bemoans' (*P*, p. 39).

A similarly ambiguous position had already been developed by Horkheimer in the 1920s towards the *Lebensphilosophie* (philosophy of life) which for Horkheimer corresponded to a new totalizing role of capitalism. With this new development in capitalism, the philosophy of life, 'had pointed an accusing finger at the gap between the promises of bourgeois ideology and the reality of everyday life in bourgeois society' (Jay, 1973, p. 48). But he also accused it of irrationalism – which involved an 'attack on the validity of scientific thought as such' (Jay, 1973, p. 49). Horkheimer's position that 'the philosophical dismissal of science is a comfort in private life, in society a lie' (Horkheimer, 1937, p. 9) later reappeared in Habermas' dualistic approach towards knowledge. Furthermore, Marxism, in its purified and intellectualized version proclaimed by Lukács and Korsch, replaced the neo-Kantian debates on welfare and social inequality. These were not times of social closure and defence of cultural hegemony. More than the Jewish cultural influence, the non-Christian background of the founders of the Frankfurt School and their spiritual roots in these times might account for their neglect of resentment morals. In contrast to the work of Weber, we do not find any systematic discussion nor any sensitive reflection of Nietzsche's critique of Christianity as fundamentally tied to the morals of resentment. Like Weber, however, the Frankfurtians stressed the social role of intellectualism in the time of an absent God.

157

Like Weber, they looked for forms of the historical foundation of this role of intellectuals in earlier stages of historical development. However, against Weber, they did not see any threat to intellectualism from resentment and, while Weber so profoundly suffered from and so brilliantly circumnavigated in his theory this threat, 'free intellectualism' to the Frankfurtians was already a taken-for-granted category. Thus, intellectualism and reason for Frankfurtians in the tradition of progressive enlightenment meant a moral stand in itself, untouchable by any fear from intellectualist resentment ethics. Weber, having lived the threat of resentment morality, responded by separating the spheres of morality and rationality (in reducing the latter to a calculated mechanism of purposive ends, and the former to a set of private beliefs). For the Frankfurt School, morality and reason were rather inseparable spheres of the intellectual enterprise. In this respect, the Frankfurtians did not neglect, suppress or avoid the Nietzschean concept of resentment ethics, but rather, in the way they understand it, they redefined it as a necessary mechanism of sociality as a whole.

Resentment and Mediation

The free intellectual, the person of independent means who selects an academic occupation out of repugnance for the ignominy of earning money, opposes the compartmentalization of mind. The instrumental reason of those who have to earn money through professional scholarship might betray their deep-seated resentment in employing well-founded suspicions against the holistic world views of the free intellectuals. The 'independence' which they despise might well be established within the ranks of domination (*MM*, 1, p. 21). Adorno, more than Weber and more than Nietzsche before him, was very well aware of this dilemma of the free intellectual. The respective intermediation of domination and reason is one of his major themes. In fact, Weber denied this mediatedness; his positivistic insistence on the value-free world of science promised to release the intellect from the destructiveness of power and the interest of instrumental usage. We can appreciate therefore the central importance of Weber's methodological and epistemological writing for his conceptualization of the role of the intellectual in contemporary capitalism. With this denial, he attempted to free intellectualism from resentment. In this respect, Weber, together with Nietzsche, was aware of the mediative forces of resentment: constitutive reason, the mediatedness of reason in domination, is resentment.

158

In opposition to Weber, Horkheimer and Adorno insisted on the mediatedness of reason; however, they denied that such mediatedness leads to resentment. Horkheimer and Adorno accepted the importance of Nietzsche's morals of resentment for any understanding of the roots of modernity; for them, resentment is the 'secret credo of the ruling classes' with which they are 'betraying the character of weakness which nature has engraved in them' and it is the 'psychology of resentment' with which Nietzsche reproaches the modern age (*DE*, p. 100). However, they denied the affinity of mediation and resentment. Mediation becomes an objective mechanism of sociality, already grounded in myth, sacrifice and reciprocity. But in historical opposition to these mechanisms, mediation becomes the basic socializing element for those to whom 'nature' has nothing left to be 'engraved in them'.

Society for the critical theorists, as for Nietzsche, consisted of a total process, as Horkheimer and Adorno made explicit in their collected essays in *Aspects of Sociology* (1973). For Nietzsche, however, resentment remained a tool of the individual revaluation of things. Similar to the 'Hiatus' (with which Jacob Burckhardt described the fundamental attitude of the civilized westener towards his surrounding), it detaches attraction, while approaching an object. In Christianity, resentment, for Nietzsche, becomes a completely new form of domination: a denial of individual will and power, while a hidden mechanism of reciprocity, employed in such a self-denial, ties the individual to a new and hidden form of domination.

The *Dialectic of Enlightenment* contributed much to an understanding of the fundamental role of resentment within the civilizing process, reduced to the 'secret credo of the ruling class' and linked to what Nietzsche called 'the terrible beauty of the deed'; however, resentment remained an actively employed tool in the hands of the ascending bourgeoisie, rather than an illness that befalls the compassionate dominators. For Horkheimer and Adorno, resentment equals simulation and mediation; it turns into a fundamental mechanism of all sociality. It is already present in Homer's Odysseus, whose spirit both organizes and contradicts the myth (*DE*, p. 43). For Horkheimer and Adorno, the history of European enlightenment starts with both the construction of myth and its betrayal. And within this dialectic between mythical reconciliation and betraying abstraction, we find the source of all European civilization, namely in Nietzsche's terminology, the artistic process to which belongs individuation. But for Horkheimer and Adorno, this human artistic process of departure from the boundaries of community and nature, even where it still depended on epic and myth, meant also 'domination and exploitation' (*DE*, p. 45). Individuation itself is linked to domination and exploitation; this is the point from where the dialectic of enlightenment departs. While for Nietzsche it is resentment ethics, which re-found all sociality in a process of departure, for the Frankfurtians, instrumental reason remains the new mechanism of evolution.

Within the patriarchal relation between the mind of man and the nature of things, there evolved the instrumental reason of the ascending bourgeoisie (*DE*, p. 4). Science precisely expresses the simultaneous domination of man and nature by bourgeois instrumental reason in the origins of western capitalism. Where myth turns into ratio, all nature turns into mere objectivity. The Frankfurtian interpretation of resentment remained tied to a Hegelian perspective of the subject-object dichotomy. It is rather its irreconcilable position in nature, which remains the intriguing point in modern humankind, rather than its 'false' psychological nature imposed on it by its resentment ethics.

It is not the falsity of the bourgeois legacy, which moves Frankfurtian thought, but rather the development of its power of domination and exploitation. For Nietzsche, this process of separation between nature and objectivity turns into an attitude of physical detachment and spiritual disinterestedness. His main concern (how to escape such destructive nihilism) can be recognized in Adorno's problem of how to create modern social life as a form of rational, humane and comfortable existence. This issue was how to reconcile rationality with homefulness. Nietzsche, however, gave more significance to the individual as a physical, a sensitive, a corporate unit of the intellect. Adorno's belief in the objective power of structures brought him to propose a theory of the 'liquidation of the individual' (Grenz, 1974, pp. 32ff). It is on this basis that Rose (1978) has argued that, unlike Nietzsche, Adorno attempted to understand these processes within a genuinely social perspective. By contrast, we argue that a life-process perspective can be, indeed must be grounded in a notion of social reciprocity.

In Nietzsche's perspective, the structure of nihilism leads to a new state of the organic, of sensitivity, valuations and interpretations of the individual, which as well could form (for the free intellect) a new stage of reversibility (of structural dominance) and of a joyful conscious rejection of given interpretations of order. With the death of God, the life-world had become open. For Nietzsche, the reification of human relations and the process of separation of nature and objectivity, with the false evaluations it creates, remains reversible for the free individual. For Horkheimer and Adorno, by contrast, it remains socially created and tied to given forms of sociality and thus unresolvable. While they saw, with Nietzsche, that the new contradiction between

160

subject and object is not purely re-mirroring a relation of meta-physical eternity, or even of 'class' or 'race', but rather a human attitude that has been created within the dialectic of enlightenment itself. Horkheimer and Adorno themselves here remained within the logic of this dialectic on the basis of two assumptions: (1) the belief in the essential and specific quality of mediation, and of the form of subject–object dichotomy in modernity brought forth by instrumental reason; and (2) they also saw its reversibility in terms of its historical factuality. In stressing the subject–object dichotomy and the social mediation within resentment, for them 'Nietzsche was one of the few after Hegel who recognized the dialectic of enlightenment' (*DE*, p. 44). While Nietzsche believed in its reversibility, Horkheimer, and more specifically, Adorno (like Weber) remained caught in the iron cage of modern civilization and thus redefined the resentment syndrome, although socially created, as a mechanism of sociality in general. For the Frankfurtians, resentment remains a means of social mediation.

Cunning and Reciprocity

Within the inner-worldly perspective of socio-historical determination of the dialectic of enlightenment, it is not resentment which takes its revenge against the departing and self-abstracting individual, as Nietzsche saw it. Nor would Horkheimer and Adorno agree with the cosmological needs of the free intellectual with which Weber once characterized the state of cognitive individuation. For the dialectic of enlightenment, artifice is the means by which the wandering self loses itself in order to preserve and rediscover itself. The seafarer Odysseus cheats the natural deities, as does the civilized trader who offers them coloured glass beads in exchange for ivory (*DE*, p. 49). Indeed the simulative, but nonetheless purposive participation in the belief of sacrificial rites becomes a powerful tool of both the allying and alienating subject. For Horkheimer and Adorno, the practice of sacrificing individuals in communities of early antiquity has to count for the social construction of an 'antithesis of the collective and the individual'. The institutionalization of sacrifice within the community turns the survival of the individual into a deceit of the collective. While 'the institution of sacrifice itself is the occasion of an historical catastrophe, an act of force that befalls men and nature alike', 'cunning is only the subjective development of the objective untruth of the sacrifice that redeems it' (*DE*, p. 51).

In a footnote then, we find a most illuminating statement: 'under the continuing jurisdiction of magic, rationality – as the behaviour of the sacrificer – becomes cunning' (*DE*, p. 50). Here certainly in a most marginal position, we find a most important and revealing statement. Horkheimer and Adorno elaborated there the dual character of sacrifice as 'the magic self-surrender of the individual to the collective' and self-preservation becomes a mere technique of this magic. The contradiction of this duality between communalization by self-surrender, and self-preservation by means of trickery, for Horkheimer and Adorno, tends to imply a development of the 'rational element in sacrifice'. If we reverse what Horkheimer and Adorno state here with 'rationality as the behaviour of the sacrificer', sacrifice becomes the mode of behaviour of the rational and there we clearly find a central feature of Nietzsche's resentment morals.

However, instead of referring to Nietzsche, Horkheimer and Adorno quote Ludwig Klages, whose *Der Geist als Widersacher der Seele* (1932) was otherwise forbidden to be quoted in Adorno's seminars. Horkheimer and Adorno present Klages' work as a testimony to the trans-historical totality of the social, implied in sacrifice and exchange. While in one respect they accepted the powerfulness of sacrifice and reciprocal exchange in the communal context, they at the same time denounced Klages, who idealized this power into a model of society. They criticized him as a reactionary romantic, 'who feels compelled to distinguish genuine communication with nature from lies' and thus does not find it possible 'to derive from magic thinking itself a counter principle to the illusion of magical domination of nature because that illusion in fact constitutes the nature of myth' (*DE*, p. 50). For Horkheimer and Adorno, cunning is the necessary tool of both, reconciliation to and at the same time abstraction from nature for the civilizing subject:

The dismissal of sacrifice by the rationality of self-preservation is exchange no less than sacrifice itself was. The identically persistent self which arises in the abrogation of sacrifice immediately becomes an unyielding, rigidified sacrificial ritual that man celebrates upon himself by opposing his consciousness to the natural context. (*DE*, p. 54)

Thus all assumptions that would lead to a purely reconciliatory understanding of sacrifice in terms of establishing a balanced and reciprocal relation (a 'genuine communication with nature') in suggesting that all that 'could have once been the truth', for Horkheimer and Adorno, descends into ideology: 'the latest ideologies are only versions of the most ancient, and revert beyond those previously known only to the same extent that the development of class society belies the previously sanctioned ideologies (*DE*, p. 53).

Horkheimer and Adorno, in following the rather lopsided perspective of the traveller and seafarer Odysseus, underestimated the binding and typifying functions of myth. In stressing the continuity of betrayal and cunning as tools of self-preservation and self-discovery of the individualising subject, they failed to elaborate the notion that this continuity might have existed in various forms. Where Horkheimer and Adorno insisted on asserting that 'cunning consists in exploiting the distinction' (*DE*, p. 60), they referred purely to the supra-cultural distinctions with which the colonizers betray the indigenous. This form of betrayal, however, differs markedly from the possibilities of exploiting the patterns of distinction entailed in a peasant-lord relationship, for example, which relies on continuity. In that relation-ship, the simulation of loyalty and solidarity (from both sides) expresses the wish for reconciliation by accepting and reaffirming the given forms of social distinction. Here the tools for the betrayal of myth and reciprocal exchange are employed to renew a given form of distinction, and the deceit, which is employed by both the peasant and the lord, appears to be a rather established way of distinction among them.

Pierre Bourdieu (1977) stressed the importance of various capacities of challenge and response in reciprocal relations in the process of an accumulation of symbolic capital. This fact reminds us of the fundamental nature of all reciprocal acts within the social process. Cunning is obviously only one tool to be employed in reciprocal games. In opposition to cunning, however, Nietzsche discovered the resent-ment morals as a totally new form in history, which arose in Judaism and Christianity; these morals could be understood as the reaction of the indigenous against the betrayals of colonizers and alien outsiders. With resentment, the simulation of self-sacrifice becomes a tool of a continuous, unstructured and unbalanced attempt of self-abstraction of the self-preserving individual. Thus, resentment appears as the cultural tool to overcome the effects of a spoiled reciprocal relation between ruler and ruled. In opposition to the pathos of distance, with which Nietzsche explored the reciprocal class relations in antiquity as a reaffirming and reassuring mechanism of distinction of both the ruled and the ruler, resentment develops as a moral mechanism which simulates the reaffirmation of reciprocity, while in fact hiding distinction, which itself becomes merely a mode of behaviour based on self-preserving ends. Resentment is the result of the challenge to and the violation of the reciprocal mechanism. Horkheimer and Adorno, in fact, failed to understand (and indeed sought to eliminate) this difference between the pathos of distance and resentment. Horkheimer and Adorno confused the self-affirmative and reconciliatory, reciprocal behaviour of distinction of a noble man with the betrayals of a colonizing seafarer:

> Deception as a mode of exchange in which everything proceeds as it should, where the contract is fulfilled and yet the other party is deceived, refers back to an economic type which if it does not occur in mythical prehistory, does so at least in early antiquity: the age-old practice of 'casual exchange' between private households. (*DE*, p. 61)

Reciprocity is challenge; gift is poison; such we hear from the anthropologists. Resentment is a construction of the betrayed to take revenge; in fact to betray better and more without moral inconvenience. Where the robber comes 'in the pathetic image of the beggar', 'feudal man retains the features of the oriental merchant' (*DE*, p. 61). There still remains measures of dealing related to the patterns of challenge and response which are entailed in the reciprocal mechanism. But resentment remains the cultural tool of the betrayed.

Horkheimer and Adorno stress the 'semitic element' in the path to modernity as they understand it, and in a way they identified Odysseus, with all his oriental features, as the first representative of modernity. In stressing the construction of sociality against the genuine character of the community, the founding fathers of the Frankfurt School focused on the trickery of world-wandering and seafaring 'nobodies', indicating the adventure of modernity. However, here they disguised and neglected the serenity into which trickery turns, when it becomes the inherent logic of a territorially-bound society. With resentment, trickery turns into a serene logic of sociality itself; however, the various layers of this logic are best studied in the unrestrained but, at the same time, socially organized hatred with which the 'equals' turn against those whom they accuse of having turned them into 'unequals' by blind forces.

Fascism and Resentment

Horkheimer and Adorno were very much aware of the relationship between fascism, the mass-culture industry and resentment. Overtly drawing on Marxist categories, in fact their understanding of fascism was based essentially on Nietzsche's resentment ethics. The fascist attempts to reconstruct a master's morality were actually described in terms of resentment, revaluating the morals of German 'barbarians' and 'slaves'. It is in this context that Nietzsche was placed in a rather close relationship to fascism:

The German Nietzsche, however, makes beauty dependent on extent; despite all the twilight of idols he cannot abandon the idealistic convention which would accept the hanging of a petty thief and elevate imperialistic raids to the level of world-historical missions. By raising the cult of strength to a world-historical doctrine, German Fascism also took it to an absurd extreme. As a protest against civilization, the masters' morality conversely represents the oppressed. Hatred of atrophied instincts actually denounces the true nature of the task-masters which comes to light only in their victims. But as a Great Power, or state religion, the masters' morality wholly subscribes to the civilizing powers that be, the compact majority, resentment, and everything that it formally opposed. The realization of Nietzsche's assertions both refutes them and at the same time reveals their truth, which – despite all his affirmation of life – was inimical to the spirit of reality. (*DE*, pp. 100–1)

While in Weber's analysis, and in most other statements by Horkheimer and Adorno on resentment morals, it is only seen to be a tool of revenge of negatively-privileged groups or classes, here in this passage Nietzsche's original argument about true Christian religion and the state culture of the late nineteenth-century German nation-state as being essentially a product of that cultural tool of resentment is fully employed and re-established against fascism. However, while for Nietzsche resentment was the unavoidable fate of modern man, for Horkheimer and Adorno it remained a mere expression of fascism and capitalist mass culture.

In *Minima Moralia* Adorno elaborated a profound insight into the nihilistic cultural productivity of resentment in modern society. The ambiguous way, however, with which Adorno shifted between master-morality, resentment and hedonism remained a barrier to any fruitful theoretical application of the concept of resentment:

It is not only the social non-conformist or even the narrow-minded bourgeois who must see restruction as superfluous in face of the immediate possibility of superfluity. The implied meaning of the master-morality, that he who wants to live must fend for himself, has in the meantime become a still more miserable lie than it was when a nineteenth century piece of pulpit-wisdom. If in Germany the common citizen was proved himself a blond beast this has nothing to do with national peculiarities, but with the fact that blond bestiality itself, social rapine, has become in face of manifest abundance the attitude of the backwoods man, the deluded philistine, that same 'hard-done-by' mentality which the master-morality was invented to combat. If Cesare Borgia were resurrected today he would look like David Friedrich Strauss and his name would be Adolf Hitler. The cause of amorality has been espoused by the same Darwinists who Nietzsche despised, and who proclaim as their maxim the barbaric struggle for existence with such vehemence, just because it is no longer needed. True distinction has long ceased to consist in taking the best for oneself, it has become instead a satiety with taking, that practises in reality the virtue of giving, which in Nietzsche occurs only in the mind. (*MM*, 60, pp. 96–7)

Here it seems that Adorno only maintained a rather materialistic understanding of resentment as he had done in *Dialectic of Enlightenment* (*DE*, p. 49, footnote 6). For Adorno, resentment turned into a master morality itself; however, it only appeared restricted to those who apply this morality to themselves. Resentment remained simply a mechanism for redefining material and social positions by deceit; it thus became merely a tool of improper social ranking. In separating it from the mechanism of the revaluation of all values under the condition of living 'without the thought of an absolute' (*MM*, no. 61, p. 97), for Adorno the resentment moral became a mechanism of mere social trickery – 'Nietzsche's theory is that the weak are guilty, for they circumvent the natural law by means of cunning' (*DE*, p. 95). Wherever Adorno admitted the possibility of resentment – as a central feature of European civilization – he immediately hits against the fascist revolt which is understood to be orientated against this hidden form of domination. 'Though he discerned both the universal movement of sovereigh spirit (whose executor he felt himself to be) and a 'nihilistic' life-force in the enlightenment, his pre-fascist followers retained only the second aspect and perverted it into an ideology' (*DE*, p. 44). Like Passolini after him, Adorno stressed the hedonistic, sexist and the 'body-power' aspects of fascism. In Adorno's criticism, the bodily strengths of slaves (celebrated a new cult of master morals which eventually takes the shape of a state ideology) are again employed as cultural tools. Thus, with fascism, the Frankfurt School denounced any theoretically fruitful attempt at a critique of resentment morals in modernity. With fascism, the Frankfurt School closed the book on resentment, civilization and European cultural criticism; they turned over to a new chapter of critique which then focussed on the 'madness of profit economy' (*MM*, no. 60, p. 97).

For Nietzsche, the destructive power in resentment morals did not lie in the psychological or instinctive fact that 'love is as cruel as hunger' (*DE*, p. 113) but rather that love becomes a means of institutional trickery against the instincts of the individual, where it had its origin. In that respect, the highest value (in religion and in ideology) is made both a tool of revenge and of social ranking. In Nietzsche, ideology and its civilizing forces, in taking away the instinctive grounds of judgement, are seen in turning the inherent structure of all civilizing processes into its false reverse. It is not the psychological and instinctive fact that love, like all human values, is subject to social trickery and social ranking in all sociality; Nietzsche's critique aimed primarily at all established mechanisms and institutional constructions related to ideology and religion which employed these values in destroying the taste of judgement on the part of the individual. Thus, more than Wagnerism, fascism would have fallen under his critical verdict. Horkheimer and Adorno, in merely criticizing false ideology, did not link resentment with ideology and thus failed to criticize the social classes that produce and reproduce it. In this manner, fascism becomes reduced to a modern revenge of nature against civilization. 'Germans' and their reactionary romanticism towards nature, linked with a culturally specific disenchantment of naturalistic hedonism, and accordingly of mechanistic and instrumental reactions, serve for a concept of fascism, which strongly denied Nietzsche's critique of Christianity, Protestantism, historicism, and the related ideologies linked with the creation of European nation-states:

It is as if the final result of civilization were a return to the terrors of nature. That fatal love which Sade highlights, and Nietzsche's ashamedly unashamed magnanimity which would go to any extreme to save the suffering from humiliation: cruelty as greatness, when imagined in play or fancy, deals harshly with man as German Fascism does in reality. (*DE*, p. 113)

With fascism, for the Frankfurt School, modernity as the age of repressive de-sublimation comes to its obvious conclusion. Hedonism in modern life, finally, signified the end of resentment as a cultural tool. The possibility that, within modern hedonism and repressive de-sublimation, resentment only takes a new and perhaps its most powerful shape as a tool of cultural nihilism, remains yet to be explored.

While for Nietzsche resentment remained a – most modern – tool of revaluation of values in the first instance, the *Dialectic of Enlightenment* employed this notion simply as a means of distinction towards nature, myth and religion. It is elaborated as a tool of socializing, as mediation in general. It is obvious that the notion – in Nietzsche, marking the essence of his critique of modernity – becomes positivistically applied and loses all its critical force against western civilization.

Horkheimer and Adorno, where they ' developed a critique of resentment, applied the notion merely in terms of inter-subjective relations, as a psychological mechanism evoking revengeful action. Thus, like Weber, they denied that resentment could become a result of the fusion of intellectualism and modern professionalism, and a tool of cultural production, which remained tied to institution formation and state functions in modern society. Furthermore, where Horkheimer and Adorno considered the relation between resentment, modern institutions and state ideology, it merely takes the form of a reflection on inter-subjective revenge-feelings in modern mass psychology, more overtly with fascism.

Nietzsche's discovery of resentment morals was intended to destroy the image of a self-sacrificing priest, whose most modern version appeared in the figure of the *Bildungsphilister* (the cultural philistine). For Weber, resentment remained a pattern of socio-psychological attitudes, exclusively reserved for negatively-privileged people and classes, and their leaders (Jews, pariah groups and the working class); Horkheimer and Adorno perceived resentment in terms of the middle and bourgeois classes of modern mass society. Like Weber, Horkheimer and Adorno denied resentment in modern intellectualism. In this respect, Nietzsche's critique of the 'theoretical man' was seen to be self-destructive and converted to a field, which was in fact quite alien: epistemology.

Intellectualism and Resistance

To establish trust in professional intellectualism, as the proper source of critique in the final instance, more than a positivistic neglect of resentment and its application to modern hedonism and state ideologies had to be achieved. Life-philosophy (and with it Nietzsche's critique) had threatened the position of intellectualism in the classical area of its intellectual legacy: the theory of knowledge. In this arena, Nietzsche, and those fundamental seducers, there departing with him, like Bergson, Klages and Heidegger, opened a new space in the battle-field of thought and progressive enlightenment. To confuse knowledge with life and the ever-increasing powers in life, for the Frankfurters, as Adorno expressed it, led necessarily to ideology. While Adorno accused Hegel on the grounds that he 'in hypostasizing both bourgeois society and its fundamental category, the individual, did not truly carry through the dialectic between the two' (*MM*, p. 17), he also criticized Nietzsche, and with him all cultural critics, who believed 'that culture creates the illusion of a society worthy of man, which does not exist' (*MM*, no. 22, p. 43). Such a notion of culture would immediately lead to ideology, 'like all expostulation about lies, has a suspicious tendency to become itself ideology' (ibid.). Thus, for Adorno, ideology remained deeply grounded in fundamental reflections on the subject, while bourgeois society has already erected itself as the society of the individual. In such an individualistic society, 'the general not only realizes itself through the interplay of particulars, but society is essentially the substance of the individual' (*MM*, p. 17).

Given the totality of the social, to depart from the individual as 'an irreducible datum' becomes an ideological enterprise:

considerations which start from the subject remain false to the same extent that life has become appearance. For since the overwhelming objectivity of historical movement in its present phase consists so far only in the dissolution of the subject, without yet giving rise to a new one, individual experience necessarily bases itself on the old subject, now historically condemned, which is still for-itself, but no longer in-itself. The subject still feels sure of its autonomy, but the nullity demonstrated to subjects by the concentration camp is already overtaking the form of subjectivity itself. (*MM*, pp. 15–16)

It was not within this concern of the subject as a base of critique that Nietzsche and life-philosophy were criticized, but within the theory of knowledge, that could not deal with the state of affairs already brought forward on the level of sociality:

Subjective reflection, even if critically alerted to itself, has something sentimental and anachronistic about it: something of a lament over the course of the world, lament to be rejected not for its good faith, but because the lamenting subject threatens to become arrested in its condition and so to fulfil in its turn the law of the world's course. Fidelity as one's own state of consciousness and experience is forever in temptation of lapsing into infidelity, by denying the insight that transcends the individual and calls his substance by its name. (*MM*, p. 16)

Grounding a theory of knowledge on the self-reflecting subject, therefore, Adorno meant to fall into the trap of the ideology of the social itself in terms of purely re-mirroring the already constructed and reconstructed subject, as an essential source of an individualistic society. Furthermore, the subjective view in the theory of knowledge would draw its 'epistemological foundation from the constancy of the thing over its appearances' (*AE*, p. 19). Adorno in this passage denied

169

the 'thing' substance in its own persistance and he saw the disintegration of the hypostasis of the 'thing', but also the fact that the 'thing' became more real, was a rather intriguing one; there was a shadow of meta-physical falsity in such a disintegration of the subject and the object. For Adorno, 'the absolutization of the schemata of conceptual order becomes as suspicious as "self-reflection of thought"' (ibid.). While Adorno's dialectics left enough space for ambiguities in his reflection on the relationship between individual and society, life and knowledge, it is primarily Habermas who remained tied to and insisted upon a rigid neo-Kantian separation between life and knowledge, which Rickert already maintained against the life-philosophers (Rickert, 1920). The notion of the subject remains closely linked with the solidity of the subjugated. Intellectualism and a theory of knowledge based on the 'objectivity of the notion' against 'mere being' are beliefs which the Frankfurtians share at large with their positivist critics.

The critical theorists of the Frankfurt School developed their theoretical position in opposition to other directions of thought, the positivists on the one hand, and the life-philosophers on the other. Although never fully or systematically elaborated in Adorno's writings, both directions were in the most part seen to be opposite sides of the same coin: the anti-intellectual feud about intellectuals, namely 'Positivism reduces the detachment of thought to a reality, that reality itself no longer tolerates.' Induced to be no more than a merely provisional abbreviation for the factual matter beneath it, thought loses, not only its autonomy in the face of reality, but with it the power to penetrate that reality. Only after its removal from life can mental life exist, and truly engage the empirical (*MM*, no. 82, p. 126). Rarely are those opponents found to be quoted by name, rarely does one find their ideas presented in detail in Frankfurtian writings, and Adorno in particular preferred a rather ambiguous and elusive metaphorical language in his critical attack on these schools.

As we have seen, there are various passages in the *Dialectic of Enlightenment* where Nietzsche was placed in a close relationship to what was then called his 'pre-fascist followers'. However, Nietzsche was also given an autonomous status within the *Dialectic of Enlightenment* and was used, specifically in terms of his genealogy, as an intellectual resource for the critique of both fascism and modern mass culture. However, when the 'subject' is tied to the creation of 'the objectivity of the notion', then it comes under attack; in life-philosophy, it was put into a lost position with society and tied to a perspective of individualistic cultural critique. Thus, Adorno writes in *Minima*

Moralia: 'Mediatedly to affirm immediacy, instead of comprehending it as mediated within itself, is to pervert thought into an apologia of its antithesis, into the immediate lie' (*MM*, no. 46, p. 73). Within this perspective, all attempts at the 'equation of the genuine and the true' (*MM*, no. 99, p. 153) become untenable. The basic reason for the untenable character of theory based on the 'genuineness of the subject' for Adorno lay in the endless mediatedness of action within modern society: 'the discovery of genuineness as a last bulwark of individualistic ethics is a reflection of industrial mass production' (*MM*, no. 99, p. 155).

Horkheimer and Adorno in the idealist tradition rest upon the specific interpretation of the subject-object relation. The project of critical theory enters there into the Marxian, not Nietzschean, problem of a reconciliation of humanity with nature:

As Habermas has noted, this was essentially a consciousness philosophy concerned with the integrated problem, so central to both the idealist and critical Marxist traditions, of how subjects relate to objects in the present world and how they might relate to them in a possible future one. (Jay, 1984, p. 58)

While Nietzsche, George and Klages were acknowledged for having discovered the nameless stupidity of modern civilization, they were also accused of having drawn the wrong conclusion: 'they did not denounce the injustice, as it in fact exists, but transfigurated and disguised the injustice as it was' (*DE*, p. 209). Modern mass culture only recreates the wish to retreat from the mechanization of life to nature, and the lost world of the soul-body identity degenerates to a flowery advertisement picture. There is no escape; there is no retreat in the Frankfurtian perspective from the drudgery of civilization. What remained for Horkheimer and Adorno was the task of criticism: 'The nature-dependency of mankind today is not to be separated from social protest' (*DE*, p. 4). Against the self-destructive results of enlightenment, which created the dichotomy between the autocratic subject on the one hand and the blind object of the natural world on the other (*DE*, p. 5), Horkheimer and Adorno maintained that the task of bringing forth change remained unchallenged. Thus, against a project of the domination of nature as a positivistic self-destruction of enlightenment, they maintained their idea of critique within enlightenment and within an enlightened tradition. Here we find their *petitio principii*: 'the liberty in societies is inseparable from enlightening thinking' (*DE*, p. 3). But liberty in society – as we have seen in the case of Odysseus – is also inseparable from falsehood, from lie and simulation. Nietzsche had formulated a truth of social existence – 'truth is the type of error without which a certain type of living being could not exist. The value of the life decides in the last instance' (*WP*, section 493); this criterion overshadowed all Frankfurtian modifications, and specifically the one, which developed a concept of knowledge, dependent on the conceptual mediation of the given. Adorno failed to develop productive arguments for his belief that reason and criticism could be used as a conceptual construction against the falsity of the social: conceptual knowledge is as much socially mediated as self-reflection. His resistance, based upon the project of liberating reason, remains also tied to what Nietzsche called the 'prejudice of reason', which 'forces us to posit unity, identity, permanence, substance, cause, thinghood, being, we see ourselves caught in error, compelled into error. So certain are we, of the basis of rigorous examination, that this is where the error lies' (*TI*, no. 71, 482). Adorno's notion of 'mediation' *Vermittlung* is a key concept for understanding his rather ambiguous position towards Nietzsche's 'theory of knowledge'. While Nietzsche is at once taken as an 'enlightened critic' (*AE*, p. 19) (and thus taken as a witness against his 'pre-fascist followers'), he was also criticized for not understanding the mediatedness of his orientation.

Much of Adorno's critique of Nietzsche goes back to an author whose philosophical essay on Nietzsche had already provided an influential perspective for accepting Nietzsche's critique of modernity, while rejecting his theory of knowledge. It was Theodor Lessing who had already argued in 1925 that the subject might have a double existence and accordingly encounters the world within a tension between the practical-sensible life and the world that is constructed consciously (Lessing, 1985, p. 85). In showing how little the scientific destruction of the notion of 'time' has contributed to changing the sensual behaviour of modern people towards time, he makes us aware of how knowledge and life in the social construction of our lives are segregated. He elaborated an old Frankfurtian idea: Nietzsche failed to understand the incongruency (*Undeckbarkeit*), or even incompatibility, of knowledge and life. For him, Nietzsche himself felt coagulated to the concretely given.

Lessing, and with him the Frankfurtians, presuming to argue against Nietzsche, posited a humanity that lives from the tension between life and truth, postulating that the idea of life should be newly realized within the sphere of life as the reality of consciousness: 'Unity would be death' (Lessing, 1985, p. 92). Lessing, furthermore, states that, although we could not destroy the 'real' world in its inaccessible to be-for-itself, with the destruction of the human-ethical meaning given to it, we would destroy any possibility of participation in what remains of our human life-world. But Nietzsche was very well aware of the incongruity between knowledge and becoming (*WP*, section 517). For example, he argued that 'a kind of becoming in itself must create the illusion of being' (*WP*, section 517), and in aphorism 518 of his *Will to Power* we find a statement to which both Lessing and Adorno would have agreed: that admitting that all is becoming, knowledge is only possible when based on a belief in being.

However, there remains the problem of the standpoint of 'unity', which 'idealism, criticism, and phenomenology' (Lessing) and 'idealism and positivism' (Adorno), speciously with Nietzsche, or departing from him, adopt as their own position. Who shall tell us about unity? Adorno insists so much on the unity of the notion and the thing, much as he laments about the discrepancies between the two, seeing reason and critique as the means of maintaining a necessarily tenuous relation. While the social-historical determination of the notion dissolves the thing in its totality, Adorno insisted:

But spirit can as little be separated from the given as the given from the spirit. Neither is a first. Since both are essentially mediated by one another, both are equally unsuitable as original principles. Were one of them to want to discover the original principle itself in such mediacy (*Vermitteltsein*), then it would confuse relational with substantial concept and reclaim the *flatus vocis* as origin.

Mediacy is not a positive assertion about being but rather a directive to cognition not to comfort itself with such positivity. (*AE*, p. 24)

The spirit, the given and mediacy – this is the holy trinity, with which Adorno intended to maintain the tensions within the subject–object dialectic, which Nietzsche himself categorized as false. While Adorno maintained Hegel's perspective, he also fully agreed with Nietzsche's 'impossibility of genuineness' and 'prejudice of reason'. Thus for Adorno, the 'problem of being today' is 'rather its absolute being-in-itself' as a 'merely absolute dillusion about its own subjective mediacy, which is imminent to the question of being itself' (*AE*, p. 22). For Adorno, 'the movement of thought which aims at knowledge of origins announces its own bankruptcy with its dogmatic and empty positing of being. It celebrates origin at the expense of knowledge' (ibid.). However, in insisting on the historical totality of mediacy, Adorno created nothing but a new bankruptcy of thought related to the relativity with which he submitted the given to the abstract and total forces of mediation.

173

Alongside this problem of the contradiction between knowledge 'in the service of life' – as Nietzsche put it in his essay on 'History and historicism' (the second of his 'Thoughts out of season') – and knowledge as a means of the self-performing individual, in contributing to the construction of a world of objective illusion for the purpose of mastering nature and preserving existence, it was Habermas who, in seeing the danger of the possible gap between natural and cultural sciences in modernity, attempted to pose the latter as the new position of developing means of communication which would allow for the explication of meaning structures as a necessary subject for the maintenance of inter-subjective relations and mutual understanding (*KHI*, p. 286). Because they mirror the structures of work and interaction (in other words, structures of life) Habermas conceived of these two transcendental viewpoints as the cognitive expression of knowledge-constitutive interests.

It would seem that Nietzsche's perspective of self-reflection, based on the unity of truth and interest, can reveal the inherent connection between science and interest in modern society, but Habermas, with Freud and the older generation of the Frankfurt School, took the position of mediacy against the 'self-denying' self-reflection of the Nietzsche-type. The theory of mediation takes into account that 'reality' is socio-historically produced and that the given organization of our mental apparatus is in itself already structured to explore the external world. But, when Habermas criticized Nietzsche on the grounds that he psychologized the connection between knowledge and interest, fearing that Nietzsche thus contributes to a 'meta-critical dissolution of knowledge as such' (*KHI*, p. 289), he, like Weber, Horkheimer and Adorno, wants to make us forget that Nietzsche's critique was essentially an attack on the types of knowledge that were developed for the foundation of institutions and institution-formation in general. Against the new class of professional state and church officials, who eat, drink and digest only through a mental apparatus which is formed and organized within institutional purposes, he posed the question: what type of knowledge is left to the individual who denies participation in the processes of institution formation, that is who fundamentally denies and criticizes the type of institution-formation and the cultural enclosures developed by western civilization? Habermas, insisted that 'the process of enlightenment made possible by the sciences' should not be criticized in a way that leads to a 'critical dissolution of dogmas' which 'produces not liberation but indifference' (*KHI*, p. 292). Habermas also feared that Nietzsche put himself into a position outside the connection between theory and practice which science dissolves.

Nietzsche indeed believed that science commits faith to a 'sovereign ignorance' and he thus developed his theory of embodiment, the little things and interpretative perspectivism. While Habermas denounced Nietzsche's attack against the institutional formation of knowledge within the process of scientification as nihilistic, he also denied the nihilistic character of the affiliation between power and reason.

In a recent reinterpretation of the *Dialectic of Enlightenment*, Habermas (1985) attempted to show how Horkheimer and Adorno remained trapped within the perspective of Nietzsche's cultural criticism. Habermas again, as in his final chapter on the 'Logic of social sciences', remained tied to his philosophical anthropology, focusing on the human capacity of cognition and on knowledge rather than on action and the bodily, organic foundations of human existence. For Habermas, Nietzsche's critique is false, because it is based on false assumptions about the character and the role of knowledge in modernity. Here again Habermas insists on a 'paradox structure' of modernity and attacks Nietzsche's theory of power as the rhetorical claims of an aesthetic fragment without commitment towards truth (1985, p. 145). According to Habermas, it is exactly the fusion of knowledge and interest, reason and power in modern society, that puts the will-to-power under constraint. Science for him is the accomplished articulation of reason and power which makes possible a process of enlightenment, thus constraining a totalizing critique of society which only glorifies a will-to-power which takes artistic production as its point of departure.

Habermas, although revising his position by considering for himself an aesthetic solution as a possibility in his *Der philosophische Diskurs der Moderne* believes that science and technology are organized to master nature. They are rather anthropologically founded in an interest of humanity to survive and to live in ever better conditions. In reversing the critical potential of Nietzsche's position, Habermas elaborates an essentially immanent affiliation between knowledge and practical interest. However, for Habermas the truth of the critique of ideology has to be exempt from critique itself. Habermas notes that 'Nietzsche invokes the argument used by Hegel against Kant in order to close off entry into the theory of knowledge' (*KHI*, p. 291). This makes the self-reflection of sciences possible. Habermas here develops an old idea from the *Dialectic of Enlightenment* in which Horkheimer and Adorno criticized the new turn that was developed by Kant, Sade and specifically by Nietzsche within the process of enlightenment, namely that enlightened thinking gains a new radicalization and reverses its subjective relativism and perspectivism against the enlightened subject

175

itself. For Nietzsche, the enlightened individual still maintains a metaphysical belief in its admiration of science (*GM*, III, p. 24), while, on the contrary, modernity has already cut away any belief in the metaphysical determination of truth. Nietzsche developed his secular radicalization of the foundation of truth and against all meta-physical pre-conditions of the critique of ideology (truth against human reality); he established the particularity and irrationality of a will-to-live. Thus, Habermas unwillingly bases knowledge on an instrumental level of institutional foundation. His problem is rather how to establish and to re-establish knowledge as a neutral power within a process of institutional formation, rather than the (Nietzschean) question: how knowledge, based on human senses and practical experience, remains possible for an individual who has been deprived of any meta-physical-ontological understanding of truth?

Nietzsche's concepts of truth must necessarily deny the technologically useful laws of the material sciences as fictions, as a 'world of objective illusion that has been produced for the purpose of mastering nature' (*KHI*, p. 295). Habermas, however, although being aware of the fact that the process of enlightenment has already brought forth a certain incongruence between humanity's reason and nature, suggests that these fictions refer to 'something' which is based in reality which then is objectified in a transcendental framework of possible technological dispositions.

However, Nietzsche (and also Horkheimer and Adorno) never denied that the methodological and instrumental fictions refer to 'something'; they rather suggest a totality of this incongruence and do believe that such fictions refer to something *wrong*, because the 'objective reality' of this type of scientific-technological-economical mastery of nature strikes back against the individual who should be – and wrongly imagines itself as – the sovereign subject of this world mastery itself (Alford, 1987). Habermas believes in the utopia of a discursive society which, by means of communicative action, bridges the gap between pure cognition and instrumental reason based on interest and mastery of nature. However, he also closes off critical theory and ends up in a position of cultural self-affirmation of the Weber-type.

Nietzsche's position was that 'no epistemological scepticism or dogmatism ever came into being without ulterior motives and that these doctrines decline in value as soon as one considers what really forced them to this position.' Nietzsche's conclusion that 'science puts faith to sovereign ignorance' is ultimately reversed by Habermas into a compartmentalizing perspective of the paradoxical structure of modernity and its affirmation. While Weber, in rejecting Nietzsche's 'empiricist misinterpretation of the connection between knowledge and interest' (*KHI*, p. 298) turned Nietzsche's critique into a positivistic and value-free foundation of science as the exploration of the 'logos of the cosmos', free from practical and utilitarian considerations, Habermas wants to rule out a situation where a critique, once evoked by science towards traditional interpretations of the 'true world', is now turned against science itself. This, for Habermas, would lead to an ironic contradiction of a self-denial of reflection which 'is so stubborn that it cannot be dissolved by arguments but only appeased by invocations' (*KHI*, p. 299).

Habermas laments the positivism of Nietzsche's position on the basis of two observations: (a) his belief in the moral origin of epistemological dogmas, and (b) his acceptance of the positivistic self-understanding of modern sciences as a monopoly of knowledge devaluing all meta-physical knowledge. This critique of Nietzsche's double positivism, however, remains untenable, and specifically his argument that the fusion of interest and power could be critically 'disintegrated' in modernity by an awareness of their given meta-historical affiliations and in more practical terms, through openly stating and not through hiding interest, remains a postulative gesture, which itself hides the fact that scientification and professionalization are continuous and evermore decisive determinants of 'interest'. Horkheimer, and more specifically Adorno, have clearly seen this fact, that science and the process of scientification prevent any self-reflection themselves; they have also seen how science is condemned to deny 'interest' and thus bound to turn reason into 'a purposeless intentionality' and into 'achievement that stakes over bodies' (*DE*, p. 93). Against this critique, Habermas' utopia leads into a perspective for a defence of the established mechanisms of a free, nature-mastering and discursive society (Maurer, 1981, p. 41).

Nietzsche's attack on the fateful amalgamation of reason and power in modern institutions was an attack on the priest and the scholar, and more specifically on their modern descendants, the *Bildungsphilister* (the cultural philistine), the new class of state officials, Protestant moralists, *Katheder*-socialists (like Dühring and others) and the 'Reich-workers' as he calls them in the *Twilight of Idols*. Against this attack, Weber evoked the picture of the value-free intellectual equipped with an ethos of responsibility and interested only in the cognitive unification of the logos of the cosmos. Horkheimer and Adorno, with the image of Odysseus, showed how betrayal and cunning remain the only tool of the 'interested' and reasonable individual to triumph over the bondage to myth and nature. For them, social trickery is an immanent mechanism

177

of all society, where sacrifice turns into a mere form of exchange. For them, the intellectual remains in a hopeless situation, evoking the desperate and paradoxical aspirations that the hopelessness could once be saved (Maurer, 1981, p. 41). Habermas, whose notion of 'knowledge-constitutive interest' was directly born in Nietzsche's epistemology, attempts to save professional science from a total critique by a conscious compartmentalization of explorative research and its legitimization by means of 'mediative reason' in *Der philosophische Diskurs der Moderne*.

We do not understand Nietzsche's critique of modernity – even where it extends to an epistemology itself – when we merely reconstruct it in the light of a basically Marxist problematic, the problem of the reconciliation between humanity and nature. Indeed, Horkheimer and Adorno attempted to reinterpret Nietzsche primarily through this perspective. Nietzsche's philosophy accomplished the process of enlightenment in that he took its claims of an identity between reason and history seriously. However, Horkheimer and Adorno understood very well that the essence of Nietzsche's question is not really about epistemology and the various human conditions of constituting knowledge. Nietzsche's true problem was about the way of life and the type of humanity that must be born in order to be able to cope with the obvious contradiction in the position of both the priest and the scholar, between morality and interest, between knowledge and power, and the formation of social institutions which they dominate. These strata became culturally productive by being fundamentally based on social trickery through auto-legitimization and through ideological claims of self-denial. Horkheimer and Adorno have understood the essence of Nietzsche's problem, but they have attempted to neutralize it. The seafarer Odysseus for them incorporates fundamentally all the elements of a modern person who is aware of the contradictions, but is at the same time able to cope with a changing set of ritualized myths threatening to colonize and to dominate his life-perspective, or even to kill him. This liberation against such myths, however, again exists in playful self-sacrifices, simulative games and symbolic exchanges. Odysseus, however, as we have to stress here, is a traveller between worlds and his simulative games are played towards those who remain locals and socially integrated by such myths. For Horkheimer and Adorno, and specifically for Adorno, Nietzsche's problem of the contradiction of reason and life in modernity led to far-reaching attempts to re-erect theory from where it once departed: from the sphere of self-reflection and teaching of life. However, while Nietzsche attacked the Socratic way of thinking (reason as virtue and virtue as happiness) as decadent and essentially negative towards life in the *Twilight of the Idols* and praised the instincts of the 'older Greeks', Adorno called himself a 'post-Socratian' and thus denounced the 'pre-Socratian' reference in Heidegger's philosophy (Mörchen, 1981).

Habermas, however, denounces Nietzsche's contradiction between 'denial of instinct' (that is, decadence) and 'increase of life' (that is, happiness) as a mere psychologistic reflection of the humanity-nature relation. Alongside reflections which were already present in Theodor Lessing's critique of Nietzsche, he develops a dualistic perspective of the different realms of knowledge. 'Habermas expresses this division in terms of his concern that social subsistence organized along functional lines and based upon money, power and technical expertise, not be allowed to intrude upon the process of communicatively based socialization' (Alfred, 1985, p. 123). With this solution, Habermas 'accepts the disenchantment of nature as the price of modernity, a price worth paying' (ibid.). With this dualistic perspective, Habermas only reaffirms a process of compartmentalization which is a product of modernity itself. Adorno argued in the dedication to *Minima Moralia* that what once was called 'life' for the philosopher has become the sphere of the private and then only the sphere of consumption, which is dragged along as a mere appendix of the material process of production, without autonomy and substance. With little instincts about the irony of 'life', Habermas quotes Nietzsche in the last passage of *Knowledge and Human Interests*, where Nietzsche ironically denied the ability of those 'psychologists of future' to self-analyze and to self-reflect on their own position of 'decadence'. Habermas as a *Virtuose einer sich selbst verleugnenden Reflexion* (a virtuoso of a reflection bound to self-denial) ends up in a position to be a prophet of a 'sad science' who remains an 'instrument of knowledge' rather than to 'instrumentalize' it.

Habermas' epistemological reinterpretation of Nietzsche falls behind the actual stage of the process of scientification of social institutions. This formation stage already combines knowledge and interest, reason and power in an indissoluble way. A defence of this prevalent combination against Nietzsche's critique leads to nothing more than the legitimation of given structures. Nietzsche's critique, however, leads much further. It attempts to show how the individual will have to re-erect *behind* these structures both given and totally new forms in intuitive knowledge in order to be able to escape the fate of the 'iron cage' of structural domination in modernity.

6

Of the Despisers of the Body – Nietzsche and French Social Theory

Résumé

It is evident that there is a significant revival of Nietzsche's philosophy in contemporary European thought and that Nietzsche has had a specific impact on aesthetics, literature and general philosophy. In particular Nietzsche is seen to be a key figure in the post-modernist debate where he has been described as a 'prophet of extremity' (Megill, 1985). Nietzsche's philosophy has become part of a broad critique of rationalism, Hegelianism and the logic of state regulation. While his philosophy has become prominent within the modernist critique, his contribution to social theory has yet to be adequately identified, discussed and developed. In this chapter we will argue that Nietzsche's position in sociology turns out to be highly problematic, since in many respects it would appear that his philosophy is an anti-sociology, or at least that Nietzsche's position may render sociology into a pre-modern discipline.

Although Nietzsche is overtly absent from social theory, throughout this study we have argued that he is the unrecognized master of social thought (the absent centre) and more particularly that his contribution to the development of the social theories of Weber, Freud, Adorno and Foucault has been neglected. For example, we have taken the position that, while the relationship between Nietzsche and Weber has been commented on, it has hardly been analysed in any systematic way. Certain superficial comparisons between Weber and Nietzsche are often noted particularly with respect to the theory of charisma, the relationship between the will-to-power and power politics, and finally the relativism of Weber's epistemology. More importantly, we have shown that Nietzsche's theme of the death of God was fundamental to Weber's emphasis on polytheistic values and ethical decisionism

(Stauth and Turner, 1986). In earlier sections of this study, we drew specific attention to the importance of the theme of resentment in the development, not only of Weber's sociology of religion, but more generally of Weber's analysis of morals, social groups and the development of modern rationalism. Furthermore, we can regard Weber's rationalization theme and the emphasis on technical rationality as an illustration of the dominance of the culture of Socratic rationality and we might also regard Weber's sociology as a rejection of Dionysian principles through the emphasis on Protestant ethical values, the ethic of world mastery and Socratic wisdom. In Nietzsche's terms, the history of the Protestant ethic and the centrality of Protestant values within Weber's sociology represent a sociological statement of no-saying philosophies. Despite the presence of these Nietzschean themes, we have demonstrated that Weber in a covert way denied the impact of Nietzsche on his sociological perspective. Weber as an individual identified personally with the professional ethics of sociological research, the importance of a strong national German state against Anglo-American imperialism, the ethic of stern responsibility and rejected all 'life-philosophies' (specifically Freudianism) as romantic reactions to the modern condition. Both his life and his sociology were a celebration of oppressive rationalism against unreflective spontaneity, the immediacy of feeling and the life-world.

Nietzsche covertly entered modern social theory through the auspices of Weber's sociology, but Nietzsche is also distinctively present in contemporary thought as a consequence of the impact of Freudianism on the post-modernist debate. As we have seen, Nietzsche sought, via the analysis of moral genealogy, to trace the origin of negative morality back to all forms of instinctual denial, standardization and rigid sublimation. Technical rationality, institutionalized through forms of industrial civilization, was a system of organized revenge against the immediacy of the life-world, pleasure and desire. In more specific terms, social life is made possible by the presence of guilt, that is, by bad conscience (Carroll, 1985). Nietzsche anticipated Freud by drawing out the crucial parallels between personal illness, language and social relations, whereby there is a sense in which getting better is related to getting better ideas. In a similar fashion, Freud was to describe hysteria as a problem of bad memory. Of course, the problem in comparing Freud and Nietzsche, as we have seen, is related to the problematic status of the 'I' in Nietzsche's thought, since his philosophy of language defined the subject as a presumption of modern thought. For Nietzsche, the individual is a construction which is peculiarly related to the grammatical structure of European languages, where the subject is the active element in relation to the predicate.

Finally, we have demonstrated that Nietzsche's presence in contemporary social thought was also fundamentally mediated by the critical theories of Horkheimer, Adorno and more recently by Habermas. There are clearly important themes from Nietzsche's philosophy in the *Dialectic of Enlightenment* and *Aesthetic Theory*. While the critical theorists sought to criticize the negative qualities of technical rationality in modern societies, they also wished to retain the notion of rationality itself as the necessary basis for the attack on modern forms of capitalist irrationality. In more general terms, the Apollo/Dionysian theme has dominated much critical social thought, especially in the work of Marcuse. It is, however, probably correct to argue that the resurrection of Nietzsche in contemporary German thought has been a resurrection of parts rather than the whole of Nietzsche (Stephens, 1986).

The presence of Nietzsche in modern social theory has consequently been mediated through these four broad strands, namely Weberian sociology, Freudian psycho-analysis, the historical de-constructions of Foucault and the work of the critical theorists. In addition, there have been certain quite specific points in contemporary thought where the key issues of Nietzsche's philosophy have, as it were, come to the surface to disturb the modern consciousness. Contemporary existential philosophy would be a case in point. Although Heidegger was obviously powerfully influenced by writers like Kierkegaard, Heidegger's analysis of being and reason was in many fundamental respects a version of Nietzsche's own critique of the pretentions of western logic (Demske, 1970). Heidegger developed this project into an anti-logical theme, since it was Heidegger who regarded reason as a tyranny over genuine forms of thought (Heidegger, 1977). Nietzsche's philosophy of being entered contemporary social thought in France via the work of Heidegger's existentialism and specifically through the work of writers like Camus and Sartre. In particular, Sartre's negative critique of language as incapable of representing reality and his analysis of bad faith were clearly within the Nietzsche tradition. The existentialism of Heidegger and Sartre was a significant development of Nietzsche in terms of the specific problems of contemporary society in the aftermath of total war.

The Peculiarities of the French

The main paradox of the recent Nietzsche revival is its location within French intellectual culture. From the early 1970s, there has been a sustained and important French debate regarding the nature of

182

Nietzsche's philosophy. In particular, we may note the contributions of Jacques Derrida who, in his study *Spurs, Nietzsche's styles*, presented an original analysis of the metaphors of Nietzsche's work with reference to the problem of women in Nietzsche's philosophy (Derrida, 1979). There is also the work of Gilles Deleuze who drew attention to the importance of the body in the work of Nietzsche and contributed a specific volume to the analysis of Nietzsche's philosophy (Deleuze, 1983). Following the reinterpretation of Freud by Jacques Lacan, Deleuze also provided an original perspective on the traditional Freudian problem of the Oedipus myth (Deleuze and Guattari, 1977). Within a wider framework the contributions of Pierre Klossowski have been important in establishing the philosophical importance of Nietzsche's work (Klossowski, 1969). The relationship between Nietzsche's treatment of nihilism and contemporary society also provided the background to the contribution of writers like J–F. Lyotard (1979, 1980). This Nietzsche revival has become the topic of some secondary commentary, analysis and translation (Allison, 1977; Burchell, 1984; Forrester, 1984; Lash, 1984; Lash, 1985). In this chapter we will be primarily concerned with the impact of Nietzsche on contemporary social thought through the work of Michel Foucault, but before turning to an analysis of Foucault, we should begin with the question of the peculiarity of the French context of the Nietzsche revival.

The growing importance of Nietzsche on post-structuralist thought has to be connected with the collapse of Marxism as the central intellectual force in the 1970s following the traumatic events of 1968 (Lemert, 1981). The Nietzsche revival is associated with the decline of the organized working class as the driving force of western politics and the emergence of new social movements which have addressed wider questions of sexuality, rights and nature. The critique of reason as an agency of repression reflects the special character of new social movements which we might describe as experiments in disordered organization. In the European context, Marxism appeared to become increasingly irrelevant to the analysis and direction of the new social movements. Marxism as a mode of analysis was unable to extract itself from the limited and specific problems of nineteenth-century capitalism and the issues which dominated Europe in the 1970s were not amenable to rigid Marxist formulation. Although writers like Louis Althusser enjoyed a certain notoriety in British social theory in the early 1970s, there was subsequently a massive and rapid decline of the influence of structural Marxism by the end of the decade. Although in recent years there have been many attempts to repossess the modern on

183

behalf of Marxism, for a variety of reasons Nietzsche appears more relevant than Marx in the era of post-modernism (Berman, 1983; Callinicos, 1985). The collapse of structuralism and the growing importance of the post-modernist debate have made Nietzsche more relevant and more attractive as a prophet of crisis. Nietzsche's emphasis on language, metaphor and perspective appears to have a specific affinity with the anxieties of the modern period. In this study we have argued that Nietzsche's social philosophy gives more space for agency, reciprocity, sensualism and affirmative philosophy which counteract the determinism of linguistic and social structuralism, naive functionalism and economistic Marxism.

It is ironic that Durkheim argued that France was the ideal cultural context for the emergence of sociology, because the French Revolution has secularized thought, making possible the emergence of a positivistic form of analysis. Cartesianism had made the rise of rational forms of inquiry possible. Because French society was Cartesian and secular, the growth of sociology as a positivistic explanation of social relations had been enhanced. St Simon and Comte both articulated this positivist utopia as the goal of social change; the engineer would replace the priest as the leading director of the new age. Cartesian rationalism came to have a particular prominence in French philosophy and social thought, but this dominance has been challenged in the post-war period. Of course, Nietzsche was very critical of Cartesian rationalism, positivism, instrumental science, and evolutionary forms of thought, especially Darwinistic science, as a consequence of his general hostility to Socratic rationality. Nietzsche's scepticism about scientific positivism, quantification and evolutionary arguments about progress is part of the general appeal of his philosophy, since there is, on both the Left and the Right, much less optimism and confidence in the scientific project, especially in a society like France which has been devastated by two world wars in the twentieth century. The celebration of the irrational and the absurd in existentialism has its roots in this tragic history of war and destruction. Nietzsche's emphasis on desire and sexuality, and his critique of the illusion of formal rationality appear to be highly compatible with the anti-rationalism and perspectivism of post-modernist theory. The seductive attraction of Nietzsche's critical treatment of rationalism may also be connected with the revival of a radical Freudianism in the work of Lacan, which challenged the dominance of institutionalized psychiatry in both France and America (Lemaire, 1977; Schneiderman, 1983). In short, Nietzsche has provided the intellectual, historical and emotional basis of post-modernism as a social problem.

184

The specific attraction of Nietzsche's philosophy in the French context does however owe a great deal to the importance of language and metaphor in Nietzsche's work. The playfulness of Nietzsche's style has proved highly congenial to the literary and aesthetic interests of French intellectuals. For Nietzsche, language is metaphorical rather than literal; its meaning rests upon the play of differences between metaphors. Language does not stand for reality, since reality is itself a metaphorical discourse. It was only by suppressing its origins in metaphor that the rational philosophy of the West, starting from Socrates, was able to maintain itself under the tyranny of reason (Norris, 1982, p. 57). Socratic reason squeezed the life out of Dionysus, by erasing our memory of the original metaphoricality of thought over experience. The consequences of Nietzsche's view of language are initially highly relativistic and threatening, leading to a radical de-construction of all taken-for-granted sense. This apparently negative approach leads eventually to a certain playfulness and to a critical response against the dominance of Cartesian thought in the form of theories of system in the modern philosophical tradition. This perspectivism in literature and politics permits a necessary distancing of ourselves from dubious commitments to oppressive institutions, language, political regulation and social movements. Nietzsche's philosophy in France has provided the basis for a sceptical questioning of commitment to capitalist culture and modern social institutions, grounded in an instrumental rationality which is life-denying.

Foucault's Nietzsche

The growing interest in Nietzsche may depend to some extent on the popularity of Foucault's analyses of language, knowledge and power. Once more we see Nietzsche mediated through the work of a contemporary social theorist. Although Foucault only occasionally made direct reference to and offered a discussion of Nietzsche (as in *Language, Counter-memory, Practice*) the impact and influence of Nietzsche on Foucault was clearly extensive.

At various times Foucault was attracted to Nietzsche's genealogy as an alternative to traditional forms of historical analysis; however, Foucault came eventually to develop his own particular views of this issue in *The Archaeology of Knowledge*. Foucault's use of Nietzsche was connected with the rejection of reductionist and deterministic theories (such as historical materialism) and also with the rejection of teleological idealism (such as Hegelianism). Foucault regarded Marx and Marxism as simply a turning point in nineteenth-century social thought and his critique of economism entailed an emphasis on the necessary connection between knowledge and power. Foucault also provided an important critique of conventional Marxist theories of power and the state. The point of Foucault's historical analysis was not to make the obscure familiar, but on the contrary to retain the sense of the bizarre, the absurd, the unexpected and the unusual as essential features of historical experience. Foucault sought to challenge our conventional and comfortable assumptions about reason and progress through a defamiliarization of history. The aim of genealogy is always to decompose, to shatter and to de-construct those elements which are held together by social convention. Nietzsche's genealogy is the antidote for all forms of historical analysis which attempt to identify and account for the development of humanity through reason and rationality. History by contrast is always an endless struggle characterized by diversity and chance, by uniqueness and unfolding in the work of Nietzsche and Foucault. History is never simply the triumph of rationality and universalism; human development has involved the institutionalization of violence in a system of rules which proceed from domination to further domination under the illusion of harmony and good will (*LCP*, p. 151). In Foucault's history, there is nothing which suggests consolation and confidence, since there are no continuities in human history; indeed, not even the body of human beings is a stable point of reference. Historical reality is simply a construction of the work of knowledge and power through a process of institutionalization. It was exactly in this manner that the discourse of orientalism constituted the East as a place of stagnation, sensuality, cruelty and despotism as the precise opposite of the rationality of the West in world history (Said, 1978).

In this respect, Foucault's notions about history are parallel to Nietzsche's treatment of western culture in *The Birth of Tragedy*. During the eighteenth century under the impact of neo-classicism, European culture came to regard the classical world as the primary criterion of excellence in art and literature. The new attitude to Greek and Roman culture was summarized by Johann Winckelmann in the phrase *eine edle Einfalt und eine stille Grösse* (noble simplicity and calm grandeur) (Honour, 1981, p. 61). Nietzsche turned this picture upside down by a genealogical analysis of th roots of Greek civilization in the fusion of Dionysus and Apollo. Behind the serenity of classical culture lay the violent ecstacies of the orgiastic sects of the god Dionysus. In a similar fashion, Nietzsche focused attention to the prominence of cruelty, violence and lust in Homer's *Iliad* in the posthumously published fragment 'Homer's contest'. Nietzsche's aim was to uncover the dynamic interaction between the principles of Dionysus and Apollo in order to condemn the shallow wisdom of Socratic rationalism. Against neo-classicism, he regarded the origins of western culture as essentially violent and vicious.

Foucault's investigation of psychiatry and the social sciences was also written against the official history of these subjects; in criticizing the pretensions of scientific discourse, Foucault attempted to present what he called a counter-memory. The provision of an alternative history was particularly important in *Madness and Civilization* where Foucault sought to show that psychiatry was not a liberating and progressive force, extracting insanity from an inappropriate cultural context. On the contrary, psychiatry was an implicit regulation of opposition under the guise of progressive reason. It involved the subjugation of individuality in the guise of folly. In general terms, we can see Foucault's work as the analysis of the rise of various forms of discipline, whereby the body and populations are regulated within an urban space (Turner, 1984). The social sciences and the specific institutions of the asylum, the factory and school were features of a general panopticism whereby bodies are regulated and contained. Official knowledge fragments and divides our experience in order to bring about greater understanding and therefore greater control: the institutional apparatus of modern society represents a sophisticated and detailed management of urban populations. Following Nietzsche, Foucault placed an important emphasis on the combination of knowledge and power as the focus of modern systems of regulation, that is the dominance of Dionysus by the Socratic institutions of reason.

The impact of Nietzsche on Foucault was closely associated with the prominence of the problem of the body in Foucault's analyses of power/knowledge. We can detect this theme at various points in Foucault's development. The target of Foucault's historical inquiry was the long term emergence of discursive and non-discursive practices by which the body of populations are organized, regulated and controlled within social spaces. The central theme of Foucault's work was the demographic transition of modern society and the necessity for rationalization. For example, Foucault claimed that

The great eighteenth-century demographic upswing in western Europe, the necessity of co-ordinating and integrating into the apparatus of production and the urgency of controlling it with finer and more adequate power mechanisms cause 'population' with its numerical variables of space and chronology, longevity and health, to emerge not only as a problem but as an object of surveillance, analysis, intervention, modification, etc. (*PK*, p. 171).

It was this 'accumulation of men' which provided the central topic of Foucault's historical inquiry, because it was this demographic issue which came ultimately to be a key factor in the proliferation of regimes and systems of control (Turner, 1985c). It was population pressures which contributed to the need for timetables, taxonomies, examinations, surveys and other forms of regulation. In *Discipline and Punish*, Foucault traced the emergence of this new type of discipline through the development of prisons, asylums, clinics and hospitals. Like Weber, he saw the problem of regulating an infantry as the modern origin of discipline. Weber had argued that 'military discipline gives birth to all discipline' (*ES*, vol. 2, p. 1155). However, it was the issue of increasing numbers of bodies within a restricted urban space which generated Foucault's concern with detailed regulation under the panoptic scheme. These issues lay behind the emergence of social medicine and sociology itself, alongside the new range of social science disciplines, especially criminology, penology and demography.

In *The Birth of the Clinic*, Foucault provided a history of the transformation of medicine and medical practice in post-revolutionary France. Once more the body became a crucial feature and topic of this analysis. This historical study was concerned in particular with the relationship between the body, knowledge and the clinic, where Foucault attempted to trace a transformation of power via an analysis of clinical medicine. In Foucault's argument, the localization of disease and illness within the singular body is an effect of modern medical classification. He wrote that

For us, the human body defines, by natural right, the space of origin and of distribution of disease: a space whose lines, volumes, surfaces, and routes are laid down, in accordance with a now familiar geometry, by the anatomical atlas. This order of the solid, visible body is only one way – in all likelihood neither the first, nor the most fundamental – in which one spatializes disease. There have been, and will be, other distributions of illness (*BC*, p. 3).

The nature of illness and disease is as a result a function of the relationship between language and body, since it is through medical discourse that we can identify, locate and understand specific combinations of disease and their relationship to the body. For Foucault, the body is constructed by discourses which constitute bodies as constellations of forces. This approach to medical history has proved to be very productive in modern medical sociology (Armstrong, 1983), in the history of insanity (Donnelly, 1983) and in the history of architecture (Evans, 1982).

The body was also central to his analysis of sexuality in which Foucault concerned himself in particular with the discourses of sexuality which emerged out of the Christian confessional and the pastoral offices of the Church (Hepworth and Turner, 1982). The issue here is that the sexual body is not, as it were, a fact of nature, but the product of specific discourses which produce the body as an effect of power practices. For example, Foucault was concerned with the contrast between the discourse of sexuality (*Ars Erotica*) and the new discourse which produces sex as a scientific topic (*Scientia Sexualis*). Foucault attempted to argue that the Victorian period had not suppressed sexuality, but on the contrary produced it as the endless topic of the sciences, religious debate and popular literature. The result is that we have become a confessing society, that is, a society which constantly produces the sexuality of the body through an endless round of discourse.

In the later volumes of the history of sexuality (*L'Usage des Plaisirs, Le Soucie de Soi* and *Les Aveux de la Chair*), Foucault turned to the problem of sexuality in Christianity and antiquity to study the development of codes of sexual behaviour which had the consequence of constituting the ethical self. In Christianity, there emerged, through a battle over celibacy for religious and chastity for lay people, a new ethical system which proscribed homosexuality, unnatural sexual acts, fornication and dangerous pleasures. The result was the emergence of monogamy and permanent wedlock as the ideal state of the laity (Ariès and Béjin, 1985). However, the main theme of Foucault's analysis was the development of a subjective moral agent, regulating sexual behaviour by codes, disciplines and practices. In order to achieve this regulation, western cultures developed three techniques – dietetics, economics and erotica. These arts or techniques defined the 'use of pleasures' for free moral beings. The creation of austerity in sexual behaviour may be associated with a new culture of the self, the rise of individualism and the discovery of the self over many centuries of western history (Abercrombie, Hill and Turner, 1986). Power over the self was consequently seen in terms of power over sexuality with the result that to know oneself was an essential aspect of the ascetic practices of Christian culture.

Modern societies are preoccupied with the regulation of the body and this gives rise to a series of disciplines which Foucault referred to in terms of the anatomo-politics of the human body and secondly to a system of regulatory control which he called a bio-politics of the population. The whole of contemporary politics bears down upon the issue of life itself as the crucial factor of modern knowledge and power.

The main emphasis therefore is on the regulation of the body and on the production of the body through administrative procedures. The central paradox of the world depicted in Foucault's analysis is that the modern growth of individual rights necessarily requires greater surveillance of persons in the interests of an abstract notion of equality (Turner, 1986c).

In this area, Foucault made a particularly important contribution to our understanding of the self and sexuality through his analysis of hermaphroditism. Foucault's argument was that it is as a result of administrative procedures that sexual identity is polarized into male and female such that one can only have one sexual identity at any given time. He argued that

Biological theories of sexuality, juridical conceptions of the individual, forms of administrative control in modern nations, led little by little to rejecting the idea of a mixture of the two sexes in a single body, and consequently to limiting the free choice of indeterminant individuals. Henceforth, everybody was to have one and only one sex. (*HB*, p. VIII)

The regulative practices of the modern state created a system of individuation which required definite sexual classification of populations.

Because Foucault was also concerned with the problem of the representation of the body, he was particularly intrigued by the work of Magritte and the surrealistic treatment of the body in contemporary art. Following the work of Ferdinand de Saussure, both Magritte and Foucault were concerned to explore the arbitrary relatinship between signifiers and signified within the world of science, literature and art. Language operates by establishing norms of difference between signified and signifier such that the relationship between an order of things and an order or words is necessarily arbitrary. As Foucault argued in *The Order of Things*, the regularity between language and reality is itself the product of discourse, which is another way of saying that all language is metaphorical. This metaphoricality of our understanding was crucial to the art of Magritte, especially in the famous painting *This is not a Pipe* which was the topic of a short but important monograph by Foucault. The paintings of Magritte are deconstructions and his treatment of the female body in *Les Liaisons Dangereuses* was an intriguing illustration of the arbitrary relationship between the sign and the signifier. Word and reality are held together by a series of arbitrary conventions.

The problem of the body and populations can be seen therefore as a continuing and central theme in Foucault's social theory. Indeed

190

Foucault claimed that the body is the crucial debate for materialistic theory when he noted that 'I wonder whether before one poses the question of ideology, it wouldn't be more materialistic to study first the question of the body and the effects of power on it' (*PK*, p. 58). Foucault was concerned with the long term rationalization and management of the body and how the body arises as the main target of contemporary politics. It is the problem of the body which lies behind his medical histories, the analysis of sexuality and his general concern with the question of disciplines. Foucault's interest in the body was related to his concern for dissent and resistance, since in Foucault's theory the body is a site of social struggle. His analysis of discipline implied a sociology of the body which would be compatible with Weber's theme of rationalization and the metaphor of the iron cage. As we have seen, Foucault throughout his work regarded the body as the effect of discourses and as the outcome of institutional-administrative practices. Just as Weber treated religious asceticism, bureaucracy and the military as a regulation of the body, so Foucault typically saw discipline as a government of the body. Indeed, it can be argued that Foucault's treatment of discipline is simply a contemporary version of Weber's analysis of rationality, especially where that rationality is institutionalized in bureaucracy and administration. The government of the body is consequently the basis for a government of society (Turner, 1982a; 1982b; 1982c; 1984; 1985a).

We may observe two problems with Foucault's treatment of the body as an effect of discourse. The first is that he wanted to write about resistance and opposition, but if the body is simply the product of discursive practices, then it is difficult to see how the body could in fact be a source of resistance. Foucault did not appear to have any genuine appreciation of the lived body within the tradition of modern phenomenology; for example,

clearly Foucault does not adope Merleau-Ponty's solution. The body of desire is not for him the phenomenal lived body. It is not a corporeal, incarnate subjectivity . . . Desire for Foucault is neither expressed in the body nor is the body the lived form of desire. (Lemert and Gillian, 1982)

In short, Foucault did not develop an explicit theory of embodiment. The second and related problem is that in the absence of a theory of resistance through embodiment, it is difficult to see how Foucault could provide a way out of the iron cage. The implication of Foucault's analysis of panopticism, discourse, power and knowledge was fatalistic; he was unable to present an alternative to pessimism and nihilism, despite many attempts towards the end of his life to provide an explanation of resistance to regulation. The theoretical necessity to avoid biologism, determinism and psychologism resulted in an anti-naturalism, which in turn precluded a phenomenology of the body.

There is a certain nostalgia surrounding classical sociology, but there is also a nostalgic theme in Foucault's emphasis on pre-conceptual experience and on his interest in madness and criminality. In *Madness and Civilization*, Foucault ascribed heroic values to the non-rational, madness and folly. Because of this nostalgia, Foucault did not offer us a way out of panopticism and his references to resistance and counter-memory were in fact descriptions of ineffectual forms of protest. In more precise terms, it is not clear that there is a strong link between his philosophy and his politics; indeed his philosophical position would appear to rule out large-scale political activity to transform social institutions. It is not clear how we get from Foucault's theory of discourse to actual politics, because he refused to offer any systematic set of alternative strategies or goals (despite constant references to the oppositional character of micro-politics). In part, Foucault's own perspectivism ruled out any privileged place for either a revolutionary or a reformist discourse and associated political practices. Rather than aggressive opposition, Foucault might at best offer a form of individualised subversion (Patton, 1984/5). In terms of Robert Merton's theory of anomie, Foucault described a strategy of retreatism as the main response to the politics of domination. Although Foucault attempted to reject the label, he never entirely escaped from the problems that surround structuralism, so that the agent or the subject in his analyses often appeared merely as the puppet of discourse or the parrot of language. Foucault's analyusis of the body involved an implicit structuralism; the body is not a site of resistance, but merely the construct of the anatomical and juridical map. The Foucaultian body is an abstract entity, the constructed effect of historical discourses.

Nietzsche's Body

This interpretation of Foucault has of course been challenged by various critics on a number of occasions. In particular, Barry Smart (1985) has provided a cogent defence of Foucault's analysis of resistance by an examination of the slogan 'where there is power, there is resistance.' Since power is only exercised over free subjects, the analysis of power must also lead to the question of freedom (to the limits of power). The existence of power necessarily involves the resistance of the will; politics therefore becomes the endless struggle between the forces of domination and the willing of the subject. In response to his critics Foucault, in the essay 'The subject and power' (Foucault, 1982), produced a statement on the nature of anti-authoritarian struggles. These political struggles have the following characteristics. They are not confined to one country or to one political system. These struggles are focused on 'power effects' rather than on the mode by which power is exercised. They are immediate, in the sense that they seek immediate change rather than some distant revolution. They are concerned with the status of the individual and they attack practices which individuate and separate the individual from the community. Modern struggles are directed against the privileges of professional knowledge and the associated institutions of government. Finally, these struggles (in asking the question, 'who are we?') are opposed to all abstract forms of knowledge which obliterate or threaten individuality.

We would welcome this statement of the character of resistance, but argue that a theory of resistance and a history of struggle were absent from Foucault's principal studies of madness, discipline and medicine. His actual studies of total rule leave little space for the struggle between freedom and power. His formal statement on the nature of struggle finds no significant counterpart in his historical studies. We conclude that Foucault was forced to make such a statement in order to satisfy his critics, but this change in emphasis did not bring him to re-analyse his earlier work on the clinic, the hospital or the penitentiary as systems of total power.

A more important issue of course is that Foucault's commentary on resistance was fundamentally a reformulation and re-statement of Nietzsche's concept of the will-to-power. The concept of will was a basic component of Nietzsche's whole philosophical perspective. He wrote that

My idea is that every specific body strives to become master over all space and to extend its force (– its will to power) and to thrust back all that resists its extension. But it continually encounters similar efforts on the part of other bodies and ends by coming to an arrangement ('union') with those of them that are sufficiently related to it: thus they conspire together for power. And the process goes on. (*WP*, section 636)

Following Schopenhauer, Nietzsche made desiring and striving the central component of his view of life, but, rather than being trapped by their willing within a fatalistic system, people become joyous in their realization and actualization of will. The embodiment of will was essential to the revaluation of values and in turn, these evaluations are features of health and healthy bodies. The result is that the analysis of struggle takes us therefore back to a theory of the body.

We are now in a position to return to the question of Foucault's relationship to Nietzsche. It can be argued that Nietzsche is too frequently treated as merely a negative and pessimistic critique of secular society who, because of his perspectivism, did not offer a significant alternative, but rather escaped into the elitist privacy of the intellectual and the irrationality of will. Nietzsche's relationship to German culture, nihilism and the death of God was of course more complex than this simple assertion would suggest. Nihilism in Nietzsche's philosophy was a challenge, especially a challenge towards the revaluation of values and the development of a form of healthy existence. Furthermore, the death of God was not a nostalgic event, but a significant feature of liberation and a necessary step towards moral autonomy. The death of God was not a tragedy, but the promise of a new modality of ethical existence. Foucault did not share this aspect of reconstruction which was part of Nietzsche's moral programme. There is nothing in Foucault's philosophy to resemble the revaluation of values, the eternal return, the celebration of the little things of everyday life, the proclamation of *amor fati*, and the will-to-power which are positive doctrines and an antidote to nihilism, retreatism and complete despair. Of course, we are not attempting to domesticate Nietzsche in the manner suggested by Walter Kaufmann (1974) who came eventually to see Nietzsche as a modern Christian philosopher of hope and altruism, but it is to suggest that Nietzsche had a philosophical programme which was committed to the reconstruction of life against the threat of negative culture and personal despair. Nietzsche's aim was to achieve a Dionysian relation to existence which he regarded as the 'highest state' a philosopher can achieve. By contrast, Foucault did not offer or indicate an alternative to the deconstruction of discourse.

We have claimed that this difference between Nietzsche and Foucault was associated with the question of the body. While Foucault saw the body as an effect of medico-sexual discourses, Nietzsche had a complicated view of the body which operated at various levels. For example, Nietzsche saw the body as a metaphor for political, social and artistic debates, but it was also the case that Nietzsche conceptualized the body in physiological terms as a real entity. Nietzsche's interest in medicine and physiology was closely associated with his own physical illness and connected with his quest for a valid form of health which would be the basis of a valid morality. Nietzsche's illness was not, as it were, an accidental feature of his life and philosophy, but a central and dominating problem within his total outlook. His letters were full of interrelated discussions of his health, philosophy, medicine and the crisis of culture (Fuss and Shapiro, 1971). Nietzsche's philosophy is deeply bound up with the problem of health. He saw German society as critically sick and interpreted his own role as a cultural psychologist of social physician whose task was to understand the social virus of his time. Much of his writing centred on this metaphor of the illness of his own body and the sickness in the social body. Within his historical writing, Nietzsche also used the metaphor of health to describe pre-modern societies; the debate about health was, for example an important feature of his analysis of Greek society. Nietzsche also used a parallel or analogy between the mind as an organ which consumes ideas and the digestive system which through physiological processes produces energy. Bad ideas in the brain are like rotten food in the digestive tract. In these references to health and illness, the metaphor of health and the physiology of the body are constantly and necessarily mixed together. In certain passages which resemble the work of Marx on religion as an opium, Nietzsche came to regard religion as a pain killer, whereby priests always made their living from the narcotizing of human ills. Religion is a palliative for those who are desperately sick, but it also actively damages the healthy when improperly administered. In addition, Nietzsche regarded illness as a form of stimulation which could lead to health. Sickness is often conceived as a desirable challenge to a healthy body which will stimulate it into new forms of action and development. Sickness in this sense is often associated with pregnancy by Nietzsche, since pregnancy is always the beginning of a new state of affairs. Nietzsche as a result often wrote about becoming a physiologist of morals and ideas. He suggested that mind and body are prone to the same type of disorders and responses to remedies. Thus it was Wagner's music which eventually made him ill and for a remedy he turned to Mozart's *Requiem*.

Digestive metaphors were important in Nietzsche's analysis and style of presentation of ideas. Nietzsche typically wrote about the advantages which came from the intestines and commented on the sluggish quality of German bowels as a consequence of eating soup before the main meal and living on over-boiled meat, greasy vegetables and soggy puddings. Poor physical digestion gave rise ultimately to mental indigestion. Like Feuerbach, Nietzsche conceived of eating as a basic appropriation of nature by human activity. Eating is a primary link between existing and thinking.

Clearly, Nietzsche's use of the term 'body' was highly complex; it was also illusive and humorous; Richard Schacht (1985, p. 270) warns us against taking Nietzsche too literally. While Nietzsche proposed to take 'the body and physiology' as 'the starting point' of his philosophy, he was obviously not a materialist in any simple fashion. He also frequently employed the reference to the body as a shock tactic. For example, he commented that 'perhaps the entire evolution of the spirit is a question of the body' (*WP*, section 676). One consistent aim was, however, to avoid the rigid dichotomization in conventional philosophy between mind/body and spirit/matter. In fact, Schacht offers a useful summary of Nietzsche's purpose. Against Spinoza's monism, Nietzsche

seeks instead to develop a naturalistic conception of human reality which takes as its point of departure our status as instances of a certain form of life among others, holds to this perspective in dealing with all aspects of our experience and activity, and shuns both the 'soul-hypothesis' *and* the 'thing-hypothesis' in doing so. (Schacht, 1985, p. 271)

To this account, we would add three qualifications. First, the body was an essential feature of Nietzsche's view of the will-to-power as embodied resistance. Second, my body is set within the everyday world of social reciprocity. Thirdly, the fact of our embodiment became an important part of Nietzsche's view of the notion of health as a moral measurement of social development. The notion of the body was not merely a convenient metaphor for Nietzsche.

However, Nietzsche saw the body, its health and its illness, in very individualized terms. It is not that I possess a body, but rather that I possess my body or in more elegant terms the issue is that I am uniquely embodied. Unlike Foucault, Nietzsche did not regard the body as the uniform product of administrative practices, since he was concerned to give an account of being an unreflective immediacy. Nietzsche's rejection of the uniform body was part of a more general hostility to quantification which in Nietzsche's terms falsely presupposed a uniformity amongst objects. For Nietzsche, the body is not uniform and more importantly my experience of my body is necessarily unique and special. Nietzsche wrote that

There is no health as such, and all attempts to define a thing that way have been wretched failures. Even the determination of what is healthy for your body depends upon your goal, your horizon, your energies, your impulses, your errors and above all on the ideals and phantasms of your soul. Thus there are innumerable healths of the body; and the more we allow the unique and the incomparable to raise its head again, and the more we abjure the dogma of the 'equality of men', the more must the concept of a normal health, along with a

196

normal diet, and the normal course of an illness, be abandoned by the medical men. (*GS*, section 120)

This notion of the unique individuality of embodiment would be quite foreign to Foucault's account of the body as an effect of anatomical maps, political practices, and juridical procedures. In short, Nietzsche's commitment to the body as a topic of analysis has a closer relationship to Epicurean materialism, the writings of the young Marx, and to Feuerbach's sensualism than to structural analysis. Nietzsche sought therefore to present an account of the lived body as the focus of moral debate rather than a history of the rationalization of the body by discipline. For Nietzsche, health is the aim of vigorous individuals and valuable societies; his philosophy was grounded in the moral values of healthy existence in opposition to dis-ease and this commitment to embodiment as a value flowed from his perception of the significance of the Dionysian principle of formless energy.

This analysis of Nietzsche and Foucault as theorists of the body is controversial. For example, Allan Megill (1985) has argued that Nietzsche and Foucault shared a common aesthetic view of the body as a construction. They are anti-naturalistic in regarding nature as the product of human subjectivity. Unlike marcuse and the critical theorists, Foucault did not celebrate the joys of instinctual pleasures, because he rejected any notion of a natural order. We might add to this interpretation the assumption that some aspects of Foucault's anti-naturalist perspective on the body were derived from Antonin Artaud's irrationalism. While Artaud had regarded the body as the seat of emotions through which life can be realized, he came to hate the body, whose unity was destroyed by its organs (Esslin, 1976, p. 105). Artaud asserted that human freedom and autonomy could only be achieved once man had been given 'a body without organs'. His revolutionary aesthetics of cruelty were part of a critique of Marxism as merely another form of rational domination. The critical edge of the view of the body in Nietzsche, Artaud and Foucault is an attempt to shock us out of a conceptual complacency with the normal and the natural. Their aesthetic doctrine was part of a Dionysian critique of systems, whether of Socrates or Hegel. Although there are similarities, we would argue that Nietzsche, in addition to a metaphorical view of the body, had a clear appreciation of instinctual life and existence as embodiment. It is difficult to understand the will-to-power in a completely anti-naturalist framework.

While Foucault belongs to a French tradition which opposes rationality as regulation through an aesthetic critique, Nietzsche's view of the body was profoundly shaped by the will-to-life philosophies of the German rejection of Hegel. As we have seen, Nietzsche's analysis of the will, tragedy and values was closely associated with the philosophy of Schopenhauer. Nietzsche derived the idea of will as ceaseless motion, which is always becoming and ceasing, from Schopenhauer. In the *Parerga and Paralipomena*, Schopenhauer described life in almost Darwinistic terminology:

Our existence has no foundation to support it except the ever-fleeting and vanishing present; and so constant *motion* is essentially its form, without any possibility of that rest for which we are longing. We resemble a man running down hill who would inevitably fall if he tried to stop, and who keeps on his legs only by continuing to run ... Thus restlessness is the original form of existence. (Schopenhauer, 1974, 2, p. 284)

This ceaseless motion is kept up by two tendencies (hunger and the sexual impulse) aided by boredom. The body is an outward manifestation of the will, but it is also the case that our moral and intellectual life is an effect of our organs. If we are angry or annoyed, this is 'an excess of bile'; if we are worried or anxious, it is 'probably the intestines' (Schopenhauer, 1974, vol. 2, p. 176). We disguise such inconvenient facts by intellectualization. This perspective was even more evident in *The World as Will and Representation* where he argued that

the parts of the body must correspond completely to the chief demands and desires by which the will manifests itself ... Teeth, gullet, and intestinal canal are objectified hunger; the genitals are objectified sexual impulse; grasping hands and nimble feet correspond to the more indirect strivings of the will which they represent. (Schopenhauer, 1969, 1, p. 108)

Nietzsche took this philosophy of will and transformed it into a joyous acceptance of our being-in-the-world. Schopenhauer's negative philosophy of will (the Buddhist acceptance of the world and aspiration for nirvana) was replaced by the pessimism of strength as the main alternative to nihilism.

Finally, there was a fundamental difference between Nietzsche and Foucault in terms of the emphasis on inter-subjectivity and reciprocity. Indeed, the nature of everyday reciprocity was largely absent from Foucault's work as a whole. We have argued throughout this study that Nietzsche placed a special emphasis on the primacy of the 'little things' of everyday life, because he saw intellectualized reasoning as derivative and parasitic upon this more significant world of experience and social reciprocity. Unlike Weber, Nietzsche had an important commitment to the value of habitual, affectual action over against instrumental rationality. Although Nietzsche's conception of a moral/healthy life was essentially aristocratic, he gave a primacy to the 'little things' of everyday interaction against the regulating superstructure of institutions. Unlike Foucault, Nietzsche gave a priority to the experiential quality of embodiment in the ordinary world of mundane phenomena. Foucault, in fact, had little conception of everyday reality as the basis for social reciprocity and as the framework for the essential flux of human experience. In this study, against Foucault's abstract notion of the body as an effect, we have focused upon the nature of embodiment, empowerment and enselfment as three dimensions of human lived experience within the everyday *habitus*. This has been the main way in which we have attempted to develop the notion of resentment, reciprocity and resistance.

Embodiment

In our view a sociology of embodiment would need to address itself to fundamental questions of phenomenology. We can best express the nature of social embodiment through a series of paradoxes and these paradoxes bring out the somewhat limited nature of Foucault's treatment of the body. As social individuals we experience our body as a natural limit and as a fixed environment which constricts and constrains our movements and our desires. This physical environment however is also my environment over which I enjoy considerable sovereignty and spontaneous control. While certain categories of persons do not own their bodies (for example, slaves), there is a phenomenological argument to the effect that we have spontaneous, immediate and sovereign grasp of our bodies. This paradox can be expressed in the notion that, while I have a body, I also am a body. My body is a lived, immediate presence rather than simply an alien, foreign and strange objective environment. In practical terms, the demise of my body is also my personal demise and the termination of my being is co-terminous with the history of my particular body. This paradox can also be rendered in the notion that, while I have a body, there is a sense in which, through body techniques, I also do a body. As writers like Erving Goffman have recognized, our embodiment requires continual and regular practices of body work whereby I constantly maintain, manage and present my physical presence within a social context, where my prestige may well hinge crucially on my embodied presence in social encounters. That is, I must undertake face-work and body-repair in order to avoid the damaging results of embarrassment and misdemeanour. My face is fundamental to my social prestige and the avoidance of stigmatization is crucial to the presentation of myself as a valued entity.

These features of our embodiment are brought into the foreground as a consequence of our experience of disease. A dis-ease is a form of alienation when we partly lose control over our bodies; our organs are experienced as things. The phenomenology of accident and disease has been brilliantly captured by Oliver Sacks in a number of volumes on specific maladies (Parkinson's disease, migraine and Anton's syndrome). Following a climbing accident, Sacks in *A Leg to Stand On* (1986) describes how he experienced his useless limb as an object and as an absence. This crisis was rather like suffering an 'internal amputation' which came ultimately to challenge his sense of reality and of being. The insanity of the amputee has been described as 'somatophrenia phantastica', in which a phantom limb brings about a confusion of reality. These crises of being raise questions about personal identity which can result in a 'neuro-existential pathology'. In the last analysis therefore, our sense of certainty is a body-experience.

Foucault's residual structuralism prevented the development of a social phenomenology of embodiment as the seat of resistance – as the locus of the will-to-power of being. By contrast, Nietzsche did anticipate an analysis of embodiment as a necessary feature of the philosophy of will. In addition, Nietzsche turned Schopenhauer's pessimistic analysis of motion into a Dionysian celebration. While we may be compelled to run down hill, running may also be an exhilarating experience – better to run than to lose a leg, better still to dance down hills.

Following this comment on the paradoxes of embodiment, we have argued that sociology has three important tasks. These are the analysis of human embodiment, which we have argued is to be combined with the notions of empowerment and enselfment. Our personal embodiment is subjective and powerful. This feature of the social world has been neglected by contemporary sociology and in this study we have taken the position that, in order to understand the agent within the sociology of action, we need a theory of the embodiment of persons. A theory of embodiment is a necessary component of a concept of resistance; it is the antidote to nihilistic determinism. Secondly, sociology addresses itself to the problem of exchange and reciprocity within the everyday life-world, which may be termed the habitus of action. This social *habitus* is immediate, practical, empirical, ongoing, dense and ever-present. We may regard reciprocity as the total range of ongoing exchanges of symbolic and non-symbolic goods, whereby our embodied existence is fundamentally and necessarily sustained only through social relations. My embodiment drives me to reciprocity to satisfy my needs and to give some satisfaction to my desires, but reciprocity also depends upon my needs which force me into social contact. Fellowship (*socius*) thus depends upon this constant and immediate exchange emerging out of the world of personalized need. Reciprocity is the place and the means of embodiment, whereby my requirements as an individual find expression through the social division of labour. My embodiment is highly individualized, but it is also simultaneously and inescapably social. Out of the everyday world of reciprocity, there emerges the potent sense of justice which is an essential component of struggle and opposition. The third task of sociology is the analysis of dominant institutions of the macro-social order. Corresponding to my embodiment, there is the economic realm of production and reproduction. Corresponding to my empowerment, there is the place of politics, which is both repressive and enabling. Related to my enselfment, there is the world of culture, consciousness and ideology which institutionalizes thought and communication through a system of sirens. Sociology attempts to comprehend the complex and difficult relations which exist between the macro-world of institutional regulation and the everyday world of reciprocity. The fact of my embodiment is an important linkage between these worlds. The sociology of the body is consequently not simply a new field of analysis, but a necessary part of all social investigation, since sociology as a discipline seeks to understand the fellowship which emerges out of the ongoing exchanges between embodied agents who seek to satisfy needs and desires within the dense everyday world of community; this is the *habitus* of the individual. Sociology should, as a consequence, be primarily concerned with the essentially practical activity of agents because, to develop a sociology of social actions, we need a theory of lived experience within the sensuous world of practical reality.

Nietzsche's Sociology

This presentation of the tasks of sociology suggests that a Nietzschean sociology would be perfectly possible. Given the emphasis on experience and Nietzsche's critical approach to formal rationality, we can argue that Nietzsche's sociology would assume a highly subjective, reflexive and personal character. Like Nietzsche's own philosophy, this sociology would be a reflection on our fundamentally personal experience of social phenomena through our embodied existence. Because the problem of the body is, in our view, crucial to an understanding of Nietzsche, we would also suggest that Nietzsche's sociology would aim at a reconciliation of being, being well and being social. That is, we should not accept or assume the natural science paradigm which sees questions of health as in some way distinct from questions of being, sociality and morality. Nietzsche's sociology involves a moral argument about personal genuineness through individual autonomy and the revaluation of values. This sociology of reciprocity and embodiment lends itself quite straightforwardly to a critique of ideology and state politics. The world of reciprocity provides an essential critique of the regulating force of the State and the mystifying impact of state ideology.

Although throughout this study we have been making certain assumptions about the possibility of a Nietzschean sociology, we have also accepted the view that there are certain irreconcilable conflicts between sociology as conventionally understood and Nietzsche's project. All sociology involves some conceptual standardization of social relations through an intellectualization of life. All sociology sees life in terms of some sort of system, however weakly and unsystematically this system is outlined. Since sociology emerged in the nineteenth century in response to problems of social control and stability in European society, it is itself part of the web of knowledge and power. Sociology in certain respects complements the work of the State in providing essential elements of social knowledge which become the basis for social control. Nietzsche, by contrast, as we have seen, argued forcefully against the very notion of the normal, the regular and the standard. Like Kierkegaard, Nietzsche was concerned to understand the extraordinary. He thought that the very process of counting was often based upon a misunderstanding, or at least that quantitative processes presuppose a certain uniformity which was taken for granted. The implication of this position is that Nietzsche's philosophy could not be reconciled with a discipline which required such notions as the 'role' and 'status'. These notions can only apply to people who are not yet free; they apply to people who have not yet learnt to resist because they are not moral agents.

A number of commentators on Nietzsche have suggested that in face he had no notion of the 'social', since his thought was fixed on the moral life of the individual. It has been claimed that

For all this talk of 'wholeness', Nietzsche is not seriously concerned to envisage a whole *society*. He envisages the whole *man*, but he shows insufficient interest

202

in the social patterns which would facilitate and sustain his wholeness. The excessive individualism of his interpretation of Greek art is matched by the nature of his concern for the creative individual and the social needs of his creative individuality at the expense of society's other members or functions. (Silk and Stern, 1981, p. 284)

Faced with the horror existence, we have three escape routes (religion, art and science), but these adaptations are also highly individualistic. Other critics have complained that Nietzsche's emphasis on artistic individuality and his critique of religious asceticism are now wholly anachronistic, providing no valuable commentary of the problems of modern society (Stephens, 1986). Other critics have claimed that the liberating social doctrine of Dionysus was limited by Nietzsche's authoritarian conception of a morality of rank (Schutte, 1984).

It is obvious that Nietzsche had no project to write a professional sociology and it is equally clear that he had no intention to provide a philosophical system of social relations. In his 'maxims and arrows' in the opening sections of the *Twilight of the Idols*, Nietzsche observed that 'the will to a system is a lack of integrity'. However, insofar as Nietzsche's philosophy is individualistic, the individualism has no relationship to utilitarian individualism. Nietzsche's 'individualism' is grounded in the affectual life – the embodiment – of the person. For Nietzsche, social institutions develop in response to affects and instincts. In particular, Greek institutions arose from the 'preventive measures' which evolved to safeguard individuals from 'their inner explosives' (*TI*, section 10, p. 3). The Socratic philosophers of ancient Greece constituted a cultural trend against the creative force of 'the agonal instinct'. He consistently emphasized the importance of sexuality as a force which overshelms individuality. However, society is only possible once a certain regularization of the person has taken place; once the free man has become standardized. In fact, to get 'into' society, there must be a profound transformation (or civilization) of the instinctual drives; in this sense, social man is a form of corruption through socialization. In *On the Genealogy of Morals*, he complained that, on entering social life, human animals

were reduced to thinking, inferring, reckoning, co-ordinating cause and effect, these unfortunate creatures; they were reduced to their 'consciousness', their weakest and most fallible organ! (*GM*, II, p. 16)

The existence of social relations requires an internalization of instinctual energies and it is this inhibition which has both positive and negative consequences. The negative included religion, asceticism and neurosis; the positive, art and music. It follows that thinking and creating are fundamentally social activities; they represent the way in which Dionysian elements have been harnessed by Apollian forms inside social relations. Society exists as a consequence of the transformation of the biological structure of the species. However, a moral person must continually rise above this standardization in order to experience moral autonomy. The main point of this commentary is, however, to note that, in writing about social institutions, Nietzsche starts with the facts of our instinctual substructure.

While Nietzsche's formulation of problems often appears to be individualistic, his analysis of moral systems, historical change and power assumes that these phenomena must be social. For example, in *Human, All Too Human*, he provided a historical account of the emergence of virtue which is a form of political sociology. Morality grows out of compulsion which eventually becomes merely conventional. Social relations which are regarded as conventional finish by assuming a natural quality. Once they are natural, they become linked to a notion of gratifications. Over a long period of time, these patterns of compulsion are regarded as virtues. The consequence is that to be moral is to be obedient to established traditions which has the paradox of undermining the moral autonomy of individuals. These moral systems are essential for the preservation of a community and moral behaviour is an effect of society. Therefore, conscience is not the voice of God in human beings, but the result of socialization which makes us feel guilt at the transgression of a norm. These moral norms make humanity calculable; they convert our untutored animality into calculated social relations. However, Nietzsche insisted that, while our instinctual equipment can be transformed, it cannot be destroyed. Social life is, as a result, a constant tension between instinctual desire, moralities, group conflicts and regulation. It is evident from this commentary that Nietzsche, far from neglecting social existence, made social phenomena a critical aspect of his understanding of history, culture and politics. Nietzsche was not primarily an anti-sociological thinker; he was a critic of system.

Traditional sociology, even when it emphasized action over system, was committed to the idea of structure, determination and constraint. It would be difficult to conceive of sociology without some reference to structural limitations on action. The moral core of Nietzsche's philosophy was by contrast centred on the overman who triumphs over these limitations on being and these determinations of existence. Nietzsche was a moral theorist of non-determination. While his philosophy would be incompatible with the notion of structural determinations of all individuals, it is not entirely clear that Nietzsche's view of the subject would be compatible with a sociology of action. It may be that the origins of the sociology of action go back to Kantian philosophy with its emphasis on the rational, subjective 'I'. For Nietzsche, however, the presumption of action is grounded in the mythical autonomy of the cognitive 'I' and therefore we might say in a Nietzschean way that 'it thinks'. Nietzsche rejected the overt universalism of Kant's moral system as merely the expression of the peculiarities of Kant's own life. On both counts, Nietzsche's project may be incompatible with the sociology of structure.

Within the framework of the post-modernist debate, one might ask whether sociology itself is a discipline limited to the modernist period, namely to the period between say 1850 and 1968. If we regard Comte as the author of the science of society as a science of constraints, then sociology must be incompatible with Nietzsche's principal assumptions, since he called into question both structure and subject. Post-modernism is attached to the notion of the triumph of subjectivity over structure, perspectivism over fixed values, contingency over determination, terror over complacency. Putting this problem in terms of Durkheim and classical sociology, we might consider the relationship between Nietzsche's notion of the death of God and the importance of causality in sociology. We have seen that Nietzsche identified the death of God positively as the discovery of personal potentiality, that is, the discovery of capacities which are not subordinated to some absolute being. The death of God is the liberation of subjectivism and individual exploration, free from conventional moral constraint. It was the great historical signal for humanity to adopt Nietzsche's moral maxim – 'Become the person you are'. These moral constraints of a religious era were in Nietzsche's philosophy conceptualised as negative and unhealthy.

In the sociology of Durkheim, it is clear that God is dead, since in *The Elementary Forms of the Religious Life* he attempted to analyse the nature of social existence without theistic presuppositions. The problem of social integration for Durkheim was linked with the absence of an absolute standard whereby the world of values could escape from the problem of relativism. However, there is in Durkheim's sociology an implicit theme that God equals society. Having analysed the death of God and the disappearance of a society based upon mechanical solidarity, Durkheim substituted 'society' for 'God' in order to explain and bring about a new integration of secular society. In this respect sociology in its conservative phase did not liberate the subjective individual from constraint, but merely rewrote the traditional theological constraints under the vocabulary of society. Insofar as 'God' now equalled 'society', we can argue that the sociology of the nineteenth century was in fact always a social theology. Nietzsche by contrast ruled out an appeal to stability, where this stability would have to rely upon some substitute for an absolute God. In this respect, Nietzsche's project was incompatible with classical sociology. Nietzsche might however provide a social theory of post-modernity as the sequel to classical sociology. To answer the question 'is sociology compatible with Nietzsche's philosophy?' we will also have to return to Simmel, since in many respects we could regard some features of Simmel's sociology as the solution to problems raised by Nietzsche about the problem of modern existence.

There are certain obvious parallels between Simmel and Nietzsche, some of which we have already alluded to in earlier sections of this study. The most obvious parallel would be between Nietzsche's perspectivism and Simmel's relativism, a relativism which is often associated with the special character of Berlin in the time of Simmel's student days. There is also the emphasis on aesthetic values in Simmel which some would regard as also crucial to Nietzsche (Megill, 1985). More importantly, there is the emphasis on the fleeting everyday world of experience as opposed to the larger structural concepts of bureaucracy, institution and society. It is well known that Simmel sought to avoid the reification of such concepts as 'society' through his emphasis on sociation. We should note that

concepts such as 'social structure', 'social systems' and even 'social institution' play a very subordinate role in his sociology. From his early work onwards, Simmel (1890) was at pains to avoid the reification or hypostatization of 'society', insisting instead that 'society is not en entity fully enclosed within itself, an absolute identity, anymore than is the human individual. Compared with the real interactions of the past, it is only secondary only the result' . . . sociology should therefore not concern itself with a reified notion of society but with social interaction and forms of sociation. (Frisby, 1985, p. 53)

This line of argument in Simmel was particularly prominent in his *The Philosophy of Money* where he saw the institutional world of monetary exchange emerging out of the life process of reciprocity and interdependence. Just as in Nietzsche's philosophy where there is the tension and contradiction between the life-force and state institutions, so in Simmel's sociology there was the more general tragedy of the contradiction between the content of action and the forms of social relationship. It is possible therefore to see Simmel's sociology as a development of Nietzsche's critique of modernity and Nietzsche's opposition to reified notions like the State and ideology. For both Nietzsche and Simmel, sociology would be a project within the wider analysis of the emergent category of 'humanity' out of animality. The argument here therefore is that the notion of society as a system of determinations is limited to a specific epoch where deterministic forms of analysis were relevant and possible. Both Marxism and sociology within this perspective would be the world-views of a specific period and relevant to a particular conjuncture of events (such as the rise of industrial capitalism). However, if we follow the position of Simmel, it may be that a form of sociology could survive which would address itself to the patterns of sociation and to the realm of reciprocity as the arena of genuine feeling and experience. While it is the case that Simmel carried out the project of Nietzsche, we would argue that Simmel's sociology does not really come to terms with the question of embodiment and with the relations which exist between embodiment, reciprocity, resentment and institutions. The importance of the revival of Nietzsche in contemporary French and German social theory is that it makes once more possible the development of a sociology of embodiment in the framework of an analysis of reciprocity in everyday life.

Conclusion: against Hegel

We can see many aspects of modern thought as a reaction against the philosophical system of Hegel. In the nineteenth century, we can identify three major alternatives to Hegelianism. First, Feuerbach rejected Hegel's idealism and developed his own version of sensualism as a moral criterion of human action. Secondly, Kierkegaard argued that Hegel's analysis of religion was actually incompatible with the nature of faith as it had developed in the Old Testament (Hohlenberg, 1954). Kierkegaard in *Fear and Trembling*, for example, showed that the religion of Abraham was not based on universalistic reason but on the absurdity of faith. Thirdly, Schopenhauer turned Hegel on his head by giving primacy to will over knowledge. By regarding all will as evil, Schopenhauer also developed a pessimistic theory of personal resignation which was completely incompatible with Hegelian teleological optimism. These reactions against the Hegelian system had a number of common dimensions. They rejected Hegel's theory of politics which saw the Prussion state as the highest achievement of universal rationalism. They emphasized the centrality of the will and spontaneous experience over abstract knowledge; they opposed the individual to the system. They were in some respects irrationalists by grasping the importance of the absurd in human life.

These critical responses to Hegel provided the context for Nietzsche's own critique of the legacy of Hegelian philosophy. Nietzsche rejected Hegelian rationalism, partly on the grounds of perspectivism whereby truths are merely interpretations. Following Schopenhauer, he gave a centrality to will over knowledge; reasoning was in fact rationalization. He regarded Hegel as a philosopher without integrity, because of the Hegelian commitment to a system. Hegelian idealism was characteristic of professional philosophers who 'are prejudiced against appearance, change, pain, death, the corporeal, the senses, fate and bondage, the aimless' (*WP*, section 407). Nietzsche placed the main emphasis on existence, not knowledge.

While Nietzsche did not read Kierkegaard, their view of philosophy was obviously similar. Karl Jaspers (1955) argued that they were both hostile to the pretensions of reasoning and therefore suspicious of professional philosophers. They were radical opponents of the 'syustem'. They both regarded existence as open to infinite interpretation, and they chose indirect rather than direct methods of communicating a new existential truth. Their thought converged on the central problem of being, and hence laid the foundation for Heidegger's *Sein und Zeit*.

This critique of Hegel from the perspective of 'existentialism' entered modern sociology, as we have seen, via Tönnies, Simmel and Weber as a critical response to the dominance of *Gemeinschaft*-relations in modern capitalism. The negative response to Hegelianism has also been a major feature of contemporary French social thought in the work of Foucault and his followers. Foucault's opposition to systems and disciplines, his celebration of existence against knowledge, and his fascination for the absurd represent a translation of Nietzsche into contemporary idioms. Foucault has used Nietzsche primarily as a criticism of the regulation of spontaneity by systems of power/knowledge and the subordination of the individual by a panoptic state.

7

The Jest of Modernity

The Absence and Return of Nietzsche

In this study of Nietzsche, we have attempted to restore the presence of Nietzsche in the origins and development of contemporary social theory by considering, in particular, the work of Weber, Freud, Adorno and Foucault. This retrieval of Nietzsche has been conducted within a debate around modernity, post-modernity and nostalgia, in which we have explored certain themes in Nietzsche as the genesis of the crisis of modern values. We have sought a solution to certain features of this problem through the analysis of the body and desire. Finally, following Nietzsche's concept of a joyful science, we have developed joyful sociology through an exploration of embodiment, reciprocity and resistance. In this conclusion, we offer a brief outline of this retrieval and reflect upon the ongoing question of modernism and post-modernism in relation to the problem of ethics and aesthetics.

In recent years, there has been a cascade of publications noting the continuing relevance and importance of the issues raised by Nietzsche for modern thought, but specifically for contemporary social theory (Dews, 1986; Deleuze, 1983; Gross, 1986; Kroker, 1985; Pütz, 1981). By giving some emphasis to Nietzsche as a positive life-philosopher, we have located him alongside Schopenhauer as philosophers of the will whose critique of culture was also largely motivated by an anti-Hegelian argument against system and systems. Nietzsche's philosophy, and especially his epistemology, ruled out any resort to system as a substitute for God, since Nietzsche, accepting the necessity of a view of reality as chaotic becoming, could not accept any analysis of being as anything other than a metaphor. Nietzsche's philosophy can, in this respect, be regarded as a critique of ideologies which provide a false comfort whether in religion, science or nationalism. While this

Nietzschean epistemology is well known and extensively commented upon, we have drawn particular attention to what we have called Nietzsche's doctorine of the little things. Nietzsche provides a philosophy of the *habitus* of the everyday world and the world of reciprocities against the larger structures of institutional formation which regulate and restrain the sensuous practicality of actions. Nietzsche was a philosopher against a repressive state-apparatus which over-regulated life, crushing all individuality. He was consequently against philosophers who were servants of the state. While Nietzsche's critique of the state and of state-ideologies has to be seen, initially within the context of German society, his perspective clearly has wider relevance. In particular, Nietzsche's perspective provides a profound criticism both of the historical process of rationalization and of instrumental reason as one of the foundations of the iron cage of bureaucratic capitalism. Nietzsche's position offers a critical account of the relationship between knowledge and power in the form of rational institutions, or at least in the form of instrumental rationalism. While our study has been primarily focused upon an attempt to elucidate this position on reciprocity, resentment and desire, we have in the process of developing that position, been forced to comment upon the suppression of Nietzsche in the perspective of twentieth-century social thought.

The presence of Nietzsche in Weberian sociology is associated with a series of tensions in Weber's work around the issues of power, economics and morality which resulted in the famous set of contradictions in his work between charisma and reason, individual and society, science and meaning. The main problem for Weber was, given the death of God proclaimed by Nietzsche, how action or science were possible in a world without guidelines, a social existence without firm directions or a personal orientation without some sense of absolutism. The absence of purpose in a world without sure moral guidelines undermined the possibility of personality in the Weberian sense. Weber's heroic attempt to construct a sociology of meaningful action in a world of secular culture was his response to the problem of meaninglessness as an effect and condition for science. Whereas Nietzsche had celebrated the end of theological absolutism, Weber confronted the gap left by God as a crisis for value freedom in a polytheistic but secular culture. This question of legitimacy lay behind the whole debate in Weber on authority and power with special reference to the state and the Church. At a more personal level, the challenge from Nietzsche was how to remain an honest man as an employee of the state, especially the state left by Bismarck's administration. In short, within Weberian sociology the impact of Nietzsche is to be seen around the unresolved questions of personal and moral authenticity, whether in politics or science. Weber's answer to Nietzsche was located in the development of a theory of the calling or vocation (*Beruf*) in science and politics.

For Nietzsche of course, knowledge was fundamentally related to human interests, since it both served interest and also helped to determine it. What was central to *The Birth of Tragedy* was the rejection of the naive rational optimism of Socratic philosophy. While Nietzsche regarded science, religion and, more generally, artistic culture as, in the last instance, illusions, they were necessary illusions. He argued, therefore, that even to survive human beings had to shape, direct and constitute reality, not simply for a personal sense of security, but on the basis of the 'utility of preservation' as he argued in *The Will to Power*. He rejected abstract theorizing insofar as it was useless from the point of view of real preservation. Against the false optimism of Darwinism and positivism, he posed the alternative in Dionysus as a direct perception into the reality of things. While Nietzsche saw knowledge forged in the conflict of interests, Weber turned Nietzsche's cultural critique into a psychology of resentment by subordinate strata. That is, he converted Nietzsche's global critique into the limited question of the religious origins of economic ultilitarianism. Nietzsche regarded resentment not simply as the basis of religious culture, but fundamental to the emergence of rationality itself as an asceticism of the mind, as the ascetic ideal.

Whereas Christianity had resolved the problem of the world through a salvation drive, Weber, in the idea of a secular ethic, transformed this quest into a political or scientific calling. By contrast, Nietzsche had regarded such intellectualism as a mere illusion, a protection against the chaotic flux of the world of becoming; intellectualism converted this problem into the conceptual apparatus of being. While this very rationalistic intellectualism in the West laid one foundation of modernity, namely its meaninglessness, Weber sought a way out of this dilemma through a vocational ethics of responsibility, thereby blocking off the challenge of Nietzsche to revalue values through a resolution of the Dionysian life-affirming principle and the Apollonian principle of form against Socrates – the final solution of Dionysus versus the Christ.

However, Weber, to some extent, shared Nietzsche's fascination for prophecy and charismatic ethical leadership. In Weber's view of the Old Testament prophet, prophecy rejected the heard in favour of a collection of enlightened disciples who, in renouncing the world, found a new form of personality. Genuine prophecy rejected the admiration of

211

the herd in favour of the solitude of the desert. Nietzsche's relationship to charismatic breakthrough remained somewhat ambiguous (Schutte, 1984). On the one hand, Dionysus provided an alternative to nihilism through the life-affirming principle of community, reciprocity and sexuality; on the other, Nietzsche's rejection of the herd and the doctrine of the Higher Man created an ethic of elitism which has proved difficult to reconcile with the doctrine of the little things. A similar tension is present in Weber's notion of domination and authority through charisma. Through the metaphor of the iron cage, Weber, almost against his secular ethics, looked towards a charismatic revival in Germany which would provide an alternative to the deadening consequences of rationalism through bureaucracy. For the heard, however, life would become increasingly subject to rationalization and disenchantment which would bring about a new regime of discipline over the body, the everyday life and mundane pleasures.

Any discussion of ethics in sociology must lead to an analysis of the person and the individual in relation to action and responsibility. While Weber's sociology was overtly based upon the methodological individualism, Nietzsche was quite sceptical of the assumption of 'the individual' as an organizing principle of experience and action. For Nietzsche, the plurality of the person could not be rendered in the unitary concept of individual. Weber also adhered to a highly rationalistic notion of action which gave a privileged position to the notions of rational choice and instrumental rationality. Thus, another conflict or tension between Nietzsche's viewpoint and Weber's rests on the relationship between experience, desire and intellectualism. The rationalization of experience by intellectualism is, for Nietzsche, yet another form of resentment and no-saying philosophy. The rationalism of the state-philosopher was merely an effect of resentment, nihilism and the ascetic ideal. We have argued in this inquiry into Nietzsche that Nietzsche's philosophy has more in common with Kierkegaard's existentialist philosophy which was critical of the notion that an intellectual could ever be an employee of the state. There were significant conflicts between Nietzsche's view of professionalism in intellectual affairs and Weber's commitment to a professional ethic in the calling of science and to the ethic of responsibility in human affairs. Nietzsche regarded all state intellectuals as necessarily a contradiction in terms.

Against these forms of rationalism, Nietzsche sought to rediscover the world of feeling, emotion and taste. He also sought to expose the strong passions behind conventional moral categories in Christianity and Kantian philosophy. There are therefore certain superficial parallels between Freudianism and Nietzsche's philosophy; for example, there is a surface relationship between Freud's personality theory in terms of the struggle between the id and the super-ego, and Nietzsche's historical analysis of desire, reason and art in the contrast between Dionysus and Apollo. In more general terms, there is an overt parallel between Freud's scientific critique of religion in relationship to libidinous forces and Nietzsche's critique of Christianity as an ascetic morality which denied an intuitive enjoyment of pleasure. More importantly, Nietzsche's notion that sickness is a consequence of the will-to-power turned against itself found its expression in Freudian psycho-analysis in the idea of the unconscious and in the theory of sublimation. Resentment is a contagion which transforms health into sickness; this condition prepares the way for the priest and the psychologist (Deleuze, 1983, p. 132). This theory of illness brings us back to the centrality of language in Nietzsche's philosophical treatment of sickness, namely that sickness is a metaphor for fundamental problems in social and personal interaction. More recent interpretations of Freud by Lacan (1977) have drawn attention to the role of language in Freudianism, namely that Freudian psycho-analytic treatment involves the analysis of the metaphors and mistakes of the language of the sick and diseased. Freud following Nietzsche rediscovered the role of the unconscious and the subconscious in personal and social relations, or at least the disguising of the role of sexuality in social relations.

We have contrasted Nietzsche's philosophical doubts with the labours of Freud and Weber as professional men of science. Nietzsche celebrated dance and laughter over laborious reasoning. While Freud and Weber were ambiguous with respect to their intellectual dependence on Nietzsche, they were also highly ambiguous as to the role of religion and civilization in the historical management of violence, desire and feeling. At one level, both Weber and Freud argued that human beings cannot be entirely happy or at home insofar as they subordinate themselves to the social requirements of discipline and order under the canopy of religion. However, it is also the case that religion makes society possible (an idea which Durkheim developed at great length). Both Weber and Freud sought a solution to the dilemma of religion and social order through the development of a scientific attitude of responsibility which involved a certain resignation to the realities of a post-God world. With the collapse of a religious vocation, the political/scientific calling became the plausible outlet for people of serious intentions. This resignation for Nietzsche was still a form of resentment and, rather than leading to an optimistic modernism, was more pessimistic in its view of the iron cage and the constant threat of irrationalism.

We can see these various options in Durkheim, Freud and Weber as scientific attempts to come to terms with certain moral problems in the modern world. In certain respects, they were themselves part of the legacy of German philosophical analysis of the problem of will and world which were perspectives which evolved through the philosophy of Schopenhauer and Nietzsche. In one sense, Weber's analysis of religious orientations to the world (that is, mysticism and asceticism) represents, in his own science, the polar positions of flight and control. Nietzsche, Weber and Freud rejected the pessimism of the will which was entailed by Schopenhauer's mystical orientation to the meaninglessness of the world as a satisfactory solution, but Weber and Freud thought that, despite the chaos of values, scientific realism and resignation would be the only possible approach to the crisis of modernism. These orientations were sharply contrasted with Nietzsche's own optimism of the will, the celebration of the everyday world of experience, the rejection of science and rationalism, the optimism of the doctrine of Eternal Return and the call for a revaluation of values.

Since Nietzsche (somewhat like Marx) saw human knowledge as serving the interests of human beings, he, in his genealogy of tragedy, identified three major and necessary illusions which make life bearable. For Nietzsche, all civilization is articulated at the higher levels of knowledge, art and faith. More specifically, these involve the Socratic commitment to knowledge and reason, the Apollonian shaping of art and the Dionysian faith in the indestructability of existence. These great cultural illusions make human existence in the world tolerable as consequences of shaping it by meaning. Corresponding to these three principles, we find different cultural systems in human history, namely the Socratic systems of knowledge, the Hellenic systems of art and the Buddhistic systems of tragic culture. For Nietzsche, the contemporary world is shaped by this Socratic impulse whereby through the 'theoretical man' all dominant human values become cognitive. This theoretical man is the isolated, competitive, contemplative hero of higher culture. While this Socratic culture is dominant, it is also permanently in a state of crisis, since reason must always discover its own limits and thereby recoil upon itself as merely a limitation, and even an illusion.

Critical theory in Germany was, in many respects, a response to the negative impact of instrumental reason which had degenerated not only through capitalist systems of exploitation, but into the gas chambers of the Nazi period. The enlightenment project had turned upon itself through the rational imposition of instrumental knowledge in the form of the administered society which precluded, not only substantive criticism, but also the autonomy of the individual. While the critical theorists overtly drew from Marx, their whole project was covertly a debate with the Nietzsche legacy. In philosophical terms, the critical theorists indirectly depended upon Nietzsche's theory of knowledge, since it was Nietzsche who undermined the possibility of an identity theory by showing that knowledge is never simply the reproduction of an external objective reality. Knowledge is always in the service of human interests and is profoundly shaped by the world of everyday requirements. Because Nietzsche felt that both the State and reason were mere illusions, his philosophy was antagonistic to the confident rationalism of the nineteenth century, especially nineteenth-century positivism. Since knowledge and being exclude each other, there can never be any simple identity between reality and the knowing subject. Because Nietzsche was so profoundly conscious of the fictional in thought, his philosophical critique lent itself naturally to a critical theory of ideology. Nietzsche's epistemology does however also give rise to serious philosophical problems, despite the power of its critique of positivism (Rorty, 1986).

Although Nietzsche was somewhat remote from the younger generation of critical theorists, his rejection of cultural philistinism was particularly influential. In particular, Nietzsche remained a profound source of opposition to the instrumental rationality which had found its ultimate nihilism in the battle-fields of northern France. Of course, the critical theorists sought in an enlightenment tradition an alternative to the instrumental rationality which had become predominant in the technical sphere of modern capitalism. For critical theorists, the progressive enlightenment project was still feasible as a moral stand against the banal consumerism of modern society and the apolitical nature of capitalist democracy. Rather like Weber, therefore, they blocked off the possibility that even moral enlightenment might be merely the resentment of politically feeble intellectuals. Nietzsche, therefore, posed a significant threat for the rational project of writers like Adorno. Resistance to the world of capitalism is still based upon reason which, in Nietzsche's view, still remains based upon the prejudices of reason which assumes unity, identity, continuity, causality, substance and being in a world which is one of becoming. In short, Adorno and other critical theorists were able implicitly to accept Nietzsche's critique of modernity while rejecting his theory of knowledge. One problem in the critical theorists' response to Nietzsche is that they failed to realize that Nietzsche was not posing merely

215

psychology of knowledge, but rather criticizing certain combinations of knowledge/power in the interests of dominant institutions such as the state and its professional strata of civil servants.

By converting Nietzsche's theory of resentment into a form of psychology, the critical theorists failed to appreciate fully that the core issue in Nietzsche's philosophy was about the way of life and the form of humanity that must be generated in order to cope with the tensions and contradictions in the relationship between knowledge, morality and power. In particular, they failed to grasp the problem of intellectualism on the part of priests and scholars towards these issues. While the parallels between Nietzsche's critical theory (both in style and method) and Adorno's 'negative dialectics' have been often recognized (Held, 1980), it is commonly thought that Adorno broke from the Nietzsche tradition to develop a more profound critique of social and economic phenomena. The assumption is that Nietzsche's critical method remained at the level of individual authenticity, providing no social framework for understanding thinking and being. However, Nietzsche's views on the body, feeling, touch, reciprocity and resentment did not in fact deny the social dimensions of experience. Furthermore, while the critical theorists often became stuck within a pessimistic perspective on modern capitalism, Nietzsche sought a revaluation of values which would go beyond the pessimism associated with the German philosophical tradition. This revaluation of values had to involve a rejection of the resentment basis of thought by state officials. Nietzsche represents a distinctive response to the crises of modernism.

Modernity and its Solutions

Nietzsche's philosophy provides an index of the modern crisis, offering a framework for the key issues which have disturbed the modern consciousness as manifest in the rational project of enlightenment. These dimensions are primarily located in the problem of the death of God, that is in the evaporation of values and the crisis of modern morality but they also raise problems about the unity of the self. Very broadly speaking, Nietzsche confronted the problem of modern nihilism as manifest in bad conscience, resentment and the ascetic ideal. The institutional framework of this crisis in the German context was the growing dominance of the State, not only in political life, but over its cultural forms. This growth of state formation was furthermore associated with the emergence of a new class of professional bureaucrats, of whom Nietzsche was specifically critical. Nietzsche

216

objected to the increasing dominance in culture of the state-philosopher as a bureaucratic employee. We can, therefore, see Nietzsche's critique as a struggle against the growth of fascism and nationalism as state-ideologies and, more generally, as a critique of rationalization as the principal process of the colonization of the life-world.

Against this crisis of nihilism, we can identify four primary solutions. One response to the modernist crisis can be defined as the aesthetic solution of passivity through artistic creation. Nietzsche often took artistic activity to be the paradigm of creative yes-saying practices, because art in its purest form (in particular music) was free from the constraints of nihilism and resentment. It is in art that we appear most fully to realize our potentialities and to break through the limitations of our circumstances, becoming the person we are. This message was particularly prominent in *Beyond Good and Evil* and in *The Birth of Tragedy*. It was crucial to Nietzsche's debate with 'Wagnerism' in western culture and his rejection of the doctrine of 'art for art's sake'. Certainly, Dionysus appears to represent artistic creativity in its fullest measure without the restraints of Socratic reason. This interpretation of Nietzsche has certainly dominated some contemporary approaches to Nietzsche's philosophy, especially by Allan Megill (1985) and Alexander Nehamas (1985). However, Nietzsche's analysis of art as a stimulant of the will-to-power was very far removed from the aestheticism of Kant, Hegel and Schopenhauer. For Nietzsche, art did not deny life by reactive critique; it opened up new possibilities for action. Art was not disinterested. The idea that an aestheticization of ethics can provide a solution to post-modernist moral dilemmas has become widespread in recent debates, because it is believed that art can enhance individual experience within the private sphere. This perspective probably requires an additional philosophical position – the unity of the self.

We have identified a second solution in the work of Weber and Freud to the crisis of modernity that is a version of the ascetic ideal, which Weber transformed into the ethic of responsibility. Given the polytheism of values, Weber sought a realistic orientation to modernity through the ethic of responsibility institutionalized in the roles of the politician and the man of science. Following the myth described in the *Dialectic of Enlightenment*, Weber metaphorically strapped himself to the mast of life in order to avoid the digressions and attractions of everyday pleasures and personal diversions. Against the crisis of morality, Weber set his stern face, embracing the life of ascetic denial within the context of the state institutions of science and political leadership. We believe a similar orientation is to be found in the work of Freud who, rejecting the life principle, identified himself with the necessities of culture against the pleasures of sexuality. This theme of denial as the basis of capitalism was also present in the work of the critical theorists who, through the work of Marcuse, attempted to develop an alternative ethic which took recognition of the liberating potential of hedonism. The ideal of a vocation in science is probably no longer available in our times, because there is profound suspicion at the popular level against the claims of science to disinterestedness. More important, there are major doubts about instrumental rationality as an orientation.

A third solution to the problem of modernism can be found in the nostalgic negation of the present in favour of some imaginary society constituted prior to the devastating effects of urbanism, industrialization and rational culture. The modern is rejected through some backward-looking reconstitution of communities prior to the destruction of the life-world by industrial capitalist systems of exploitation. The nostalgic metaphor dominated classical sociology which, through a series of dichotomies, celebrated the simplicity and coherence of the rural past. These metaphorical dichotomies converged on the basic distinction between *Gemeinschaft* and *Gesellschaft* which combined the primary contrasts between rural and urban, magical and rational, traditional and modern. The dichotomy was essentially a distinction between two forms of will. This metaphor of nostalgic times was, in classical sociology, often the expression of a somewhat conservative evaluation of the present in favour of status, sacred and community over the anonymous world of the contemporary city.

It is possible to detect certain nostalgic themes in Nietzsche which were associated with the legacy of Hellenism, despite the fact that Nietzsche was highly critical of the contemporary view of Greek culture as tranquil, orderly and secure. Nietzsche gave a special emphasis to the violence and contradictions of classical pre-Socratic Greece. The conflicts on the sports-field and in the polis were institutionalized forms of violence which, in Nietzsche's view, kept Greek society healthy. The expression of this violence was consequently turned outwards as a healthy form of the will-to-power, rather than turned inwards producing sickness and neurosis. Sport was an institution against decadence. We might detect within the positive view of pre-Socratic culture a form of nostalgia for a society of healthy men. We have, however, argued against such an interpretation of Nietzsche on the grounds that he gave far more emphasis to the importance of the revaluation of values, that affirmation of life and the celebration of moral development in the post-God world. Nietzsche's view of contemporary nihilism did not as a result lead to a backward-looking commitment to pre-modern societies.

There are, in addition, some theoretical reasons from Nietzsche's view of history for rejecting a nostalgic interpretation of Nietzsche where nostalgic memory formed the basis for a solution to the crisis of modernity. These theoretical reasons can be derived from *On the Advantage and Disadvantage of History for Life* which was originally published in 1874 in which Nietzsche reflected upon the inevitability of a sense of history for all conscious creatures who are historical beings. The point about animals is that they cannot experience nostalgia, since they have no conscious sense of history. Nietzsche identified three forms or kinds of history, namely the monumental, the antiquarian and the critical. Nietzsche saw monumental history as a negative critique of contemporary conditions against the constructed images of the past. Monumental history is a form of disguise which negates the present. By contrast, antiquarian history represents a form of negative nostalgia in which again the present is buried in a mythical past in what Nietzsche called the odour of decay. By contrast, critical history would be in the service of life as a positive reflection upon the content and forms of culture which give an affirmation to human existence. The underlying issue in this argument is that knowledge should always be in the service of life, in the service of the will-to-power. Therefore, a negative nostalgia was ruled out by Nietzsche's own interpretation of the social functions of the sense of history for the preservation of life and culture. Given this interpretation of Nietzsche, it is possible to perceive a continuity between Marx's view of the potentiality of the modern as against the stagnation of past, a perspective on Marx most recently defended by Marshall Berman in *All That is Solid Melts into Air* (1983). It is perhaps not surprising, therefore, that recent commentators on Nietzsche and Marx with respect to modernity have perceived a convergence in their mutual critique of the falsity of the modern experience as organized around an abstract unity which is fundamentally illusory (Kroker, 1985). Nietzsche's response to the modernist crisis can also be understood in terms of a denial of illusions of traditional metaphors of unity, progress and identity, combined with a positive affirmation of the 'little things' of the everyday world of reciprocity against the regulating institutions of nihilistic culture with a positive assessment of the bodily basis of experience and thought. Nietzsche often called, not for a new idea, but for a new way of feeling. Nietzsche pointed towards a fourth solution, which we may regard as partly aesthetic. This fourth solution was through the pessimism of strength towards an affirmation of life-enhancing experience – the will to power which is a will to strength, truth, autonomy and meaning through an expansion of desire.

The Body-Pleasure

The contemporary restoration of the purpose of Nietzsche's critique of culture via an appreciation of the body depends, to a considerable extent, on Deleuze's *Nietzsche and Philosophy* which was first published in France in 1962. In that study of Nietzsche, Deleuze emphasized the centrality of the will-to-power in Nietzsche's philosophy, and recognized in Nietzsche's philosophical perspective an anti-dialectical attack on the Hegelian legacy. This critique of everything which smelt of Hegel was not a nostalgic search for a coherent past. The tragic is not nostalgic because it does not involve a search for some lost unity. For Nietzsche, the point of the rediscovery of Dionysus was not to reconstruct some lost harmony, but to rediscover dancing as affirmation.

Deleuze saw the importance of the body in Nietzsche's philosophy as an aspect of the philosophical tradition which went back to Spinoza. In this tradition, the body is seen as a quantity of forces in relations of mutual tension. The problem of the body as flesh in western culture is that it was appropriated by scientific discourses which exaggerated the reactive character of the body, seeing the body in largely negative and critical terms. The body became dominated by mechanistic metaphors which described bodily processes in terms of reaction. On a more general level, this growth of science was part of a cultural denial of life as essentially involving difference. Reasoning involved standardizing. From the Nietzschean perspective according to Deleuze, the health of the body is measured in terms of the active side of the will-to-power. The ascetic discipline exercised over the body by religion was thus simply one feature of regulation and control, limiting the life-force through the discipline of sense and feeling. The regulation of the body through science and religion finds its high point in the doctor/priest who infects humanity with nihilistic sickness. Responsibility and guilt are forms of moral infection and, therefore, there is a considerable difference between Kant's disinterested moral universalism or Weber's response through the ethic of responsibility and Nietzsche's response through joyous affirmation and renewal. This negative regulation of feeling through Christian practice had found its modern expression in German philosophy with its emphasis on reason and disinterest.

These developments in French social theory are extremely helpful in developing not only a new appreciation of Nietzsche, but a new perspective on modern institutions and practices. However, in this study of Nietzsche, we have departed significantly from some aspects of these interpretations of Nietzsche and the body, since in our view, they often fail to break out of a structuralist dilemma. In more specific terms, they fail to develop a theory of resistance because the body is seen to be either an effect of discourse, a construction of culture or merely a site of active forces. The concept of the 'lived body' from phenomenology found no significant place in the works of Derrida, Deleuze and Foucault. Therefore, we utilize Nietzsche's general views on the will-to-power as a foil to develop and expand more general notions concerning the relationships between resentment, reciprocity and resistance as a framework for an approach to the general problem of modernity through feeling, touch, movement and sense.

We have employed the notion of social embodiment as the focus of an argument about resistance to the regulation of larger institutions and as the place for individual difference and opposition to the dominating regularity of institutions and state formations. By this emphasis on resistance and its site in the body, we have avoided any analytic nostalgia which would conceptualize the social as an integrated unity. By contrast, we have seen the social as an endless set of conflicts and tensions within the loose framework of institutional life. This institutional life is, however, ultimately grounded in the *habitus* of everyday interactions. In most classical social theories (Hobbes, Weber, Durkheim and Freud), the body enters society through the denial and negation of pleasure in the form of institutionalized regulation of sexuality. This trend leads eventually to a positive theory of sacrifice.

These social reflections on a theory of the social concentrates on certain positive attitudes towards life. However, these reflections do not attempt to provide a philosophy for eternal values, or meta-physical properties, or some notion of the essence of human kind. It is in this respect, misleading to regard our theory as an ontology in the traditional sense. The construction of this modern world supports the changing of such attitudes towards life. The theory of modernity is constructed upon the assumption that there is a major gap between certain institutional-functional necessities and moral interests. This separation belongs to a form of social theory which remains under the enduring legacy of the death of God in searching ut substitutes for a divine absolute and in searching for a redemption. More specifically, the theory of modern society depends on a set of contradictory perspectives, such that individuals may only be 'liberated' through their sacrifice to institutional requirements. The anthropological argument, so characteristically rephrased in the notions of instrumental and substantive rationalism, created a notion of sociality which committed all interpretations of modernity to the simple dichotomy between the regulation of the self and the necessity for institutional control. Institutionalization appears to be simply a matter of regulating individuation. In this framework, the discourse of modernity turns in fact into a conservative ideology, providing an apologetic defence of traditional forms of regulation through institutions in the ultimate interest of official orders. The problem then is how to avoid the conventional distinction between the individual and society, that is to avoid the epistemological problem of treating the socialized self as an aspect of the subject-object relationship. Clearly, all social attitudes towards life are indeed socially constructed in a dialectic of life, reality, its valuation and revaluation.

If we attempt to speak of a joyful sociology, we have in mind a theory of the self, developing within the patterns of various distinctive mechanisms of appreciation and evaluation. Since Kant's philosophy, the philosophical debate on modernity has been connected with the issue of hierarchy, universality and the meta-physical foundations of such mechanisms of appreciation and valuation of moral attitudes. This joyful sociology, however, does not seek to create epistemological grounds for a hierarchy or universality of attitudes which would console us and reconcile us to social reality. While life needs no account or justification for its existence, happiness does not merely depend upon the satisfaction of needs. The utilitarian principle as a foundation for the understanding of needs, is based upon fundamental attitudes of sacrifice and discomfort (the pleasure and pain principle) as necessary features of human existence. These rationalist approaches have done little to develop human techniques of life-ability or capacity as the basis for an art of joyful existence. The professional man, turning himself into a modern intellectual, has made the ethic of resentment a necessary tool of personal excellence and cultural distinction. The uncultured, disprivileged, marginal and racially excluded are socially stigmatized and regulated by the institutions which professional men control and deploy for their own selfish benefits under the legitimizing slogans of economic efficiency. Resentment is *par excellence* the ethos of the professional man of public institutions. By contrast, the ethos of resistance is most closely associated with the morals of the working class and other subordinate groups. Working-class attitudes have been created and recreated as a modern morality of resistance fundamental to the language of survival against capitalist exploitation and political regulation. This is the attitude of how to survive the threat of institutional exploitation and economic regulation based on the modern enterprise and the modern State. The ethos of resistance was employed by the working class as a mechanism of defence, as a protection of their social life based upon traditional notions of reciprocity and exchange. Historically, the ethos of resistance has nothing to do with psychological resentment, but is rather a language of immediate survival; it is a body language against that of bodily pain, threats of extinction and of disembodiment. On the psychological level, the ethos of resistance has to be seen as an ethos of bodily display, the sign of territoriality and locality, a language of defence in general.

Action, Community, Nature

Following Nietzsche's philosophical discourse, we may distinguish two fundamental forms of human activity, that is between aesthetic and moral action. The dilemmas and ambiguities which are involved in passing from one type to another results in a floating pattern which underlies all forms of social ranking and social distinction. Aesthetic action is fundamentally affective, immediate and direct action. If I wish something I may try to transmit my will immediately and I have then to enter into a power game with others for which this transmission at least brings change to their situation within the existing status quo. We should take note here that Nietzsche was particularly aware that aesthetic action is not simply the transmission of affective will. In the dialectical relationships between Dionysus and Apollo, Nietzsche observed a profound and significant feature of the floating, interchanging and continuously transforming relations between the need for reconciliation with and the separation from both community and nature. However, the world of art remained defined through the predominance of the affective form of action against the tradition of Kant which emphasized the disinterested quality of artistic behaviour and passive evaluation.

From this type of action, the immediate affective form, we have to identify and distinguish a second mode of transforming one's will into action. In this second type, the will becomes separate from action and, indeed, will is denied within action. Only if the will is denied can such an agent feel strong enough to act. This is the case that innocence is felt to be only possible in the denial of will and personal interest. In addition, the success of action as an intended action has also to be denied or to be disguised. Success has to be demonstrated as a result of a will-less historical development. More directly, this form of denial of

223

the will in action takes the form of a moral transfiguration of will in terms of a masking or disguising of human intention. It is indeed a specific form of articulation of will in action insofar as the individual will is denied, but on the other hand, will in general remains present. These types of action do not refer to personal interests, but on the contrary, designate the interests of the general population and the universal community so moral action is not simply a denial of the will. This camouflage of the will is what Nietzsche called the 'holy lie' in *The Anti-Christ*. Through these moral notions and this masking of intention, the specific individual interests are transfigured and transposed, appearing as merely elements within a general will. Morality, therefore, within Nietzsche's philosophy may be regarded as a form of simulation. Moral behaviour as social behaviour implies a mechanism of simulation which derives from the attribution of meaning to action. We may call this simulative mechanism 'the organization'.

In communities which are based upon co-residence and kinship, the social ecology of the life-world creates basic principles of common action which relate to and are connected with the foundations of social cohesion within the community. These are the social principles of solidarity, community, reconciliation and reciprocity. These fundamental principles provide the operating criteria by which all action is ultimately measured and evaluated, even where this action is aimed at a social ranking and differences of prestige between persons. Both magical and mythological symbolism define such regulations of solidarity, reconciliation and reciprocity. These mythical imaginations are transmitted into rule-determined behaviour where a variety of interdicts bring about a separation of the internal and external, the sacred and the profane, and between human beings and the natural world. These separations and interdictions are the result of a dualistic vision of the world. These dichotomous models of reality and symbolism in primitive society form a constraint with respect to social ranking. In general, in these societies, signs and meanings have a fixed and permanent character, being legitimized by various forms of tradition and conventional reciprocity. In their unreflective application, there is little potential for a redefinition of communal norms through endless reinterpretations. The growth of social distance, rank and the economic division of labour are only possible if they are defined within the existing framework grounded upon solidarity and reciprocity. The emergence of social stratification, distance, distinction and prestige are closely connected by the world of symbols, by principles of reciprocity within the community and by a larger framework of myth which emphasize social balance. Social rank, where it takes place, is connected to certain functions of administration and interpretation of these mythical realities. It is as a result of this functional separation that a simulative mechanism appears: the way of life of social distance has to stimulate a way of life of solidarity, reconciliation and reciprocity. The world of social distance is thus parasitic upon the world of reciprocities. There are, however, within the distributive patterns of reciprocity, a number of mechanisms which entail the possibility of social distance. There are certain forces of social imbalance between response and non-response which emerge out of the very process of symbolic exchange. Various anthropological studies have brought this to our attention.

In modern society, social ranking and social distance based upon hierarchy are only possible for those members of the society who pretend to be separated from persons by means of a service to the community by showing the submission of their own private interests to the general interest. This is the problem of claims to professionalism via credentials. These claims to service involve the subordination of particular to universal commitments. We may define this as a game of moral pretence which we regard as a form of simulation. The morally correct man in the modern world is one who 'sacrifices' his personal interest to the generality and welfare of the whole. This gains an even wider significance if we consider the consumer element of modern society, where the disillusion of the moral man with the total system can be closely and clearly observed.

Simulation is determined through culturally specific discourses which attribute meaning to persons, things and beings. It was originally religion which determined the specific pattern in which simulation would develop, but in the new dimension of technology, there are new channels for these processes in modern conditions. The simulative mechanism has transformed technology into a cultural superstructure. Religion, ideology and technology are now the most significant mechanisms of simulation. The greater the possibilities of simulation offered by an organization, the more variation in attribution and distribution of societies can be developed, the less meaning has to be implied and the more power can be acquired by the organization. The result is the reduction of meaning in power. Religion, ideology and technology suspend and dissolve all given appearances; they develop and attribute entirely new meanings to things and persons. Thus, the powerful can be made weak, the ugly can be rendered beautiful, and the honest made dishonest. The more striking the reversal, the more forceful the necessity for a ruling immediacy.

However, we do find religions, ideologies and technologies which provide some outlet for the expression of instinctive and affective

225

interests and activities. But these forms of organization then leave little scope for the redefinition and resettlement of social attribution and distribution. In this case, symbolic accumulation, distance and elevation remain wedded to inter-subjective discourses. The reference to principles of domination, which are external to the main spheres of immediate interests and which acquire legitimation only from outside these spheres, appear to employ more regulation and organization for the defence of real power than for immediate coercion. However, the elimination of sense and meaning in organizations also leads to a destruction of all forms of subjective will. Finally, the active individual also has to refer to simulative discourses to put will into action. These simulative discourses are regulating organizational discourses and they also generate forms of social regulation. In simulative discourses, the basic principles of the relation between individual and institution in modern society are represented.

Because there is no fundamental system of meaning embedded in powerful organizations at the societal level within contemporary social systems, the acting individual is confronted by a range of problems. One solution is to create a new simulative discourse both within and about these organizations which we shall refer to here as the rehabilitation and 're-enthronization' of archaic morals. Professions, functions or services derived from the necessity to administer simulative discourses, or from the given necessity of general integration of the individual into these simulative discourses, have been described and analysed extensively in the work of Jean Baudrillard (1975; 1981). He had demonstrated how simulation becomes a fundamental aspect of the totality of modern society; this involves the collapse of political economy through the transformation of work and labour into various categories of simulation. The production of the sign becomes the basis of production in modern systems. All decisions and executions in professions, functions or services are no longer to be regarded as necessities of 'economic' objectivity. As a consequence of these developments, a new moralization of systematic functions in organizations may be observed. Public services, works and activities are now legitimized as an individual sacrifice for the common benefit. Nothing which is done within the public arena can any longer be regarded as simply an outcome of egoistic interest. Public functions are to be legitimized by various criteria: as a sacrifice for a friend, for a new feeling of communal obligation, or even for an idea of inter-personal sensation for the consumption of some beautiful object. It is only through the illusion of a new inter-subjectivity by which we can manage to execute these difficult simulative services for public works.

Systematic action is moral action involving the denial and reversal of individual will in the 'general interest'. It is on this basis that self-denial and sacrifice becomes an organizational principle of modernity.

The specification of reason in these organizational systems (the reduction of institutions to mere functioning molecules) leads eventually to a reduction of the systematically active human being to a merely simulative functionary. Reason is thus reduced to a defence of life alone and the question emerges as to whether the destruction of reason in morals could, in fact, lead to a new morality.

With the development of religion in history, social action in general was gradually transformed into merely simulative action. Society cannot be understood as an order of objects and goals, since society is not a system of reference for meaningful action. Moreover, society has to be perceived and understood as a floating order of references, symbols, intentions, simulations and anticipation through which the basic principles of various morals have been and will be channeled.

The mechanism of regulative distribution of these principles is simulated in a continuous process with reference to the most elementary lines of connection and distribution which pure nature has to offer. The rapid development of genetic and cybernetic systems of regulation is a striking example of this more general social development. The more elementary the mechanisms which are produced in a self-referential process of regulation, the more complex is the development of moral levels of reference in which the individual defines action and existence. In this respect, the highest values are mobilized to execute the simplest forms or terms of action. The heroic historical programme of scientific Marxism (that is, to understand the existence of apes through the development of mankind) is to be replaced by an understanding of modernity through its archaic traits: the most fundamental forms of contemporary behaviour are, in many ways, very similar to the behaviour of apes. Pure life as the only valid moral principle, death as the real subversion, as the subversion of life against the system. Are these the alternatives which are left to us?

Having developed this framework, we are now in a position to consider Nietzsche's treatment of morals which has been transformed into sociological categories such as the notion of meaningful social action in Weber and the ideas of reason and critique in Adorno. Nietzsche identified four types of morality and our basic argument is that this distinction has not been fully grasped or developed by subsequent theory. By focusing on any one of these types, theory has become fundamentally reductionist in its approach to the analysis and understanding of modern society. In Nietzsche's system, the first moral of order is the most abstract sense of rhythm and ritual. This particular form of moral activity comes closest to the natural order with respect to the will-to-power. Secondly, there are moral principles which are connected with the system as such and which emanate from the system in its specific historical form and in its concrete form as a system. The moral of organizational structure, we shall call here an institution. This, in Nietzschean terms, is the morality of the pathos of distance; in our terminology or discourse, this is the moral of the system itself. Thirdly, we may designate, following Nietzsche, the everyday moral as the morality of lowest association, the morality of the defence of the basic necessities of everyday life; that is, a morality of basic utilitarianism. Finally, there is a fourth moral (which was referred to only on very rare occasions in Nietzsche's work) which we shall call in this context, the morals of utopia. With an allusion to some of Nietzsche's writing, we might call this form the extra-moral morality. This moral is the morality of the egoistic and non-egoistic individual, the moral system of the calculating and distancing individual, the moral system of the passionate and the significant; finally, it is the moral form of art and aesthetic behaviour. In order to clarify this moral system, we should concentrate for a moment on Nietzsche's own work and, in particular, on *Beyond Good and Evil* and *The Genealogy of Morals*.

In various contexts, Nietzsche referred to morality as obviously neutral and formalized in its regulation of relations as a self-referential, formalized or formalizing mechanism; that is, as a system of reference which is to be distinguished from the execution of individual will. In the most general perspective, morality transfigures itself into the will-to-power which is then identified with real consequences in the organic world. Symbolic occurrences assimilate this to the material and to the organic. It is this very important idea which becomes a new dimension in the notion of simulation which we have already developed, following the work of Baudrillard. In another context, Nietzsche spoke of morality as the language of signs of affects in which the symbolic occurrences are differentiated from the material and organic ones. Within this language of signs and its formalization, there is the tyranny against nature. This tyranny can also be seen as a means of generating meaning and sense. Obviously, it is this penetration of formalization in human life which leads to the formalization which Nietzsche referred to as a formal consciousness. This refers to the simplest, most repetitive and submissive ideas which are necessary for organizing everyday life. We should emphasize the fact that Nietzsche had an unambiguous and distinctive conception of what he meant by formalization, namely the arbitrary character of rhythms, repetition and regulation which exists both in nature and in human behaviour.

From the coercive necessity of this formalization, there developed two different types of morality which Nietzsche referred to in terms of a pathos of distance. The distinction evolved from the confrontation between the formal element of a language of signs and human instincts and emotional effects. While the warrior-aristocrat emerged from the low morality of everyday life by affect and power, it is the priestly stratum which administered the formality of everyday life and the elementary necessity for survival. Here we discover the resentment of utilitarianism and slavery in human history. It was the priestly stratum and the warrior group which distanced themselves from others through this pathos. The moral grounds by which they distinguished themselves from other people were extremely different. Within this context, we could refer to Nietzsche's notion of the noble morality which developed on the basis of affirmative joy. It is a mode of noble valuation which implies a feeling of happiness for oneself. We could define this type of moral as the morality of the system, because it is so closely tied to the construction of separating institutions from the place and control by individuals.

Nietzsche elaborated a continuity of ritualized everyday morality through history. Ritualization in this context was linked to the whole development of utilitarian forms of thought. There is a utilitarian aspect in non-egoistic action and there is a continuity of the utilitarian aspect involved here; this continuity is linked within the necessity for the organization of everyday life. It is exactly the conversion of this morality of low instincts to a ruling morality, to a moral of systems and institutions, against which Nietzsche was particularly critical. It was exactly this development which he referred to in terms of the necessity for the revaluation of all values in a process of rebellion in morality. The success of this rebellion is unthinkable without resentment. In this rebellion of slavery, the resentment itself becomes creative and the most wicked and weak ideals are transformed into tools of culture. This is the primary scandal in history which Nietzsche lamented that the instincts of resentment of the non-egoistic, of the mediocre, of the disinterested became the reason of every culture. For Nietzsche, it is the representation of base morality in institutions which led to the decadence and nihilism of European culture in history. It was exactly on this level of the mechanism of transformation and transfiguration of the instincts of resentment into systematic rules where the cucle of simulative order is developed and reproduced. Continuous liberation was finally transformed into a continuity of manipulation; these are the morals of an anti-system transformed into the system itself.

229

In various passages, Nietzsche attempted to formulate the Utopia of an anti-system morality which would not be transformed into an institution, system of social order. For example, in *The Genealogy of Morals*, Nietzsche attempted to demonstrate the necessity for a reconversion, a new reversion of values through a self-reflection of mankind to create a new epoch which would be a period of extra-moral morality and in which the immoralists could hope for a real or true action which would lie in its non-intentionality. The intentional moral has always been a pure prejudice, a mere preliminary in history and Nietzsche saw the potential of history in the overthrowing of morals and in a self-overcoming of moral systems. In a passage from *The Anti-Christ*, Nietzsche lamented the pure egoism of Christianity which was only interested in the construction of institutional frameworks; he expressed his wish for genuine charity and true love between one's fellow human beings without the intervention of rigid institutional frameworks. There is also a passage in *The Gay Science* in which he expressed the moods of an artistic inspiration of science, philosophy and morality based upon inter-subjectivity which could provide the basis for a critique of institutional and public functions. In this regard, Nietzsche's moral system of utopia is a form of affirmative aestheticism against the routinization of system by instrumental reason.

For Nietzsche, the main scandal of history lies in the fact that this lowest type of morality found ways and means to establish itself as the ruling or dominant morality of society in contemporary historical development. Weber established, through a cynical reading of Nietzsche, utilitarianism as the basic principle of modern society. The privatization of norms into an inner subjectivity indicated the helplessness of Weber's position in confronting the totality of objectification within the systematic development of social institutions. Adorno and Horkheimer's criticism of modern systems was equally limited. That reason and identification of individuality could become part of the pattern of simulation within the system was not fully understood by Adorno and Horkheimer. Nietzsche's idea of non-intentional action seems to indicate a far deeper critique of modernity and a more secure insight for a utopian critique of the impact of instrumental reason on everyday reciprocity. With reference to Nietzsche's typology of morals, we have argued that this typology provides a very broad spectrum for the analysis of modern social systems and for a critique of social theory. In particular, the typology draws our attention to the need for repetition and formalization, the requirements for distance, resentment and abstraction, the necessity of utilitarianism in everyday life, and finally the need for non-intentional being. These provide the dynamic elements of the will for power in history.

Decadence/Nihilism

While a number of writers (Rorty, 1986) have seen the impact of Nietzsche on contemporary thought and culture as a negative and largely distructive intervention, we have attempted to focus on what we regard as the more positive, yes-saying dimensions of Nietzsche's attempt to recover the everyday world of sense as the object of activity and theory. In terms of the theory of knowledge, Nietzsche's contribution to epistemology has been analysed in terms of a theme of de-construction; by contrast, our own perspective on reciprocity, the *habitus* and feeling has departed from this philosophical orientation to reassert sensuous experience and the lived body over rationalized abstraction. It is interesting to note, furthermore, that other comment-ators (Jay, 1986) have drawn attention to the prominence of vision, abstraction and male sexuality within instrumental rationality in the history of western thought. Here again, we have suggested that Nietzsche's doctrine of the 'little things' provides a new emphasis on touch, sense, feeling and emotion; this is an assertion of the voice and the hands over the eye. The main thrust of these observations is that Nietzsche, rather than providing a negative response to the problem of modernism, offered a positive diagnosis in opposition to the pessimism of will characteristic of nineteenth-century romanticism. In short, Nietzsche provides an antidote to decadence which we may regard as a general description of the total problem of nihilism.

This issue of decadence became particularly prominent in some of Nietzsche's final contributions to the analysis of modernity, namely in *The Case of Wagner* and *Nietzsche contra Wagner*. These texts have exercised a long and haunting impact on contemporary thought, especially in the realm of musical criticism and literary analysis (Foster, 1981; Mann, 1985). Observing Wagner and commenting on Baudelaire, Nietzsche proclaimed that he had developed a nose for decadence and decay. The odour of decay was particularly heavy around Wagnerian music which expressed the impoverishment of life, the negation of health and a general weariness; Wagner, according to Nietzsche, virtually summed up the problems of modernity, but Wagner stood in a particularly complex relationship to that culture of nihilism, because to understand modernism one has to become a Wagnerian. Nietzsche condemned Wagner's romanticism, his backward-looking attachment to medieval culture and his deployment of a worn-out Christian symbolism in his major operas, especially in *Parsifal*. In *The Case of Wagner* Nietzsche treated Wagnerism as a form of contemporary illness, particularly a neurological illness. He wrote:

Precisely because nothing is more modern than this total sickness, this lateness and overexcitement of the nervous mechanism, Wagner is the modern artist *par excellence*, the Cagliostro of modernity. In his art all that the modern world requires most urgently is mixed in the most seductive manner: the three great *stimulantia* of the exhausted – the brutal, the artificial, and the innocent (idiotic). (*CW*, p. 166)

For Nietzsche, if Schopenhauer represented decadence in thought, then Wagner represented it in music. Once more, Nietzsche constantly mixed observations on sickness at the level of the body with social criticism of the political role of Wagner's music with social observations on the problem of German culture, given the particular development of the State in Germany. For example, he condemned Wagner's music as a form of hysteria; Wagner's style involved what Nietzsche called the hallucination of gestures.

The aesthetics of decadence appealed to the lowest values, to the values of brutal nationalism and the herd morality of state-dominated culture. Wagner's notion of the total work of art (*Gesamtkunstwerk*) perfectly expressed this politicization of music in the interests of a base value which was in Thomas Mann's view a bourgeois ethic.

It is quite clear that Nietzsche saw art in principle as a life affirmative process, in some respects the perfect expression of a positive will-to-power. In *The Birth of Tragedy*, he had regarded the aesthetic principle as a justification for life, indeed its only justification. We have noticed that a variety of recent writers on Nietzsche have emphasized this aesthetic solution to the crisis of modernism (Nehamas, 1985). However, in the work of Wagner and Badelaire, Nietzsche argued in *Ecce Homo* that the world-transfiguring and affirmative character of art had been corrupted into a new form of decadence, thereby silencing the flutes of Dionysus. In part, this was the consequence of the underlying nationalism and anti-semitism of Wagnerism with its peculiar mixture of Christianity, paganism and 'democratic' components.

The argument against Wagner, therefore, lends further evidence to support the view that one of the principal features of Nietzsche's philosophy was its anti-nationalistic character and its opposition to anti-semitism. It may also be taken as evidence that Nietzsche's aesthetic views are not, in any direct fashion, examples of anarchic anti-rationalism. In arguing against Baudelaire, Nietzsche opposed the principle of art for art's sake. In some respects, Nietzsche regarded Baudelaire (with his emotional instability, his stuttering and his neuroses) as the physical and cultural embodiment of stylistic decadence. The Nietzsche legacy has been too quickly and too easily

232

associated with romanticism, elitist culture and aesthetic decadence, especially by writers within a braodly Marxist tradition (Lukács, 1964; Lukács, 1974). Nietzsche did not see art as an inward or self-justifying activity, devoted to its own specific ends and internal discourse. Art is less about bourgeois comfort and more concerned with development and enhancement of life as Nietzsche attempted to assert in *The Will to Power*. For Nietzsche, all great art involved the unification of the positive features of both the Dionysian and Apollonian principles.

The prominence of the debate about art in Nietzsche's philosophy has been clearly recognized by modern writers on Nietzsche's philosophy (Schacht, 1983; Stern, 1979). We do not deny the importance of this aesthetic dimension in Nietzsche's philosophy. However, we have attempted to balance this emphasis against Nietzsche's claim to take seriously the 'little things' of the everyday world of reciprocity, interaction and exchange. The life-enhancing feature of art lies in the fact that it is not in opposition to life, because it is not primarily an abstract and abstracting feature of rationalization. Decadent art is associated with decadent society, and both are taken to be forms of sickness. The aesthetic response to modernistic nihilism is, therefore, simply one dimension of a broader affirmative approach to the 'little things' against the revenge of reason as represented by the 'theoretical man'. Nietzsche despised the despisers of the body: the divines, the theologians, the philosophers, the state officials, the cultural philistines and above all 'the Germans'. Nietzsche's message, therefore, in the last analysis was emphatic, affirmative, and clear:

My formula for greatness in a human being is *amor fati*: that one wants nothing to be other than it is, not in the future, not in the past, not in all eternity. Not merely to endure that which happens of necessity, still less to dissemble it – all idealism is untruthfulness in the face of necessity – but to *love* it. (*EH*, p. 68)

Bibliography

For works by T. W. Adorno, M. Foucault, S. Freud, J. Habermas, F. Nietzsche and M. Weber see Abbreviations, pp. vii–ix.

Abercrombie, N. (1980), *Class Structure and Knowledge*, Oxford, Basil Blackwell.

Abercrombie, N., Hill, S. and Turner, B. S. (1980), *The Dominant Ideology Thesis*, London, George Allen and Unwin.

Abercrombie, N., Hill, S. and Turner, B. S. (1986), *Sovereign Individuals of Capitalism*, London, George Allen and Unwin.

Alexander, J. C. (ed.) (1985), *Neofunctionalism*, Beverly Hills, Sage Publications.

Alexander, J. C. (1985), 'The individualist dilemma in phenomenology and interactionism'. In S. N. Eisenstadt and H. J. Helle (eds), *Macrosociological Theory, perspectives in sociological theory*, vol. 1, Beverly Hills, Sage Publications, pp. 25-57.

Alford, C. (1987), 'Habermas, post-Freudian psychoanalysis and the end of the individual', *Theory Culture and Society*, 4 (1), pp. 3-29.

Allison, D. B. (ed.) (1977), *The New Nietzsche. Contemporary styles of interpretation*, New York, Delta Books.

Althusser, L. (1969), *For Marx*, Harmondsworth, Penguin.

Althusser, L. (1971), *Lenin and Philosophy and Other Essays*, London, New Left Books.

Althusser, L. and Balibar, E. (1970), *Reading Capital*, London, New Left Books.

Anderson, L. (1980), 'Freud, Nietzsche', *Salmagundi*, 47-8, pp. 3-29.

Ariès, P. and Béjin, A. (eds) (1985), *Western Sexuality. Practice and precept in past and present times*, Oxford, Basil Blackwell.

Armstrong, D. (1983), *Political Anatomy of the Body, medical knowledge in Britain in the 20th century*, Cambridge, Cambridge University Press.

Aron, R. (1971), 'Max Weber and power politics'. In O. Stammer (ed.) *Max Weber and Sociology Today*, Oxford, Basil Blackwell, pp. 83-100.

Bibliography

Atoji, Y. (1984), *Sociology at the Turn of the Century*, Tokyo, Dobunkan.
Avineri, S. (1970), *The Social and Political Thought of Karl Marx*, Cambridge, Cambridge University Press.
Badcock, C. R. (1980), *The Psychoanalysis of Culture*, Oxford, Basil Blackwell.
Baier, H. (1982), 'Die Gesellschaft – ein langer Schatten des toten Gottes. Friedrich Nietzsche und die Entstehung der Soziologie aus dem Geist der decadence', *Nietzsche-Studien*, 10-11, pp. 6-22.
Bakhtin, M. (1968), *Rabelais and his World*, Cambridge, The MIT Press.
Barker, F. (1984), *The Tremulous Private Body. Essays on subjection*, New York and London, Methuen.
Bataille, G. (1982), *The Story of the Eye*, Harmondsworth, Penguin.
Baudrillard, J. (1975), *The Mirror of Production*, St Louis, Telos.
Baudrillard, J. (1981), *Critique of Political Economy of the Sign*, St Louis, Telos.
Bell, D. (1976), *The Cultural Contradictions of Capitalism*, London, Heinemann.
Berger, P. L. (1969a), *A Rumor of Angels*, New York, Doubleday.
Berger, P. L. (1969b), *The Social Reality of Religion*, London, Faber and Faber.
Berger, P. L. (1974), 'On the Obsolescence of the Concept of Honour' in P. L. Berger, B. Berger and H. Kellner (eds) *The Homeless Mind*, Harmondsworth, Penguin, pp. 79-89.
Berger, P. L. and Kellner, H. (1965), 'Arnold Gehlen and the theory of institutions', *Social Research*, 32, pp. 110-15.
Berger, P. L. and Luckmann, T. (1967), *The Social Construction of Reality. Everything that passes for knowledge in society*, London, Allen Lane.
Berger, P. L. and Pullberg, S. (1966), 'Reification and the Sociological Critique of Consciousness', *New Left Review*, 35, pp. 56-71.
Berman, M. (1982), *All that is Solid Melts into Air. The experience of modernity*, London, Verso.
Bernstein, R. J. (1979), *The Restructuring of Social and Political Thought*, London, Methuen.
Binswanger, L. (1955), *Le rêve et l existence*, Paris, Desclee de Brouwer.
Bocock, R. (1983), *Freud*, London, Tavistock.
Bottomore, T. and Goode, P. (1978), *Austro-Marxism*, Oxford, Clarendon Press.
Bourdieu, P. (1977), *Outline of a Theory of Practice*, Cambridge, Cambridge University Press.
Breger, L. (1981), *Freud's Unfinished Journey, conventional and critical perspectives in psychoanalytic theory*, London, Routledge and Kegan Paul.
Brown, J. A. C. (1961), *Freud and the Post-Freudians*, Harmondsworth, Penguin.
Brubaker, R. (1984), *The Limits of Rationality. An Essay on the Social and Moral Thought of Max Weber*, London, George Allen and Unwin.
Bucher, B. (1981), *Icon and Conquest, a structural analysis of the illustrations of de Bry's Great Voyages*, Chicago and London, University of Chicago Press.
Burchell, G. (1984), 'Introduction to Deleuze', *Economy and Society*, 13, pp. 43-51.

Bibliography

Cabanis, G. P-J. (1981), *On the Relations Between the Physical and Moral Aspects of Man*, Baltimore, The John Hopkins University Press, 2 vols.

Callinicos, A. (1985), 'Post-Modernism, Post-Structuralism and Post-Marxism?', *Theory, Culture and Society*, 2, pp. 85-102.

Carroll, J. (1985), *Guilt – The Grey Eminence Behind Character, History and Culture*, London, Routledge and Kegan Paul.

Carter, A. (1979), *The Sadeian Woman*, London, Virago.

Cassirer, E. (1981), *Kant's Life and Thought*, New Haven and London, Yale University Press.

Cipolla, C. M. (ed.) (1973a), *The Industrial Revolution*, London, Collins/Fontana.

Cipolla, C. M. (ed.) (1973b), *The Emergence of Industrial Societies*, London, Collins/Fontana.

Dallmyer, F. R. (1981), *Twilight of Subjectivity, contributions to a post-individualist theory*, Amherst, Mass., University of Massachusetts Press.

Danto, A. C. (1965), *Nietzsche as Philosopher*, New York, Macmillan.

Davis, F. (1974), *Yearning for Yesterday. A sociology of nostalgia*, New York, Free Press.

Deeken, A. (1974), *Process and Permanence in Ethics, Max Scheler's moral philosophy*, New York, Paulist Press.

Deleuze, G. (1983), *Nietzsche and Philosophy*, London, The Athlone Press.

Deleuze, G. and Guattari, F. (1977), *Anti-Oedipus, Capitalism and Schizophrenia*, New York, Viking Press.

Demske, J. M. (1970), *Being, Man and Death. A key to Heidegger*, Kentucky, University Press of Kentucky.

Derrida, J. (1979), *Spurs, Nietzsche's Styles*, Chicago, University of Chicago Press.

Dews, P. 1986), 'Adorno, Post-structuralism and the critique of Identity', *New Left Review*, 157, pp. 28-44.

Dodds, E. R. (1951), *The Greeks and the Irrational*, Berkeley, University of California Press.

Donnelly, M. (1983), *Managing the Mind. A study of medical psychology in early 19th century Britain*, London and New York, Tavistock.

Donzelot, J. (1979), *The Policing of Families*, New York, Pantheon Books.

Dreyfus, J. L. and Rabinow, P. (1982), *Michel Foucault, beyond structuralism and hermeneutics*, Brighton, Harvester Press.

Dreyfus, H. L. and Rabinow, P. (1986), 'What is maturity? Habermas and Foucault on "What is enlightenment"' In David Couzens Hoy (ed.) *Foucault, a reader*, Oxford, Polity Press, pp. 109-47.

Durkheim, E. (1912), *The Elementary Forms of the Religious Life*, London, Allen and Unwin.

Durkheim, E. (1960), *The Division of Labour in Society*, Glencoe, Free Press.

Eden, R. (1984), *Political Leadership and Nihilism. A study of Weber and Nietzsche*, Tampa, University Presses of Florida.

Elias, N. (1978), *The Civilizing Process, the history of manners*, Oxford, Basil Blackwell.

Elias, N. (1982), *The Civilizing Process, state formation and civilization*, Oxford, Basil Blackwell.

Elias, N. (1983), *The Court Society*, Oxford, Basil Blackwell.

Engels, F. (1954), *Dialectics of Nature*, Moscow, Progress Publishers.

Esslin, M. (1976), *Artaud*, London, Fontana.

Evans, R. (1982), *The Fabrication of Virtue, English prison architecture 1750-1840*, Cambridge, Cambridge University Press.

Faust, B. (1982), *Women, Sex and Pornography*, Harmondsworth, Penguin.

Firth, R. (ed.) (1957), *Man and Culture, an evaluation of the work of Bronislaw Malinowski*, London, Routledge and Kegan Paul.

Fleischmann, E. (1964), 'De Weber à Nietzsche', *Archives Européennes de Sociologie*, 5, pp. 190-238.

Forrester, J. (1984), 'Who is in analysis with whom? Freud, Lacan, Derrida', *Economy and Society*, 13, pp. 153-77.

Foster, J. B. (1981), *Heirs to Dionysus, a Nietzschean current in literary modernism*, Princeton, Princeton University Press.

Fox, R. (1966), 'Totem and Taboo Reconsidered'. In E. Leach (ed.) *The Structural Study of Myth and Totemism*, London, Tavistock, pp. 161-78)

Frankfurt Institute for Social Research (1973), *Aspects of Sociology*, London, Heinemann.

Freund, J. (1968), *The Sociology of Max Weber*, London, Allen Lane.

Freund, J. (1979), 'German sociology in the time of Max Weber'. In T. Bottomore and R. Nisbet (eds) *A History of Sociological Analysis*, London, Heinemann, pp. 149-86.

Freund, P. E. S. (1982), *The Civilized Body, social domination, control and health*, Philadelphia, Philadelphia Press.

Frisby, D. (1981), *Sociological Impressionism. A re-assessment of Georg Simmel's social theory*, London, Heinemann.

Frisby, D. (1984), *Georg Simmel*, Chichester and London, Ellis Horwood and Tavistock.

Frisby, D. (1985), 'Georg Simmel, sociologist of modernity', *Theory, Culture and Society*, 2, pp. 49-68.

Fromm, E. (1980), *Greatness and Limitations of Freud's Thought*, London, Jonathan Cape.

Fuss, P. and Shapiro, H. (eds) (1971), *Nietzsche – A Self-Portrait from his Letters*, Cambridge, Mass., Harvard University Press.

Gane, M. (1983a), 'Durkheim: woman as outsider', *Economy and Society*, 12, pp. 227-70.

Gane, M. (1983b), 'Human nature and perspective of sociology', *Social Research*, 30, pp. 300-18.

Gehlen, A. (1965), *Theorie der Willensfreiheit und frühe philosophische Schriften*, Berlin, Neuwide.

Giddens, A. (1972), *Politics and Sociology in the Thought of Max Weber*, London, Macmillan.

Giddens, A. (1984), *The Constitution of Society, outline of the theory of structuration*, Oxford, Polity Press.

Goldmann, L. (1964), *The Hidden God*, London, Routledge and Kegan Paul.

Goudsblom, J. (1980), *Nihilism and Culture*, Oxford, Basil Blackwell.

Grenz, F. (1974), *Adornos Philosophie in Grundbegriffen: Auflösung einiger Deutungsprobleme*, Frankfurt, Suhrkamp.

Gross, L. (1986), 'Derrida and the limits of philosophy', *Thesis Eleven*, 14, pp. 26-43.

Gurevich, A. J. (1985), *Categories of Medieval Culture*, London, Routledge and Kegan Paul, pp. 42-3.

Haar, M. (1977), 'Nietzsche and metaphysical language'. In D. B. Allison (ed.), *The New Nietzsche. Contemporary styles of interpretation*, New York, Delta Books, pp. 5-36.

Habermas, J. (1984), *The Theory of Communicative Action, vol. 1, Reason and the Rationalization of Society*, Boston, Beacon Press.

Hamilton, P. (1983), *Talcott Parsons*, Chichester and London, Ellis Horwood and Tavistock.

Harries, K. (1978), 'Ontology and the search for man's place' in M. Murray (ed.), *Heidegger and Modern Philosophy, Critical Essays*, New Haven and London, Yale University Press, pp. 65-79.

Heidegger, M. (1959), *An Introduction to Metaphysics*, New Haven, Yale University Press, pp. 37-8.

Heidegger, M. (1962), *Being and Time*, New York, Harper and Row.

Heidegger, M. (1966), *Discourse on Thinking*, New York, Harper and Row.

Heidegger, M. (1977), *The Question Concerning Technology and Other Essays*, New York, Harper and Row.

Held, D. (1980), *Introduction to Critical Theory, Horkheimer to Habermas*, London, Hutchinson.

Heller, A. (1978), *Renaissance Man*, London, Routledge and Kegan Paul.

Heller, A. (1984), *Everyday Life*, London, Routledge and Kegan Paul.

Heller, E. (1961), *The Disinherited Mind*, Harmondsworth, Penguin.

Heller, P. (1966), *Dialectics and Nihilism: essays on Lessing, Nietzsche, Mann and Kafka*, Amherst, Mass.

Hennis, W. (1963), 'Max Weber's central question', *Economy and Society*, 12, pp. 135-80.

Hennis, W. (1986), 'Die Spuren Nietzsches im Werk Max Webers', *Nietzsche-Studien*, 16, pp. 382-40.

Hennis, W. (1987), *Max Webers Fragestellung*, Tübingen, J. C. Mohr.

Hepworth, M. and Turner, B. S. (1982), *Confession, studies in deviance and religion*, London, Routledge and Kegan Paul.

Hirst, P. Q. (1975), *Durkheim, Bernard and Epistemology*, London, Routledge and Kegan Paul.

Hohlenberg, J. (1954), *Søren Kierkegaard*, London, Routledge and Kegan Paul.

Hollingdale, R. J. (1973), *Nietzsche*, London, Routledge and Kegan Paul.

Bibliography

Holton, R. J. (1984), *The Transition from Feudalism to Capitalism*, London, Macmillan.

Holton, R. J. and Turner, B. S. (1986), *Talcott Parsons on Economy and Society*, London, Routledge and Kegan Paul.

Honour, H. (1981), *Neo-Classicism*, Harmondsworth, Penguin.

Horkheimer, M. (1934), reprinted in Horkheimer, M. (1968), *Kritische Theorie, eine Dokumentation*, Frankfurt, S. Fischer Verlag, vol. 1, pp. 118-74.

Horkheimer, M. (1937), reprinted in Horkheimer, M. (1968), *Kritische Theorie, eine Dokumentation*, Frankfurt, S. Fischer Verlag, vol. 2, pp. 2-136.

Hudson, L. (1982), *Bodies of Knowledge. The psychological significance of the nude in art*, London, Weidenfeld and Nicholson.

Hughes, H. S. (1959), *Consciousness and Society, The reorientation of European social thought 1890-1930*, London, MacGibbon and Kee.

Jackson, S.W. (1981), 'Acedia, the sin and its relationship to sorrow and melancholy in medieval times', *The Bulletin of the History of Medicine*, 55, pp. 172-85.

Jaspers, K. (1955), *Reason and Existence*, New York, The Noonday Press.

Jay, M. (1973), *The Dialectical Imagination, a history of the Frankfurt School of the Institute of Social Research 1923-1950*, London, Heinemann.

Jay, M. (1986), 'The Empire of the gaze: Foucault and the denigration of vision in twentieth-century French thought'. In David Couzens Hoy (ed.) *Foucault, a critical reader*, Oxford, Basil Blackwell, pp. 175-204.

Johnson, D. (1983), *Body*, Boston, Beacon Press.

Kaufmann, W. (1974), *Nietzsche, Philosopher, Psychologist, Anti-Christ*, Princeton, Princeton University Press.

Kent, S. A. (1983), 'Weber, Goethe and the Nietzschean allusion: capturing the source of the iron cage mataphor', *Sociological Analysis*, 44, pp. 297-320.

Kent, S. A. (1985), 'Research note: Weber, Goethe, and William Penn: themes of marital love', *Sociological Analysis*, 46, pp. 315-20.

Kierkegaard, S. (1985), *Fear and Trembling*, Harmondsworth, Penguin.

Kilminster, R., (1979), *Praxis and Method, a sociological dialogue with Lukács, Gramsci and the Frankfurt School*, London, Routledge and Kegan Paul.

Klages, L. (1929-32), *Der Geist als Widersacher der Seele*, Bonn, Bouvier.

Klibansky, R., Panofsky, E. and Saxl, F. (1964), *Saturn and Melancholy. Studies in the history of natural philosophy, religion and art*, New York, Basic Books.

Klossowski, P. (1969), *Nietzsche et le Cercle Vicieux*, Paris, Mercure.

Korsch, K. (1970), *Marxism and Philosophy*, London, New Left Books.

Krell, D. F. (1975), 'Nietzsche in Heidegger's Lehre', *The Southern Journal of Philosophy*, 13, pp. 197-204.

Kroker, A. (1985), 'Baudrillard's Marx', *Theory, Culture and Society*, 2(3), pp. 69-84.

Kronman, A. T. (1983), *Max Weber*, London, Edward Arnold.

Kurzweil, E. (1980), *The Age of Structuralism, Levi-Strauss to Foucault*, New York, Columbia University Press.

Bibliography

Lacan, J. (1977), *Écrits, A Selection*, London, Tavistock.

Lash, S. (1984), 'Genealogy and the body, Foucault-Deleuze-Nietzsche', *Theory, Culture and Society*, 2, pp. 1-18.

Lash, S. (1985), 'Post-modernity and desire', *Theory and Society*, 14, pp. 1-33.

Lefebvre, H. (1968), *The Sociology of Marx*, London, Allen Lane.

Leiss, W. (1972), *The Domination of Nature*, New York, George Braziller.

Lemaire, A. (1977), *Jacques Lacan*, London, Routledge and Kegan Paul.

Lemert, C. C. (ed.) (1981), *French Sociology, rupture and renewal since 1968*, New York, Columbia University Press.

Lemert, G. C. and Gillan, G. (1982), *Michel Foucault, social theory as transgression*, New York, Columbia University Press.

Lepenies, W. (1985), *Die Drei Kulturen, Soziologie Zwischen Literatur und Wissenschaft*, München, Carl Hanser Verlag.

Lessing, T. H. (1985), *Nietzsche*, Münich, Matthes and Seitz.

Levin, D. M. (1985), *The Body's Recollection of Being. Phenomenological psychology and the deconstruction of nihilism*, London, Routledge and Kegan Paul.

Levin, K. (1978), *Freud's Early Psychology of the Neuroses, A historical perspective*, Brighton, Harvester Press.

Lloyd-Jones, H. (1971), *The Justice of Zeus*, Berkeley, University of California Press.

Löwith, K. (1967), *From Hegel to Nietzsche*, New York, Holt, Rinehart and Winston.

Löwith, K. (1982), *Max Weber and Karl Marx*, London, George Allen and Unwin.

Luckmann, T. (1967), *The Invisible Religion. The problem of religion in modern society*, New York, Macmillan.

Luhmann, N. (1984), *Religious Dogmatics and the Evolution of Societies*, New York, The Edwin Mellen Press.

Lukács, G. (1964), *Realism in Our Time*, New York and Evanston, Harper and Row.

Lukács, G. (1967). In Abendroth, Holz, Klopfer, *Gespräche mit Lukács*, hg von T. Pinkus, Reinbek bei Hamburg, Rowohet.

Lukács, G. (1971), *History and Class Consciousness*, London, Merlin Press.

Lukács, G. (1974), *Soul and Form*, London, Merlin Press.

Lukes, S. (1975), *Emile Durkheim, His life and work*, Harmondsworth, Penguin.

Lyotard, J. F. (1979), *La Condition Post-moderne*, Paris, Editions de Minuit.

Lyotard, J. F. (1980), *Des Dispositifs Pulsionnels*, Paris, Editions de Minuit.

MacIntyre, A. (1958), *The Unconscious, A conceptual study*, London, Routledge and Kegan Paul.

MacIntyre, A. (1967), *A Short History of Ethics*, London, Routledge and Kegan Paul.

MacIntyre, A. (1967), *Secularization and Moral Change*, London, Oxford University Press.

MacIntyre, A. (1969), *Marxism and Christianity*, London, Duckworth.

MacIntyre, A. (1971), *Against the Self-Images of the Age, essays on ideology and philosophy*, London, Duckworth.

Bibliography

MacIntyre, A. (1981), *After Virtue, a study in moral theory*, London, Duckworth.
MacIntyre, A. and Ricoeur, P. (1969), *The Religious Significance of Atheism*, New York and London, Columbia University Press.
MacRae, D. (1974), *Weber*, London, Fontana.
Macpherson, C. B. (1962), *The Political Theory of Possessive Individualism, Hobbes to Locke*, Oxford, Clarendon Press.
Malinowski, B. (1927), *Sex and Repression in a Savage Society*, London, Routledge and Kegan Paul.
Mann, M. (1986), *The Sources of Social Power*, Cambrdige, Cambridge University Press.
Mann, T. (1948), *Nietzsche's Philosophie im Lichte Unserer Erfahrung*, Berlin, Kuhrkamp.
Mann, T. (1985), *Pro and Contra Wagner*, London, Faber and Faber.
Mannoni, M. (1973), *The Child, His Illness and the Others*, Harmondsworth, Penguin.
Marcuse, H. (1955), *Eros and Civilization*, Boston, Beacon Press.
Marcuse, H. (1964), *One Dimensional Man*, London, Routledge and Kegan Paul.
Marcuse, H. (1968), *Negations*, London, Allen Lane, Penguin.
Marcuse, H. (1969), *Eros and Civilization*, New York, Sphere Books.
Markus, G. (1978), *Marxism and Anthropology*, Assen, van Gorcum Press.
Marsella, A. J., Devos, G., Hsu, F. L. K. (eds) (1985), *Culture and Self. Asian and western perspectives*, New York and London, Tavistock.
Martin, D. (1969), *The Religious and the Secular*, London, Routledge and Kegan Paul.
Marx, K. (1968), *Theories of Surplus Value*, Moscow, Moscow Foreign Publishing House, 3 vols.
Maurer, R. K. (1981-2), 'Nietzsche und die kritische Theorie', *Nietzsche-Studien*, 10-11, pp. 34-58.
McCarthy, T. (1978), *The Critical Theory of Jurgen Habermas*, London, Hutchinson.
McGill, V. J. (1931), *Schopenhauer, Pessimist and Pagan*, New York, Brentano.
McNeil, J. T. (1932), 'Medicine for sin as prescribed in the penitentials', *Church History*, 1, pp. 14-26.
Meek, R. L. (ed.) (1971), *Marx and Engels on the Population Bomb*, Berkeley, Ramparts Press.
Megill, A. (1985), *Prophets of Extremity, Nietzsche, Heidegger, Foucault, Derrida*, Berkeley, University of California Press.
Mennell, S. (1985), *All Manners of Food, Eating and Taste in England and France from the Middle Ages to the Present*, Oxford, Basil Blackwell.
Menzies, K. (1976), *Talcott Parsons and the Social Image of Man*, London, Routledge and Kegan Paul.
Merton, R. K. (1964), *Social Theory and Social Structure*, New York, Free Press.
Miller, J. (1979), 'Some implications of Nietzsche's thought for Marxism', *Telos*, 58, pp. 22-41.
Mitchell, J. (1975), *Psychoanalysis and Feminism*, Harmondsworth, Penguin.

Bibliography

Mitzman, A. (1971), *The Iron Cage, a historical interpretation of Max Weber*, New York, The University Library.

Mommsen, W. J. (1974), *The Age of Bureaucracy, perspectives on the political sociology of Max Weber*, New York, Harper and Row.

Mommsen, W. J. (1985), *Max Weber and German Politics 1890-1920*, Chicago University of Chicago Press.

Mörchen, H. (1981), *Adorno und Heidegger, Untersuchung einer philosophischen Kommunikationsverweigerung*, Stuttgart, Kleft-Cotta.

Muller, G. J. (1986), 'Weber and Mommsen: non-Marxist materialism', *The British Journal of Sociology*, 37(1), pp. 1-20.

Nehamas, A. (1985), *Nietzsche, life as literature*, Cambridge, Mass., Harvard University Press.

Nisbet, R. A. (1953), *The Quest for Community, a study in the ethics of order and freedom*, New York, Oxford University Press.

Nisbet, R. A. (1967), *The Sociological Tradition*, London, Heinemann.

Norris, C. (1982), *Deconstruction, Theory and Practice*, London, Methuen.

O'Flaherty, J. C., Sellner, J. C. and Helm, R. M. (1976), *Studies in Nietzsche and the Classical Tradition*, Chapel Hill, North Carolina, North Carolina University Press.

O'Neill, J. (1985), *Five Bodies. The human shape of modern society*, Ithaca and London, Cornell University Press.

O'Neill, J. (1986), 'The disciplinary society', *The British Journal of Sociology*, 37(1), pp. 420-60.

Parkin, F. (1982), *Max Weber*, Chichester and London; Ellis Horwood and Tavistock.

Parsons, T. (1937), *The Structure of Social Action*, New York, McGraw-Hill.

Parsons, T. (1949), *Essays in Sociological Theory*, New York, Glencoe.

Parsons, T. (1951), *The Social System*, New York, Free Press.

Parsons, T. (1963), 'Christianity and modern industrial society'. In E. A. Tiryakian (ed.) *Sociological Theory, Values and Sociocultural Change*, New York, Free Press, pp. 33-70.

Parsons, T. and Shils, E. A. (eds) (1951), *Toward a General Theory of Action*, New York, Harper Torch Books.

Parsons, T., Bales, R. F. and Shils, E.A. (1953), *Working Papers in the Theory of Action*, New York, Free Press.

Pasley, M. (1978), 'Nietzsche's use of medical terms' in M. Pasley (ed.) *Nietzsche: Imagery and the Thought. A collection of essays*, London, Methuen, pp. 123-58.

Patton, P. (1984-5), 'Michel Foucault, the ethics of an intellectual', *Thesis Eleven*, 10/11, pp. 71-80.

Pivcevic, E. (1970), *Husserl and Phenomenology*, London, Hutchinson.

Pruyser, P. W. (1973), 'Sigmund Freud and his legacy: psychoanalytic psychology of religion'. In C. Y. Glock and P. E. Hammond (eds) *Beyond the Classics? Essays in the scientific study of religion*, New York, Harper and Row and Harper Torch Books, pp. 243-90.

Pütz, P. (1981-2), 'Nietzsche and critical theory', *Telos*, 50, pp. 103-14.

Rabil, A. (1967), *Merleau-Ponty, existentialist of the social world*, New York and

242

London, Columbia University Press.
Reich, W. (1975), *The Mass Psychology of Fascism*, Harmondsworth, Penguin.
Reiff, P. (1966), *The Triumph of the Therapeutic. Uses of faith after Freud*, London, Chatto and Windus.
H. Rickert, *Die Philosophie des Lebens: Darstellung und Kritik der philosophischen Modeströmungen unserer Zeit*, Tübingen (Mohr), 1920.
Ringer, F. K. (1969), *The Decline of the German Mandarins, the German academic community 1890-1933*, Cambridge, Mass., Harvard Univeristy Press.
Robertson, R. (1978), *Meaning and Change, explorations in the cultural sociology of modern societies*, Oxford, Basil Blackwell.
Roderick, R. (1986), *Habermas and the Foundations of Critical Theory*, Basingstoke, Macmillan.
Rorty, R. (1986), 'Foucault and epistemology'. In David Couzens Hoy (ed.) *Foucault, a critical reader*, Oxford, Basil Blackwell, pp. 41-9.
Rose, G. (1978), *The Melancholy Science, an introduction to the thought of Theodor W. Adorno*, London, Macmillan.
Rose, G. (1984), *Dialectic of Nihilism, post-structuralism and law*, Oxford, Basil Blackwell.
Rotenstreich, N. (1965), *Basic Problems of Marxist Philosophy*, Indianapolis, The Bobbs-Merrill Company.
Roth, G. and Schluchter, W. (1979), *Max Weber's Vision of History, Ethics and Methods*, Berkeley, University of California Press.
Sacks, O. (1986), *A Leg to Stand On*, London, Pan Books.
Sahlins, M. (1977), *The Use and Abuse of Biology. An Anthropological Critique of Socio-Biology*, London, Tavistock.
Said, E. W. (1978), *Orientalism*, London, Routledge and Kegan Paul.
Scaff, L. A. (1984), 'Weber before Weberian sociology', *The British Journal of Sociology*, 35, pp. 190-215.
Schacht, R. (1983), *Nietzsche*, London, Routledge and Kegan Paul.
Scharf, B. R. (1970), 'Durkheimian and Freudian theories of religion: the case for Judaism', *The British Journal of Sociology*, 21, pp. 151-63.
Scheler, M. (1961), *Ressentiment*, New York, Free Press.
Scheler, M. (1962), *Man's Place in Nature*, New York, The Noonday Press.
Scheler, M. (1970), *The Nature of Sympathy*, Connecticut, Archon Books.
Schelsky, H. (1957), 'Ist die Dauerreflektion institutionalisierbar?', *Zeitschrift für evangelische Ethik*, 1, pp. 153-74.
Schluchter, W. (1981), *The Rise of Western Rationalism: Max Weber's development history*, Berkeley, University of California Press.
Schmidt, A. (1971), *The Concept of Nature in Marx*, London, New Left Books.
Schneiderman, S. (1983), *Jacques Lacan, the death of an intellectual hero*, Cambridge, Mass., Harvard University Press.
Schopenhauer, A. (1969), *The World as Will and Representation*, 2 vols, New York, Dover Publications.
Schopenhauer, A. (1974), *Parerga and Paralipomena*, 2 vols, Oxford, Clarendon Press.
Schutte, O. (1984), *Beyond Nihilism. Nietzsche without masks*, Chicago and London, University of Chicago Press.

Bibliography

Schutz, A. (1971), *Collected Papers*, 3 vols, The Hague, Martinus Nijhoff.

Shaw, M. (ed.) (1985), *Marxist Sociology Revisted, critical assessments*, London, Macmillan.

Sheridan, A. (1980), *Michel Foucault, The Will to Truth*, London, Tavistock.

Shorter, E. (1977), *The Making of the Modern Family*, London, Collins/Fontana.

Sigrist, C. (1971), 'The problems of pariahs'. In O. Stammer (ed.) *Max Weber and Sociology Today*, Basil Blackwell, pp. 240-50.

Silk, M. S. and Stern, J. P. (1981), *Nietzsche on Tragedy*, Cambridge, Cambridge University Press.

Simmel, G. (1907), *Schopenhauer und Nietzsche*, Liepzig, Duncker and Humbolt.

Simmel, G. (1978), *The Philosophy of Money*, Boston, Routledge and Kegan Paul.

Skultans, V. (1979), *English Madness, ideas on insanity 1580-1890*, London, Routledge and Kegan Paul.

Slater, P. (1977), *Origin and Significance of the Frankfurt School: a Marxist perspective*, London, Routledge and Kegan Paul.

Smart, B. (1985), *Michel Foucault*, Chichester and London, Ellis Horwood and Tavistock.

Smith, J. W. and Turner, B. S. (1986), 'Constructing social theory and constituting society', *Theory, Culture and Society*, 3, pp. 125-34.

Sontag, S. (1969), *Illness as Metaphor*, New York, Farrar, Straus and Giroux.

Stauth, G. and Turner, B. S. (1986), 'Nietzsche in Weber oder die Geburt des modernen Genius im professionellen Menschen', *Zeitschrift fur Soziologie*, 15(2), pp. 81-94.

Stephens, A. (1986), 'Nietzsche: the resurrection of parts', *Thesis Eleven*, 13, pp. 94-109.

Stern, F. (1961), *The Politics of Cultural Despair*, Berkeley and Los Angeles, University of California Press.

Stern, J. P. (1978), *Nietzsche*, London, Fontana.

Stern, J. P. (1979), *A Study of Nietzsche*, Cambridge, Cambridge University Press.

Tenbruck, F. H. (1980), 'The problem of thematic unity in the work of Max Weber', *The British Journal of Sociology*, 31, pp. 316-51.

Therborn, G. (1976), *Science, Class and Society. On the formation of sociology and historical materialism*, London, New Left Books.

Therborn, G. (1980), *The Ideology of Power and the Power of Ideology*, London, Verso.

Thomas, J. R. (1984), 'Weber and direct democracy', *The British Journal of Sociology*, 35, pp. 216-40.

Thomas, R. H. (1983), *Nietzsche in German Politics and Society, 1890-1918*, Manchester, Manchester University Press.

Thulstrup, N. (1980), *Kierkegaard's Relation to Hegel*, Princeton, Princeton University Press.

Timpanaro, S. (1975), *On Materialism*, London, New Left Books.

Bibliography

Tönnies, F. (1955), *Community and Association*, London, Routledge and Kegan Paul.

Tribe, K. (1983), 'Prussian agriculture – German politics: Max Weber 1892-1897', *Economy and Society*, 12, pp. 181-226.

Turner, B. S. (1977), 'Class solidarity and system integration', *Sociological Analysis*, 38, pp. 345-58.

Turner, B. S. (1978), *Marx and the End of Orientalism*, London, George Allen and Unwin.

Turner, B. S. (1981), *For Weber, essays on the sociology of fate*, Boston, Routledge and Kegan Paul.

Turner, B. S. (1982a), 'Nietzsche, Weber and the devaluation of politics: the problem of state legitimacy', *The Sociological Review*, 30, pp. 367-91.

Turner, B. S. (1982b), 'The government of the body. Medical regimens and the rationalisation of diet', *The British Journal of Sociology*, 33, pp. 254-69.

1982c), 'The discourse of diet', *Theory, Culture and Society*, 1(1), pp. 23-32.

Turner, B. S. (1983), *Religion and Social Theory. A materialist perspective*, London, Heinemann.

Turner, B. S. (1984), *The Body and Society, explorations in social theory*, Oxford, Basil Blackwell.

Turner, B. S. (1985a), 'More on "the government of the body"', *The British Journal of Scoiology*, 36, pp. 151-4.

Turner, B. S. (1985b), 'State, religion and minority status', *Comparative Studies in Society and History*, 27, pp. 304-11.

Turner, B. S. (1985c), 'The practices of rationality: Michel Foucault, medical history and sociological theory'. In Richard Fardon (ed.) *Power and Knowledge: anthropological and sociological approaches*, Edinburgh, Scottish Academic Press, pp. 193-213.

Turner, B. S. (1986a), 'Simmel, rationalisation and the sociology of money', *The Sociological Review*, 34(1), pp. 93-114.

Turner, B. S. (1986b), *Citizenship and Capitalism, the debate over reformism*, London, George Allen and Unwin.

Turner, B. S. (1986c), *Equality*, Chichester and London, Ellis Horwood and Tavistock.

van den Berg, J. H. (1966), *The Psychology of the Sickbed*, Pittsburgh, Dunquesne University Press.

Warnock, M. (1965), *The Philosophy of Sartre*, London, Hutchinson.

Warren, M. (1984), 'Nietzsche's concept of ideology', *Theory and Society*, 13, pp. 541-65.

Weber, M. (1926), *Max Weber – ein lebensbild* Tübingen, Mohr.

Wellmer, A. (1984-5), 'Adorno's aesthetic redemption of modernity', *Telos*, 62, (Winter), pp. 89-116.

White, H. (1979), 'Michel Foucault'. In J. Sturrock (ed.) *Structuralism and Since, from Levi-Strauss to Derrida*, Oxford, Oxford University Press.

Wiggershaus, R. (1987), *Die Frankfurter Schule, Geschichte, theoretische Entwicklung Politische Bedeutung*, München, Carl Hauser Verlag.

245

Bibliography

Wilson, B. (1982), *Religion in Sociological Perspective*, Oxford, Oxford University Press.

Wilson, B. R. (ed). (1970), *Rationality*, Oxford, Basil Blackwell.

Wilson, J. D. (1935), *What Happens in Hamlet*, Cambridge, Cambridge University Press.

Winch, P. (1958), *The Idea of a Social Science and its Relation to Philosophy*, London, Routledge and Kegan Paul.

Wollheim, R. (1971), *Freud*, London, Fontana.

Wouters, C. (1986), 'Formalization and informalization: changing tension balances in civilization processes', *Theory, Culture and Society*, 3, pp. 1-18.

Wrong, D. H. (1961), 'The oversocialized conception of man in modern sociology', *American Sociological Review*, 26, pp. 183-93.

Wrong, E. H. (1963), 'Human nature and perspective of sociology', *Social Research*, 30, pp. 300-18.

Wrong, D. H. (1977), *Skeptical Sociology*, London, Heinemann.

Zeitlin, I. M. (1984), *Ancient Judaism*, Oxford, Polity Press.

Index

Index

248

Index

249

Index

252

Index

Index by Keith Seddon